UNICOMPARTMENTAL ARTHROPLASTY WITH THE OXFORD KNEE

UNICOMPARTMENTAL ARTHROPLASTY WITH THE OXFORD KNEE

John Goodfellow

John O'Connor

Hemant Pandit

Christopher Dodd

David Murray

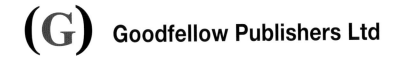

(G) Goodfellow Publishers Ltd

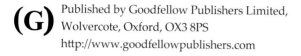

(G) Published by Goodfellow Publishers Limited,
Wolvercote, Oxford, OX3 8PS

http://www.goodfellowpublishers.com

British Library Cataloguing in Publication Data: a catalogue record for
this title is available from the British Library.

Library of Congress Catalog Card Number: on file.

ISBN: 978-1-910158-45-6

First published by Oxford University Press, 2006

Published by Goodfellow Publishers, 2011

Reprinted 2012, 2013 (twice), 2014, 2015

This edition 2015, reprinted 2016

Typeset by P K McBride, Southampton

Cover by Cylinder

Printed by Short Run Press Ltd., Exeter, England

Preface

A whole book, about one knee prosthesis! And only half a knee prosthesis at that!

The scope of this book is, actually, a little wider than the exclamations above suggest, but some excuse is surely required. We have written, in fact, about unicompartmental arthroplasty, an intellectually exciting and technically demanding subject for which the authors have a shared enthusiasm. However, since surgical expertise is gained slowly, most practitioners learn only one way of dealing with a particular clinical problem, and we are no exceptions. Our experience of treating unicompartmental arthritis over the last 25 years has been almost exclusively with our own invention, the Oxford Unicompartmental Knee, and we can only write with first-hand authority about that. We have, of course, tried to make good this deficiency from the published reports of other surgeons (whose experience, although different, is usually similarly limited); but, as with other history books, the realistic reader will expect only an *attempt* at a balanced view, and not necessarily an unbiased attempt.

Until very recently, unicompartmental arthroplasty itself was something of a niche activity. Most orthopaedic surgeons in the world did not use the method at all, and even its champions thought it appropriate for no more than a small proportion of arthritic knees in need of surgery. As will appear, we believe that as many as one-third of those who currently undergo total knee replacement may be better treated by unicompartmental arthroplasty. Soon, a million total knee arthroplasties will be performed in the world each year, and so this book is offered for the consideration of all practising knee surgeons.

The challenge of unicompartmental replacement is nothing less than to replace the deformed surfaces of one compartment of the knee so effectively that the soft tissues of the whole joint, and the retained articular surfaces of the other compartments, can all resume their physiological functions. This is a more difficult task than that confronted by total knee replacement, and it is anomalous that most prosthetic designs and methods of implantation for unicompartmental replacement have remained so unsophisticated during the three decades in which the technology of total replacement has (perhaps unsteadily) advanced.

The undertaking of a unicompartmental arthroplasty requires knowledge of the mechanics of the normal knee, and of the pathological anatomy of the arthritic knee. The prosthesis used must impose no unphysiological limits on the function of the retained structures and therefore it must be implanted in a unique relationship to the ligaments of the individual knee. This may only be consistently achieved if the instruments allow measured intraoperative adjustment of the components to match the particular anatomy. The components need to be sufficiently wear resistant to function for the expected lifetime of the patient, which is usually much longer than 10 years.

Lastly, the surgeon needs to have gained the *appropriate* skills and experience. Even long familiarity with other procedures on the knee does not, it seems, suffice to avoid the consequences of the 'learning curve' for unicompartmental arthroplasty.

John Goodfellow
John O'Connor
Christopher Dodd
David Murray

Preface to the second edition

Since the publication of the first edition, several things have happened. We have greatly missed the contribution of John Goodfellow who died in August 2011. He was the main driving force behind the writing of the first edition, as indeed he was behind the original development of the Oxford Knee. We have retained his name as first author because, although there are substantial additions of new material, quite a lot has remained unchanged. Readers will be able to detect the points at which the smooth flow of John's writing stops and another hand takes over.

Also, there have been further developments in the instrumentation, the introduction of cement-less components and of components specifically designed for use in the lateral compartment. Finally, a substantial body of new clinical and scientific evidence has been gathered, evidence which further encourages us to recommend the use of the Oxford Knee to our surgeon colleagues.

We dedicate this edition to the memory of John Goodfellow.

John O'Connor
Hemant Pandit
Christopher Dodd
David Murray

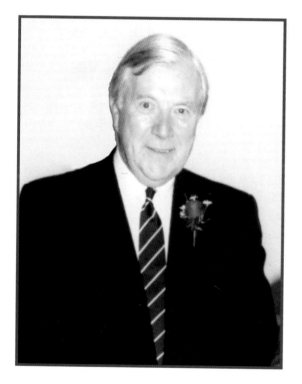

John Goodfellow, FRCS, M.S. (1927-2011).
Photograph of John when he was President of the British Orthopaedic Association. In his presidential address, he repeated his view that engineering is the basic science of orthopaedic surgery, a view which had led to the start of his collaboration with John O'Connor, Department of Engineering Science, in 1966.

Acknowledgements

Many people have assisted us with the work on which the book is based and deserve our thanks. In particular Barbara Marks without whose endeavours the book and its second edition would not have happened. We would like to acknowledge the contribution of Cathy Jenkins and Jo Brown who expertly gather the clinical data that underpins our research.

We acknowledge the help and support of our surgeon colleagues and, in particular, Andrew Price, William Jackson and Max Gibbons, who continue to participate actively in our instructional courses. We are also grateful to Peter McLardy-Smith, Roger Gundle, David Beard and Karen Barker for their contributions over the years.

We are grateful for the help and support of all the following research fellows who have gained, or are working on, a thesis around the Oxford knee: Russell Miller, Adrian Weale, Brett Robinson, Jonathan Rees, David Isaac, Paul Monk, Aashish Gulati, Ben Kendrick, Luke Jones, Nick Bottomley, Alexander Liddle, Abtin Alvand, and Thomas Hamilton.

We thank our anaesthetist colleagues Mansukh Popat, Matthew Sainsbury, Peter Hambly and Graham Burt for their contributions both in the operating theatre and with optimising early discharge. None of the clinical work would have be possible without the help of the nurses, physiotherapists, radiographers and the other staff of the Nuffield Orthopaedic Centre and we are grateful to them all, particularly Vicky Flanagan, Heather Topf, Yvonne Attwood and Paul Cooper.

The theoretical modelling of the human knee and associated experimental work has been improved by several 'generations' of engineers and their work is frequently cited in this book. Particular mention is made of Amy Zavatsky, David FitzPatrick, Richie Gill, David Wilson, Jennifer Feikes, Danielle Toutungi, Tung-Wu Lu, and Ahmed Imran. We are also grateful to Ben van Duren, David Simpson, Stephen Mellon and Elise Pegg for their invaluable engineering input.

Since 1984, the technical skills to make the implants and instruments we describe were provided by the engineers and craftsmen of Biomet. We especially record the contributions of Russell Lloyd and the late Ron Bateman. David Moorse, Kit Pitman and especially Keith Thomas have helped in innumerable ways, as did Amanda Rogers. We are also grateful for the contribution of the following Biomet development engineers – Mona Alinejad, Duncan Ridley, Tim Lawes and Jim Truscott.

In the past forty years, very many professional colleagues have contributed to our studies at Oxford, as consultants, surgical trainees or engineering students, and several of their names appear as authors of papers referred to in this book. We are also grateful to the many surgeons worldwide who have shared their insights on the Oxford Knee with us.

John Goodfellow
John O'Connor
Hemant Pandit
Christopher Dodd
David Murray

Contents

Additional material to accompany this book, including animated computer models and surgical videos, can be found at: www.oxfordpartialknee.com.

1

Introduction and Historical Overview

Osteoarthritis of the knee is one of the most common causes of painful loss of mobility in middle-aged and elderly people in many populations and is the main indication for knee replacement surgery. From the early days of arthroplasty, it was recognised that arthritis was often limited to the medial (or lateral) compartment of the knee and, in the pioneering operation of MacIntosh [1], metal spacers could be used in one compartment or both. Gradually, however, as the advantages of bicompartmental arthroplasty were appreciated, unicompartmental (or partial) replacement was less and less practised, and in some countries almost disappeared. With the introduction of tricompartmental replacement, a large body of surgical opinion concluded that osteoarthritis of the knee was a disease of the whole joint (like osteoarthritis of the hip) and that common sense required the replacement of all the articular surfaces to provide long-term relief of symptoms.

The attention of designers and manufacturers focused on the improvement of implants and instruments for total replacement, and the gap between the survival rates of unicompartmental knee arthroplasty (UKA) and total knee arthroplasty (TKA) widened, reinforcing the prevailing opinion of their fundamental merits.

Popular neglect of the unicompartmental alternative is reflected in a lack of innovation. The St Georg (1969) is still in use today, and most designs developed since are similar to that. Until recently, the components were implanted largely 'by eye', as in the early days of total replacement.

A further consequence of the success of TKA was loss of interest in the natural history and pathological anatomy of the osteoarthritic knee. Since total replacement is equally applicable, and almost equally successful, over the whole range of manifestations of that disease, there was no longer much point in its further analysis. However, the longitudinal studies by Ahlback [2] had already suggested that unicompartmental osteoarthritis does not inevitably spread to other parts of the knee. In addition, numerous post-mortem descriptions published in the 1970s and 1980s had revealed the almost universal presence of cartilage lesions in some parts of the joint in middle-aged and elderly people, implying that their presence is consistent with normal knee function. These observations challenge the common-sense conclusion that replacement of all the articular surfaces is a necessary requirement for a clinically successful arthroplasty.

UKA versus TKA

A few surgeons have been able to report clinical results and cumulative survival rates after UKA to match those of total replacement, but the general opinion, led by National Registers, is that the failure rate of UKA is not only much higher than TKA; but also is unacceptably high. If the failure rate is so high, why should surgeons bother with UKA? It may, of course, offend one's sense of economy to replace more of a damaged joint than is necessary, but there are more practical reasons as well. The function following UKA tends to be better than following TKA; successful UKA is even more effective than successful TKA. Many surgeons who have performed both procedures have found that the range of flexion is greater and gait is more nearly normal, particularly with demanding activities like stair descent, because the biomechanics of the knee are more completely restored [3, 4].

However, it is on the grounds of safety, with reduced morbidity and mortality, that unicompartmental replacement most strongly recommends itself. To examine rare events such as mortality, large data sets are necessary. As unicompartmental replacement tends to be used more in younger active patients than total knee replacement, it is essential that patients are carefully matched so as to achieve a fair comparision. Based on data from the National Joint Register of England and Wales (NJR) and other large data sets, 25,000 UKA were matched with 75,000 TKA [5]. While the revision rate of UKA was 2.4 times higher at eight years than TKA, there were many advantages of UKA. The hospital stay was shorter and readmission within one year was less. The incidence of major medical complications such as myocardial infarction, stroke, thromboembolism and deep infection was about half and the death rate was lower. During the first thirty days post-operation, the death rate was about one quarter, and even out to eight years it was 13% less. If 100 patients had a unicompartmental knee rather than a total, over an eight-year period, one life would be saved at the expense of three revisions. On the basis of these results, Cobb concluded that UKA is "unequivocally safer" than TKA [6]. Even taking into account the higher revision rate, UKA is still more cost effective than the TKA option [7, 8]. A large study by Willis-Owen et al. showed nearly 50% of knees presenting with end-stage arthritis are suitable for a UKA and UKA offers a substantial cost saving over TKA (£1761 per knee) [9].

Revision tends to be easier after UKA than TKA as it usually involves a simple conversion to a TKA. The results of revisions of UKA are better than those of revised TKAs and nearly as good as those of primary TKA [8]. As a result, the threshold for revision of UKA is lower than that of TKA. Following a UKA, about 60% of patients with very poor results have revisions whereas only about 10% of TKA with similarly poor results have revisions [10]. Therefore, even though UKA tend to have fewer poor results than TKA, they have a higher revision rate. If the possibility to rectify a problem following a joint replacement can be considered to be an advantage, the higher revision rate of UKA, which is a manifestation of its ease of revision, should not be considered to be a disadvantage.

Unicompartmental implant design

The first 'modern' designs, the St Georg (1969) and the Marmor (1972), had poly-centric metal femoral condyles articulating on flat (or nearly flat) polyethylene tibial components, both cemented to the bones [11, 12] (Fig. 1.1). The stated principles of Marmor's design were to reproduce as accurately as possible the polycentric form of the natural femoral condyles; and to avoid constraint of the articulation by employing a non-conforming tibial plateau [13]. Most of the models introduced since were designed on the same principles.

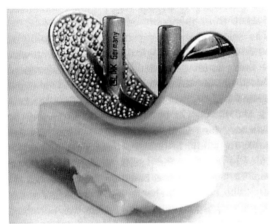

Figure 1.1 St Georg unicompartmental prosthesis.

Initially, problems were caused by loosening following distortion of the thinnest polyethylene components (6 mm thick), which were abandoned in favour of thicker ones [14]. The persisting problem of deformation of the all-polyethylene component led to the use of metal-backed tibial implants, but this, in turn, resulted in diminished thickness of polyethylene and sometimes further problems with wear [15]. However, the fundamental problem remained. A round femoral component makes contact with a flat tibial component on a very small contact area, with high contact stresses, so that problems of wear and deformation were inevitable [16, 17]. Using a more conforming tibial component introduces constraints which may not be compatible with ligament function (see Chapter 3).

The Oxford Knee

Phase 1

In 1974, two of the authors (JWG and JJOC) introduced congruous mobile bearings for knee prostheses [18]. The first 'Oxford Knee' had a metal femoral component with a spherical articular surface, a metal tibial component which was flat, and a polyethylene mobile bearing, spherically concave above and flat below, interposed between them (Fig. 1.2). The device was fully congruent at both interfaces throughout the range of movement (to minimise polyethylene wear) and fully unconstrained (to allow unrestricted movements and minimise the risk of loosening). These features of the Oxford Knee have remained unchanged to the present day.

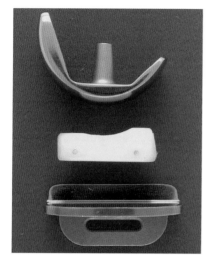

Figure 1.2 The Oxford Knee (Phase 1) (1978).

At first, the implant was used bicompartmentally, as a total joint replacement, with two sets of components inserted one medially and one laterally. The non-articular surface of the femoral component of the original design (Phase 1) had three inclined facets and was fitted to the femur by making three saw-cuts as shown in Figure 1.3. Many surgeons found it difficult to locate the femoral component accurately in relation to the ligaments and, therefore to match the extension gap to the flexion gap.

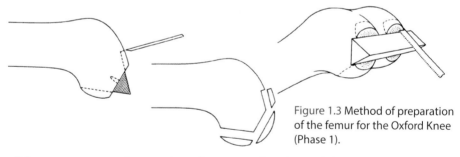

Figure 1.3 Method of preparation of the femur for the Oxford Knee (Phase 1).

It became apparent that good results were only achieved if the ACL was intact [19]. Another observation was made, that if the ACL was intact, then the arthritis tended to be confined to the anteromedial part of the tibia and the distal part of the medial femoral condyle. In these cases, all ligaments were functionally normal. This disease was called Anteromedial OA (AMOA) [20]. On the basis of these two observations, in 1982 the device began to be used unicompartmentally and the primary indication was AMOA.

Phase 2

In 1987, the Phase 2 implant was introduced specifically for unicompartmental arthroplasty [21]. The non-articular surfaces of the femoral component had a flat posterior facet and a spherically concave inferior facet (Fig. 1.4). The posterior femoral condyle was prepared by a saw-cut and its inferior facet was milled by a spherically concave bone-mill rotating round a spigot in a drill- hole in the condyle (Fig. 1.5). By shortening the spigot, measured thicknesses of bone could be milled incrementally from the inferior surface of the condyle, allowing the gaps in flexion and extension to be balanced intraoperatively and simultaneously shaping the bone to fit the implant [21]. This accurate system for restoring ligament tension to normal not only decreased the bearing dislocation rate to very low levels but also restored knee kinematics, and thus function, to normal. The 10 year results of the Phase 1 and 2 Oxford Knee were published by the designers in 1998 [22] and by an independent surgeon, Dr Svard in 2001 [23]. These two studies demonstrated, for the first time, that the long term survival of UKA can be as good as that achieved by TKA. Similar results were also shown by Barrington and Emerson in 2010 [24].

Phase 2
8 fill 1 femoral
Size +
universal tibiae

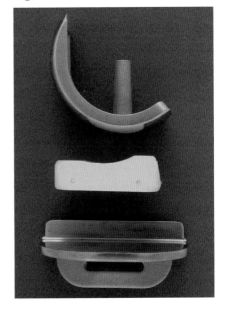

Figure 1.4 The Oxford Unicompartmental Knee Arthroplasty (OUKA (Phase 2)) (1987).

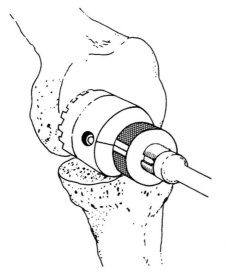

Figure 1.5 Method of preparation of the femur for the OUKA (Phase 2) with a concave rotary mill turning around an adjustable spigot.

Phase 3

The Phase 1 and Phase 2 prostheses were implanted through an open approach with dislocation of the patella, as in TKA. In 1998, the Phase 3 prosthesis was introduced specifically for medial unicompartmental use with a minimally invasive approach (Fig. 1.6). The single size of femoral component (used in all the Phase 1 and 2 implants) was replaced by five parametric sizes, the universal tibial plateau was replaced by right- and left-handed tibial components and the bearings were modified to diminish the likelihood of impingement and rotation. The instruments were miniaturised to facilitate their use through a small parapatellar arthrotomy. The functional results and speed of recovery of Phase 3 were found to be better than those of Phase 2 [25].

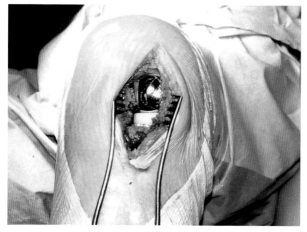

Figure 1.6 The OUKA (Phase 3) (1998) implanted through a small incision.

In 2004, cementless components based on the Phase 3 were first used (Fig 1.7). Apart from having a porous titanium and hydroxyapatite coating, the main difference between the cementless and the original Phase 3 was that the cementless femoral component had two pegs. Because, generally, cementless TKA have not performed as well as cemented [26], the cementless OUKA was carefully assessed. Randomised controlled trials with clinical and Radiostereometric (RSA) outcome measures were used to assess fixation, and a large multicentre cohort study was used to assess complications and contraindications [27]. Because the results of cementless have proved to be at least as good as those of cemented, many experienced surgeons now just use the cementless OUKA.

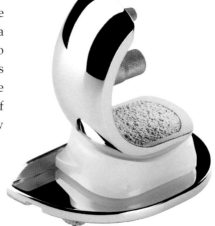

Figure 1.7. The cementless components.

It was clear from the cementless experience that a two peg femoral component was preferable to a single peg. Therefore, a two peg cemented component, that was similar to the cementless, was introduced (Fig 1.8). A clinical study has shown that the two peg cemented component performs well [28].

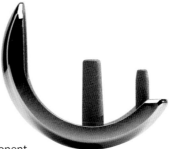

Figure 1.8 The two peg cemented femoral component.

Instrumentation

In 2012, a new set of instruments, called Microplasty (Fig 1.9), was introduced so as to make the operation more reliable. They are a substantial improvement compared to the original Phase 3 instrumentation. For example, they help with achieving the correct tibial resection height; they facilitate positioning of the femoral component and have a system for preventing impingement. The instruments have been optimised for use with the two peg cementless as well as the two peg cemented component.

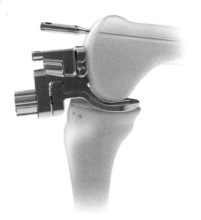
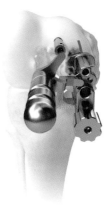

Figure 1.9. The Microplasty femoral drill guide.

Also in 2012, the Signature patient specific instrumentation for the Oxford Knee was introduced. An MRI scan is obtained pre-operatively and, based on this, the provisional position of the components is determined. The surgeon then has the opportunity to adjust the positioning. Once the correct positioning is confirmed, patient specific guides are produced. During the operation, these are applied and control the positioning of the components although final balancing is achieved using traditional instrumentation. The Signature instruments currently are not as reliable as Microplasty so are not recommended for inexperienced surgeons [29, 30]. However, it is expected that with time they will improve.

Lateral arthroplasty

Initially the same components were used for both medial and lateral unicompart-mental replacement. The results on the lateral side were, however, disappointing with a dislocation rate of about 10% [31]. The reason for the high dislocation rate was that the lateral collateral ligament is loose in flexion (Fig 1.10). In contrast, the medial collateral ligament is tight in all positions. Over the years, many improvements to the implants and the surgical technique for lateral arthroplasty have been introduced with a steady improvement in results. The current iteration (Fig. 1.11), which involves a convex domed tibial plateau and biconcave bearing implanted through a lateral parapatellar approach, has reduced the dislocation rate to a level that is acceptable although it is still higher than that achieved on the medial side and is therefore only appropriate for surgeons experienced with the Oxford Knee. Less experienced surgeons are advised to use fixed bearing UKA laterally. The surgical technique is very different from that used on the medial side. Because lateral unicompartmental replacement is less common than medial UKA, the domed lateral Oxford Knee is only performed by a limited number of surgeons. However, with further improvements, we expect the dislocation rate to decrease further and the use of the domed lateral to increase.

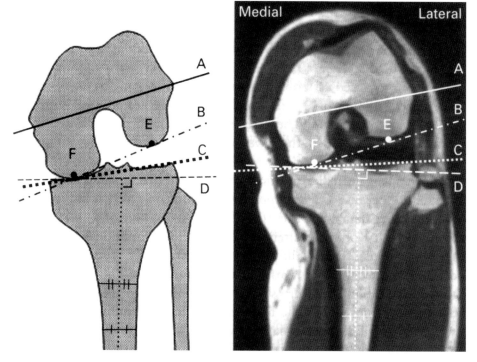

Figure 1.10 Distraction of the lateral compartment in normal flexed valgus-stressed knee. (Reproduced with permission and copyright © of the British Editorial Society of Bone and Joint Surgery [Tokuhara Y, Kadoya Y, Nakagawa S, Kobayashi S and Takaoka K. The flexion gap in normal knees. An MRI study. *J Bone Joint Surg [Br]* 2004; **86-B**: 1133–6].)

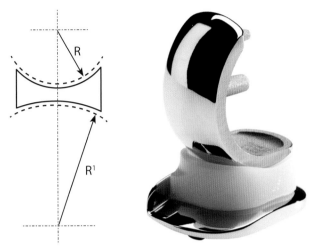

Figure 1.11 Diagram and photograph of the Oxford Domed Lateral Unicompartmental Knee, with spherical femoral and tibial convex components and a biconcave meniscal bearing.

Fixed Bearings

In 2003, a fixed bearing tibial component, known as the Vanguard M, that could be used with the Oxford instrumentation was introduced (Fig. 1.12). The reason this was introduced was to allow surgeons in the United States of America to use the Oxford instrumentation as the mobile bearing version was not yet FDA-approved. Prior to the approval of the mobile bearing Oxford in the United States, large numbers of Vanguard Ms were implanted. The use of the device has since decreased; however, it is still available and can be used by surgeons who have worries about stability of the mobile bearing or if there is a problem with recurrent dislocation. The device, which was initially designed for the medial compartment, can also be used in the lateral compartment. For the surgeon who is not very experienced with the OUKA, it is probably preferable to use a fixed bearing device rather than a mobile on the lateral side. However, the Vanguard M was designed for the medial side and is not the optimal shape for the lateral side. To address this issue, a fixed bearing lateral Oxford (FLO) has been introduced. This is interchangeable with the mobile lateral arthroplasty and the combination should allow surgeons of all levels of experience to use an OUKA on the lateral side.

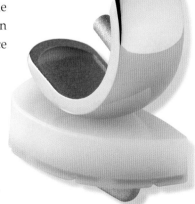

Figure 1.12 Vanguard M fixed bearing Oxford Knee.

Indications

Over the years, the indications and contraindications for the Oxford Knee used medially have become more clearly defined. The main indication is AMOA although Spontaneous Osteonecrosis of the Knee (SONK) is also a good but rare indication. The key criteria that need to be satisfied to make the diagnosis of AMOA is that there is bone-on-bone medial OA, the ACL is functionally intact, there is full thickness cartilage laterally and the intra-articular deformity is correctable, but not over correctable, indicating that the MCL is functionally normal. If a patient has severe symptoms, if these criteria are satisfied and there are no general contraindications for arthroplasty, then an Oxford Knee is indicated. All the specific contraindications for UKA defined by Kozinn and Scott [32], and others, do not apply. In particular, patient age, activity level and obesity are not contraindications; nor are site of pain, the state of the PFJ (except for severe lateral OA), chondrocalcinosis or lateral osteophytes. The indications for the Oxford Knee are satisfied in about 50% of knees needing replacement. However, when surgeons start using the Oxford, they are often concerned about ignoring the Kozinn and Scott contraindications, particularly the PFJ, so their usage is lower. With time and development of confidence, usage tends to increase.

In the published or presented series of the Phase 3 Oxford Knee with 10 year results which together include about six thousand patients, the survival is about 95% [33]. The surgeons involved tended to adhere to the recommended indications and use the Oxford Knee in at least 20% and commonly 50% of their knee replacements. In contrast, the National Registers report a ten-year survival of about 85%. The main reason for the high failure rate in the National Registers is that most surgeons do very small numbers. In the UK, the commonest number of UKA done by surgeons doing this procedure is one per year and the average is about five per year [34]. Analysis of NJR data showed that the survival rate was lowest among surgeons doing small numbers and increases as surgeon numbers increased. It is suggested that surgeons should perform more than 12 per year to achieve results comparable to those of the high volume operators. The only way surgeons can easily increase their numbers of UKA is to increase the proportion of their knee replacements that are UKA. Analysis of NJR data would suggest that to get good results, surgeons should do at least 20% and ideally 50% of their knee replacements as OUKA. If surgeons want to use the Oxford Knee, they should therefore adhere to the recommended indications and ignore the unnecessary contraindications. They will then do at least 20% of their knees as Oxfords and should achieve good results.

Purpose of this book

The main aim of this book is to advise surgeons on the choice of patients appropriate for treatment with OUKA (Chapters 4 and 5), and to guide them on the performance of the operation (Chapters 6 and 7) and the management of complications (Chapter 11). In addition we have chapters about the design of the OUKA (Chapter 2), knee kinematics (Chapter 3), post-operative management (Chapter 9), and results (Chapter 10). We also have chapters about the rare medial indications (Chapter 8) and lateral OUKA (Chapter 12).

The reader may wish to view the website for this book, where there are animations of the surgical technique and videos of the operation:

www.oxfordpartialknee.com

References

1. MacIntosh DL. Hemiarthroplasty of the knee using a space occupying prosthesis for painful varus and valgus deformities. *J Bone Joint Surg [Am]* 1958; **40-A**: 1431.

2. Ahlback S. Osteoarthrosis of the knee. A radiographic investigation. *Acta Radiol Diagn (Stockh)* 1968: Suppl 277:7-72.

3. Laurencin CT, Zelicof SB, Scott RD, Ewald FC. Unicompartmental versus total knee arthroplasty in the same patient. A comparative study. *Clin Orthop Relat Res* 1991; (**273**): 151-6.

4. Rougraff BT, Heck DA, Gibson AE. A comparison of tricompartmental and unicompartmental arthroplasty for the treatment of gonarthrosis. *Clin Orthop Relat Res* 1991; (**273**): 157-64.

5. Liddle AD, Judge A, Pandit H, Murray DW. Adverse outcomes after total and unicompartmental knee replacement in 101,330 matched patients: a study of data from the National Joint Registry for England and Wales. *Lancet* 2014; **384**(9952): 1437-45.

6. Cobb JP. Patient safety after partial and total knee replacement. *Lancet* 2014; **384**(9952): 1405-7.

7. Andrews B, Willis-Owen CA, Aquil A, Cobb JP. A cost-utility analysis of knee arthroplasty using data from three national registries Paper #668. AAOS. New Orleans; 2014.

8. Robertsson O, Borgquist L, Knutson K, Lewold S, Lidgren L. Use of unicompartmental instead of tricompartmental prostheses for unicompartmental arthrosis in the knee is a cost-effective alternative. 15,437 primary tricompartmental prostheses were compared with 10,624 primary medial or lateral unicompartmental prostheses. *Acta Orthop Scand* 1999; **70**(2): 170-5.

9. Willis-Owen CA, Brust K, Alsop H, Miraldo M, Cobb JP. Unicondylar knee arthroplasty in the UK National Health Service: an analysis of candidacy, outcome and cost efficacy. *Knee* 2009; **16**(6): 473-8.

10. Goodfellow JW, O'Connor JJ, Murray DW. A critique of revision rate as an outcome measure: re-interpretation of knee joint registry data. *J Bone Joint Surg Br* 2010; **92**(12): 1628-31.

11. Marmor L. Unicompartmental and total knee arthroplasty. *Clin Orthop Relat Res* 1985; (**192**): 75-81.

12. Neider E. Schlitten prothese, Rotations knie und Scharnierprothese modell St. Georg and Endo-Modell. *Orthopade* 1991; **20**: 170-80.

13. Marmor L. Preface. Prothese Unicompartimentale du Genou. Paris: Expansion Scientifique; 1998.

14. Marmor L. The Modular (Marmor) knee: case report with a minimum follow-up of 2 years. *Clin Orthop Relat Res* 1976; (**120**): 86-94.

15. Palmer SH, Morrison PJ, Ross AC. Early catastrophic tibial component wear after unicompartmental knee arthroplasty. *Clin Orthop Relat Res* 1998; (**350**): 143-8.

16. Ashraf T, Newman JH, Desai VV, Beard D, Nevelos JE. Polyethylene wear in a non-congruous unicompartmental knee replacement: a retrieval analysis. *Knee* 2004; **11**(3): 177-81.

17. Collier MB, Engh CA, Jr., McAuley JP, Engh GA. Factors associated with the loss of thickness of polyethylene tibial bearings after knee arthroplasty. *J Bone Joint Surg Am* 2007; **89**(6): 1306-14.

18. Goodfellow JW, O'Connor JJ, Shrive NG, inventors; Endoprosthetic knee joint devices. British Patent Application 1534263. 1974.

19. Goodfellow J, O'Connor J. The anterior cruciate ligament in knee arthroplasty. A risk-factor with unconstrained meniscal prostheses. *Clin Orthop Relat Res* 1992; (**276**): 245-52.

20. White SH, Ludkowski PF, Goodfellow JW. Anteromedial osteoarthritis of the knee. *J Bone Joint Surg Br* 1991; **73**(4): 582-6.

21. Goodfellow JW, O'Connor JJ, inventors; Oxford Knee (femoral). UK, French, German, Swiss Patent EP 0327397, Irish Patent 62951, US Patent 5314482. 1989.

22. Murray DW, Goodfellow JW, O'Connor JJ. The Oxford medial unicompartmental arthroplasty: a ten-year survival study. *J Bone Joint Surg Br* 1998; **80**(6): 983-9.

23. Svard UC, Price AJ. Oxford medial unicompartmental knee arthroplasty. A survival analysis of an independent series. *J Bone Joint Surg Br* 2001; **83**(2): 191-4.

24. Barrington JW, Emerson RH. The Oxford Knee: First report of 20-year follow-up in the US. AAOS. New Orleans; 2010. Paper no 422.

25. Price AJ, Webb J, Topf H, Dodd CA, Goodfellow JW, Murray DW, Oxford Hip & Knee Group. Rapid recovery after Oxford unicompartmental arthroplasty through a short incision. *J Arthroplasty* 2001; **16**(8): 970-6.

26. Forsythe ME, Englund RE, Leighton RK. Unicondylar knee arthroplasty: a cementless perspective. *Can J Surg* 2000; **43**(6): 417-24.

27. Liddle AD, Pandit H, O'Brien S, Doran E, Penny ID, Hooper GJ, Burn PJ, Dodd CA, Beverland DE, Maxwell AR, Murray DW. Cementless fixation in Oxford unicompartmental knee replacement: a multicentre study of 1000 knees. *Bone Joint J* 2013; **95-B**(2): 181-7.

28. White SH, Roberts S, Jones PW. The Twin Peg Oxford partial knee replacement: the first 100 cases. *Knee* 2012; **19**(1): 36-40.

29. Alvand A, Khan T, Jenkins C, Rees J, Jackson W, Dodd C, Price A. (2015). The impact of patient-specific instrumentation (PSI) on surgical accuracy and functional outcome during unicompartmental knee replacement (UKR): A prospective randomised

controlled study. British Association for Surgery of the Knee (BASK) Annual Meeting, Telford, UK.

30. Barrington JW, Emerson RH. What is the most accurate insertion platform for a mobile-bearing UKA? A case-control, blinded radiographic analysis. Annual Meeting of the American Association of Hip and Knee Surgeons. Dallas, Tx, USA; 2013.

31. Gunther T, Murray DW, Miller RK, Wallace D, Carr AJ, O'Connor JJ, McLardy-Smith P, Goodfellow JW. Lateral unicompartmental arthroplasty with the Oxford meniscal knee. *Knee* 1996; **3**(1-2): 33-9.

32. Kozinn SC, Scott R. Unicondylar knee arthroplasty. *J Bone Joint Surg Am* 1989; **71**(1): 145-50.

33. Murray DW, Marks BE, Kontochristos L, Dodd CA, Pandit H. The Oxford unicompartmental knee replacement: long term results. *Chin J Joint Surg* 2013; **7**(4): 540-4.

34. Liddle AD. Failure of unicompartmental knee replacement [DPhil]. Oxford: University of Oxford; 2014.

35. Baker P, Jameson S, Critchley R, Reed M, Gregg P, Deehan D. Center and surgeon volume influence the revision rate following unicondylar knee replacement: an analysis of 23,400 medial cemented unicondylar knee replacements. *J Bone Joint Surg Am* 2013; **95**(8): 702-9.

2

Design and Biomechanics of the Oxford Knee

The description of the Oxford Knee starts with an explanation of the function of mobile bearings in knee prostheses. An obvious advantage is that the areas of contact between the joint surfaces are maximised. In this chapter, we shall show that wear at the polyethylene surfaces is thereby minimised and that optimal kinematics can be achieved with minimal risk of loosening. We will discuss the biomechanics of the cementless components and problems that may occur with the tibia.

Designing against wear

Articular surface shapes and contact pressures

Most surface replacements of the knee, total as well as unicompartmental, have articular surfaces like those shown in Figure 2.1, approximating to the shapes of the ends of the human femur and tibia. The metal femoral surfaces are convex and the polyethylene tibial surfaces are flat or shallowly concave. These shapes do not fit one another, in any relative position, and so only parts of their articular surfaces are in contact and able to transmit load.

Most prosthetic femoral condyles attempt to mimic nature and are polyradial, with the shortest radius posterior. Thus the area of contact is smaller in flexion than in extension (Fig. 2.1). However, the compressive loads transmitted across the interface are potentially greatest in flexion, attaining up to six times body weight during stair ascent and descent [1]. For a given load, the average contact pressure (load per unit area) at the articular surfaces is inversely proportional to the area of contact; therefore the less congruous the surfaces, the higher is the average pressure at their interface. The wear rate of ultra-high-molecular-weight polyethylene (referred to hereafter as 'polyethylene') is said to increase exponentially with increasing contact pressure, rather than linearly as would be expected from classical wear theory [2]; conversely, wear rate has been found to decrease with increasing contact area [3].

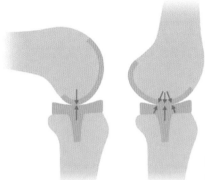

Figure 2.1 Typical polycentric incongruous knee replacement with a smaller contact area in flexion.

The natural knee

The presence of the cartilaginous menisci in the knee of humans (and of all other mammals) gives rise to an entirely different regime of contact (Fig. 2.2). Instead of one incongruous interface, two congruous interfaces are created, with much better distribution of load.

Fairbank, in 1948, first deduced that the human meniscus had a load-bearing function and suggested the mechanism of load transmission shown in Figure 2.3 [4]. The menisci consist mainly of collagen fibres disposed circumferentially to withstand the tensile hoop stresses engendered by load bearing; these stresses are resisted at the anterior and posterior horns by their attachments to the tibia [5]. The proportion of load transmitted indirectly by the menisci in human (and animal) joints has been estimated as between 45 and 70% of the applied load [6]. The remaining 30 – 55% is carried by the articular cartilage of the femoral and tibial surfaces within the embrace of the meniscus through their direct contact in the middle third of each plateau.

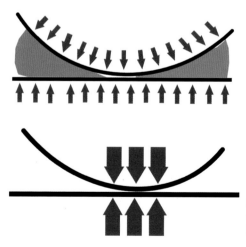

Figure 2.2 Load-sharing function of the meniscus, increasing effective contact area and reducing contact pressure. Loss of a meniscus reduces contact area and increases contact pressure.

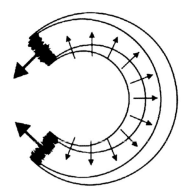

Figure 2.3 Mechanism of load transmission: the radially outward component of applied pressure is resisted by hoop stresses in the circumferential fibres of the meniscus. (Adapted from and reproduced with permission from Lippincott Williams & Wilkins [Shrive NG, O'Connor JJ and Goodfellow JW. Load-bearing in the knee joint. *Clin Orthop* 1978; **131**: 279–87].)

Mobility of the natural meniscus

Anteroposterior movements of the femoral condyles on the tibia during flexion–extension and axial rotation (Fig. 2.4) have to be accommodated by movements of the menisci. In 1680, Borelli [7] noticed that '*they are pulled forward when the knee is extended and backwards in flexion*'. Various estimates and measurements of these movements during flexion have been reported: 6 mm medially and 12 mm laterally [8]; 5.1 mm (SD 0.96) medially and 11.2 mm (SD 2.29) laterally [9]; medial anterior horn 7.1 mm (SD 2.49), medial posterior horn 3.9 mm (SD 1.75), lateral anterior horn 9.5 mm (SD 3.96), and lateral posterior horn 5.6 mm (SD 2.76) [10]. Freeman and his group suggest that the knee is a medial pivot with no movement medially; however, even Freeman's data suggests that there is movement of about 8 mm (Fig 2.4).

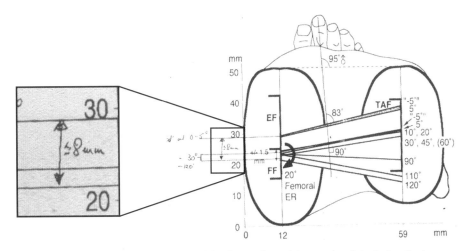

Figure 2.4 Anteroposterior movements of the femoral condyles on the tibia during flexion–extension and axial rotation, with annotations by Mr Michael Freeman.

Compliance of the natural meniscus

During flexion–extension and axial rotation, the natural meniscus not only changes its position on the tibial plateau, as the movements of the femoral condyle dictate, but also changes shape to fit the various curvatures of the polyradial femoral condyle (Fig. 2.5). In full extension, the large radius of the inferior surface of the condyle forces the limbs of the meniscus apart in an anteroposterior direction. As the knee flexes, and the smaller radius of the posterior condyle is offered, the anteroposterior measurement of the meniscus diminishes appropriately, possibly because divergence of the tibiofemoral contact areas forces the two menisci apart, drawing their anterior and posterior limbs closer together (Fig. 2.6) [6]. Changes in the shapes of the menisci are reflected in the differences in anteroposterior movements of the anterior and posterior horns and in the mediolateral movements of the medial and lateral edges of the two menisci observed by Vedi *et al.* [10].

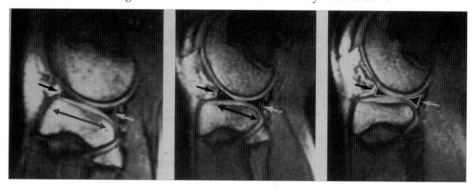

Figure 2.5 Magnetic resonance images demonstrating changes in the anteroposterior span of the meniscus during flexion. (Adapted from and reproduced with permission and copyright © of the British Editorial Society of Bone and Joint Surgery [Vedi V, Williams A, Tennant SJ, Spouse E, Hunt DM, Gedroyc WM. Meniscal movement. An in vivo study using dynamic MRI. *J Bone Joint Surg [Br]* 999; **81-B**: 37–41].)

Discussion

The meniscus is an integral part of the tibial articular surface, serving to maximise the contact area without limiting angular and translational movement between the bones. Therefore, load is transmitted at an average pressure that the articular cartilage can withstand. Evidence of the importance of this mechanism is provided by the observation that excision (or dysfunction) of a meniscus results in osteoarthritic degeneration of the remaining cartilage surfaces in the affected compartment [4].

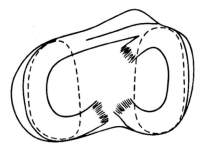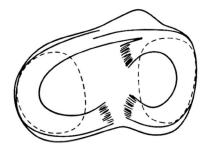

Figure 2.6 Shape changes of the meniscus during flexion-extension. Dotted curves outline contact areas in extension (left) and flexion (right) (diagramatic). (Reproduced with permission from Lippincott Williams & Wilkins [from Shrive N G, O'Connor JJ, and Goodfellow JW. Load-bearing in the knee joint. *Clin Orthop* 1978; **131**: 279–87].)

The Oxford 'Meniscal' Knee

The mechanical advantages conferred by the natural meniscus can be enjoyed by an artificial knee if it is provided with two joint interfaces instead of one. The design of the articular surfaces of the Oxford Knee has not changed since its first implantation in 1976 (Fig. 2.7). The femoral component made of metal has a spherical surface, the metal tibial component is flat. The polyethylene meniscal bearing has a spherical upper surface and a flat lower surface. The meniscofemoral interface (ball-in-socket) allows the angular movements of flexion–extension, the meniscotibial interface (flat-on-flat) allows translational movements (Fig. 2.8), and axial rotation is allowed by a combination of translation and spinning movement at both interfaces. The unconstrained mobile bearing does not resist the movements demanded by the soft tissues, muscles, and ligaments. Restoration of natural mobility and function may be expected (Chapter 3). The surfaces of the prosthesis experience mainly compressive forces, features which should minimise component loosening[11]. A low loosening rate is reflected in a high long-term survival rate (Chapter 10).

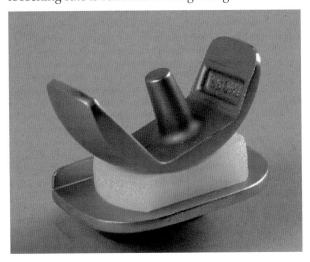

Figure 2.7 Components of the Oxford Knee (Phase 1).

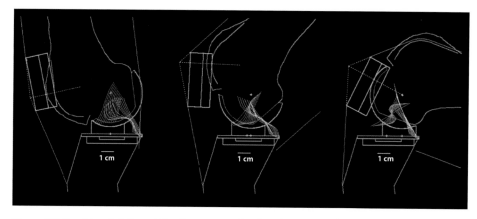

Figure 2.8 Combined sliding at the femoro-meniscal and menisco-tibial interfaces during flexion–extension allow anteroposterior translations of the femur on the tibia under the control of the ligaments while maintaining full conformity between the components in all positions (see Chapter 3).

The method of load transmission through the polyethylene bearing is, of course, quite different from that through the natural meniscus, but the functions of the two structures are analogous. The prosthetic bearing converts one incongruous interface into two congruous interfaces, maximising the area available for load transmission without limiting the freedom of joint movement, a feature which should minimise polyethylene wear while restoring physiological function. These are the justifications for calling the Oxford Knee a 'meniscal bearing' implant.

Why use a spherical not a polyradial femoral condyle?

A rigid polyethylene bearing can model only the mobility of the natural meniscus, and not its compliance. It cannot change shape and therefore cannot fit more than one of the several radii offered by a polyradial condyle. The only pairs of shapes that can maintain congruity in all relative positions of the components are a sphere in a spherical socket and a flat surface on a flat surface. Figure 2.9 shows the medial half of a specimen of a distal femur, sectioned through the sulcus of the trochlear groove. A circle fits the cartilage surface at the base of the trochlear groove quite well. Another circle fits the posterior facets of the femoral condyle, although it does not match its most distal facet. Therefore, a spherical femoral prosthesis attached to the posterior condyle can reproduce the shape of all but the most anterior part of the medial condyle.

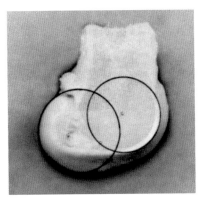

Figure 2.9 Sagittal section of the distal femur demonstrating that the sulcus of the trochlea and most of the medial condyle are circular. (This material has been reproduced from the Journal of Engineering in Medicine: Proceedings of the Institution of Mechanical Engineers Part H. 1989 Vol 216 Issue H4 pp 223–233. The geometry of the knee in the sagittal plane. O'Connor J, Goodfellow J, Shercliff T, Biden E. Permission is granted by the Council of the Institution of Mechanical Engineers.)

Other mobile-bearing designs

Since 1978, several designers have used mobile bearings in total and unicompartmental knee prostheses but with polyradial femoral condyles [12, 13]. In such implants, the concavity on the upper surface of the bearing must have a radius of curvature large enough to accommodate the largest radius of the femoral condyle (offered in extension) and therefore too large to match the smaller radii (offered in all positions of flexion when the compression forces between the components are greater). The contact pressures in flexion are likely to be large. Thus the function of such a mobile bearing is not analogous to that of the natural meniscus and is unlikely to minimise wear. Non-conforming mobile-bearing prostheses offer little theoretical advantage over non-conforming fixed-bearing designs.

Polyethylene wear in the Oxford Knee

The following studies have demonstrated that the theoretical expectation of a low polyethylene wear rate has been fulfilled in practice.

Retrieval studies

Twenty-three bearings were retrieved from 18 failed bicompartmental Oxford arthroplasties, 1–9 years after implantation [14]. The minimum thickness of each was measured with a dial gauge (Fig. 2.10) and compared with the mean thickness of 25 unused bearings. The mean penetration rate was very low; calculated by two methods, it was either 0.043 or 0.026 mm/year. There was no correlation between the initial minimum thickness of the bearings (range 3.5–10.5 mm) and their rate of wear.

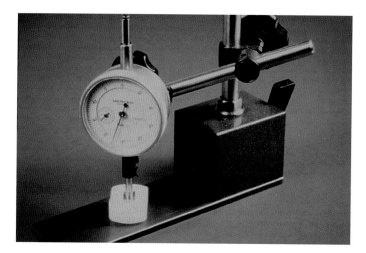

Figure 2.10 Dial gauge used to measure the thickness of a bearing at the bottom of the spherical socket.

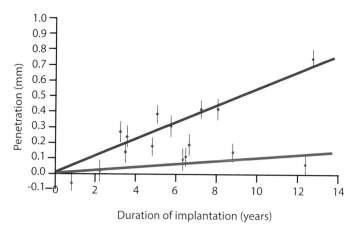

Figure 2.11 Retrieval studies. Measured penetration into the bearing plotted against duration of implantation. Bearings without impingement shown in blue and with impingement shown in red. The vertical line through each data point represents one standard deviation of the mean of the measured thickness of unused bearings obtained direct from the manufacturer. The regression lines through the data give the penetration rates (mm/year). (Reproduced with permission and copyright © of the British Editorial Society of Bone and Joint Surgery. [Psychoyios V, Crawford RW, O'Connor JJ, Murray DW. Wear of congruent meniscal bearings in unicompartmental knee arthroplasty. A retrieval study of 16 specimens. *J Bone Joint Surg [Br]* 1998; **80-B**: 876–82].)

The same method was used to study 16 bearings retrieved from failed OUKA (Phase 2) medial arthroplasties, 0.8–12.8 years after implantation [15]. The mean penetration rate was 0.036 mm/year (maximum 0.08 mm/year). Again, there was no correlation between the rate of wear and the initial bearing thickness (range 3.5–11.5 mm).

Ten bearings had erosion of their non-articular surfaces, caused by impingement against bone or cement. The most common site was anterior, produced by impingement in extension against bone in front of the femoral component (Fig. 2.12). The six bearings without impingement had a mean penetration rate of 0.01 mm/year compared with 0.054 mm/year for the 10 bearings with impingement (P < 0.0001) (Fig. 2.11). It was observed that there was a strong correlation between impingement and mechanical causes of failure such as loosening or lateral OA, suggesting that impingement may cause failure. It was also found that, in three quarters of cases revised for pain with no mechanical problem, the pain did not improve.

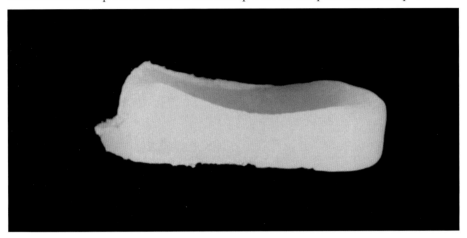

Figure 2.12 Retrieved bearing showing damage due to anterior impingement. (Reproduced with permission and copyright © of the British Editorial Society of Bone and Joint Surgery [Psychoyios V, Crawford RW, O'Connor JJ, Murray DW. Wear of congruent meniscal bearings in unicompartmental knee arthroplasty. A retrieval study of 16 specimens. *J Bone Joint Surg [Br]* 1998; **80-B**: 876–82].)

Kendrick *et al.* [16] used the same method to study a further 47 Phase 1 and Phase 2 bearings retrieved after OUKA at a mean time to revision of 8.4 years (SD 4.1). Twenty had been implanted for more than 10 years (maximum 17 years). Thirty-one of the 47 bearings showed evidence of impingement, and the mean penetration rate in these was 0.07 mm/year. The rate for the 16 bearings without impingement was 0.01 mm/year, the same as that found by Psychoyios *et al.* [15]. The penetration rate of Phase 1 bearings (machined from blocks of Hostulen RCH1000 polyethylene) was about double that of Phase 2 bearings (individually compression moulded from Montel Hifax 1900H powder). However, the impingement rate in Phase 1 implants (91%) was also much higher than in Phase 2 implants (58%).

Kendrick *et al.* [16] further stratified the impinged bearings into a group showing evidence only of extra-articular impingement damage and those also showing intra-articular surface damage (Fig. 2.13). Those showing intra-articular impingement had a penetration rate 2.5 times that of the group with extra-articular surface damage alone, while the latter had a penetration rate five times higher than those (0.01 mm/year) free of impingement damage.

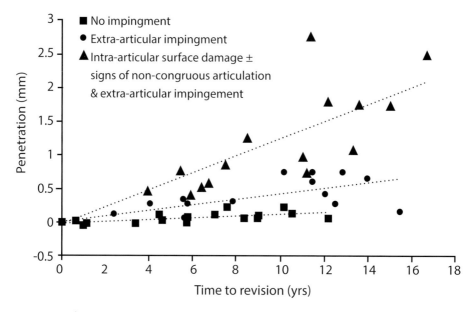

Figure 2.13. The penetration (mm) for different subgroups: no impingement; and a normal articular surface; abnormal macroscopic wear and normal articular surfaces with extra-articular impingement; abnormal macroscopic wear and abnormal articular surfaces with intra-articular impingement ± signs of non-congruous articulation (mm/year). (Reproduced with permission and copyright © of the British Editorial Society of Bone and Joint Surgery [Kendrick BJ, Longino D, Pandit H, Svard U, Gill HS, Dodd CA, Murray DW, Price AJ. Polyethylene wear in Oxford unicompartmental knee replacement: a retrieval study of 47 bearings. *J Bone Joint Surg JBr]* 2010; **92**(3): 367-73].)

In vivo penetration studies using Röntgen stereometric analysis

We have developed a method of measuring wear *in vivo* using Röntgen stereometric analysis (RSA), and have applied it to patients following OUKA [17–18]. The method does not require markers attached to the components or implanted in the patient's bones and therefore can be used retrospectively. Penetration of the bearings was measured in eight controls (three weeks after OUKA) and in seven patients in whom the prosthesis had been implanted about 10 years previously [17]. The mean penetration for the control group was 0.1 mm, demonstrating the accuracy of the method. The mean penetration rate for the 10-year group was 0.02 mm/year, similar to that observed in retrieved bearings without impingement (0.01 mm/year).

Kendrick *et al.* applied the same RSA technique to 13 knees in nine patients treated by JWG for AMOA [19, 20]. The mean follow-up at the time of examination was 20.9 years (range 17.2 to 25.9). The range of penetration rates for the six Phase 1 knees in the cohort was 0.023 to 0.099 mm/year (Fig 2.14), whereas that for the seven Phase 2 knees was 0.016 to 0.030 mm/year, with a mean value of 0.022 mm/year, a value similar to those observed in non-impinging bearings in the retrieval studies. We infer that the Phase 2 design was more successful in minimising impingement and its effects and that any oxidation of the polymer after 20 years *in vivo* had not accelerated the wear rate.

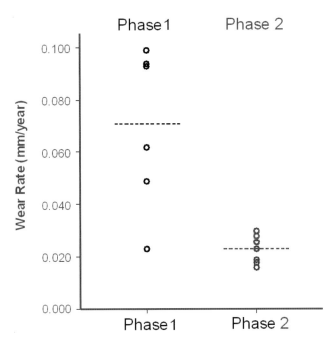

Figure 2.14. Scatterplot showing the distribution of rates of linear wear by Phase. The horizontal dashed lines indicate the mean wear rate for each phase [19].

Wear simulation studies

Retrieval and *in vivo* studies are the 'gold standard', providing evidence of actual performance of components in the infinitely varied circumstances of real life. Simulation studies have the disadvantage that the tests may be so far from lifelike as to invalidate the results. However, they are useful for longitudinal measurement of wear, for comparison of competing designs and materials under similarly controlled conditions, and for simulating the effects of years of natural wear in a few months.

A Stanmore knee simulator [21] was used to test a group of OUKA bearings over 3 million cycles [22]. During the first million cycles (thought to represent one year of normal activity), the bearings had a measured penetration of 0.05 mm (Fig. 2.15). Thereafter, the penetration rate was steady at 0.019 mm/year. The early higher rate of penetration was attributed to creep of the viscoelastic polyethylene which ceased once the bearings had bedded in after about a million cycles. The wear rate thereafter was similar to that observed in non-impinging retrieved bearings and in the *in vivo* studies of Phase 2 bearings.

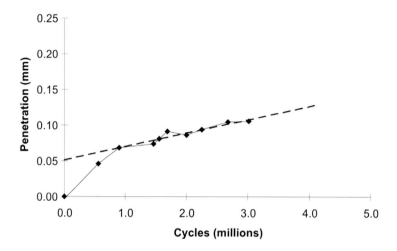

Figure 2.15 Simulator studies. Measured penetration plotted against millions of cycles of movement and load, with a regression line through the >1 million cycle data. (Reproduced, with permission, from Scott R, Schroeder D. Correlation of knee simulation to in-vivo use: evaluating the Oxford Unicompartmental knee. Transactions of the Orthopaedic Research Society **vol. 25**, Orlando, Florida, 2000; 434.)

Finite-element analysis

Morra and Greenwald [23] carried out a finite-element stress analysis of four uni-compartmental prostheses, two fixed-bearing and two mobile-bearing (the OUKA and an implant with a polycentric femoral component). The shapes of the surfaces of the components were determined using a coordinate measuring machine. They modelled three instants in the normal walking cycle with the knee near extension, and calculated surface contact areas and pressures and the maximum value of the von Mises stress, said to be a measure of the tendency for delamination.

As expected, the fixed-bearing designs both had small contact areas, high contact stresses, and von Mises stresses significantly in excess of the material damage threshold (9 MPa). Both mobile-bearing knees had contact areas at least three times larger than the fixed-bearing designs but smaller than their nominal values because of manufacturing tolerances. The contact areas of the OUKA implant varied from 284 to 346 mm², compared with the nominal value of 580 mm² for ideally shaped components. Both mobile-bearing designs exhibited '... *very low contact stress and an absence of von Mises stress above the material damage threshold*' (Fig. 2.16(b)). No calculations were performed for knees flexed to 90°–100°, when the loads can be larger and the contact areas of the polycentric mobile bearing prosthesis would have been smaller than those of the congruent OUKA.

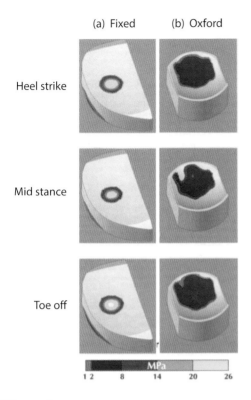

(a) Fixed   (b) Oxford

Heel strike

Mid stance

Toe off

MPa
1 2   8   14   20   26

Figure 2.16 Contact stresses (a) fixed flat bearing, (b) mobile fully congruous bearing (courtesy of A Seth Greenwald, DPhil (Oxon)) [23].

Discussion

The gradual diminution of bearing thickness over time is due to a combination of **creep** (bulk cold-flow of the viscoelastic polymer) and loss of material due to **wear** at its two articular surfaces. Penetration measurements of retrieved bearings do not allow an estimate of the relative contributions of these two processes, but the simulator studies suggest that creep only occurs initially and that, thereafter, penetration can be attributed entirely to surface wear.

Penetration rate

There was a significantly higher penetration rate in bearings with evidence of impingement, possibly because bone and polyethylene debris in the joint acted as third bodies between the articular surfaces. Impingement can be avoided by appropriate surgical technique, and a properly implanted bearing should not impinge against bone or cement. The latest instrumentation sets (Microplasty, Chapter 7) include an anterior mill specifically designed to remove potentially impinging bone from the front of the femoral component.

The mean rate of penetration of the 22 medial bearings with no evidence of impingement, the rate measured *in vivo* at 10 years and 20 years in clinically successful patients, and the rate in the simulator studies were all very small (0.01–0.02 mm/year). They are an order of magnitude lower than the mean rate of 0.15 mm/year reported for 19 retrievals of the St Georg fixed bearing prosthesis [24].

They are also much lower than the mean rate of 0.49 mm/year reported for 81 retrievals of various round-on-flat fixed bearing designs by Collier *et al.* [25] who attributed these high wear rates to the use of sterilisation by gamma irradiation of the polyethylene in air. This ignores the low penetration rates which we have reported for fully conforming meniscal bearings [14, 15], all of which were made of polyethylene which had been irradiated in air. We think that the low contact stresses associated with the large contact areas of the Oxford prosthesis can protect even a vulnerable material from excessive wear (if impingement is avoided). The high contact stresses associated with a round femoral component in contact with a flat or nearly flat tibial component common in fixed bearing designs may yet prove to be beyond the capacity of modern highly cross-linked polyethylene, particularly in view of the known reduction in fracture toughness which has been associated with cross-linking [26]. However, doping cross-linked UHMWPE with Vitamin E offers the exciting prospect of a material with low wear rate and high fatigue resistance [27].

It is not wise to extrapolate long-term wear rates from short-term measurements because the polymer may degrade and oxidise, but, at the rates reported, the OUKA bearings would lose 1 mm of thickness in 50–100 years. The high survival rates of the OUKA up to 20 years after implantation demonstrate (Chapter 10) that, in congruous articulation, polyethylene can survive as long as the patient even when used in thin components [28].

The rate of penetration of the Oxford bearings was also much lower than that reported by Wroblewski [29] for the acetabular component of the fully congruous Charnley hip (0.19 mm/year). This is not surprising as the projected area of contact is larger in the OUKA than in the Charnley hip, and the contact stresses are correspondingly lower.

A similarly low rate of penetration (0.026 mm/year) was found for a fixed-bearing total knee prosthesis with fully congruent cylindrical articular surfaces [30], suggesting that it is congruity, rather than the use of mobile bearings, that allows the transmission of high loads with little wear.

Similar data have not been published for mobile bearings articulating with poly-radial femoral condyles, but they may not enjoy such low wear rates as they cannot be congruent throughout the range of movement. In one such device, the most frequent cause for revision was bearing failure, and bearing exchange for wear is a well-recognised procedure [31, 32].

Bearing thickness

In incongruent articulations, the wear rate of polyethylene is greater when it is used in a thin layer [33]. Perhaps the most important observation made during our retrieval studies, with particular significance for unicompartmental arthroplasty, is that polyethylene used in congruent articulation has a wear rate that is independent of its initial thickness, at least down to 3.5 mm. This fact is less important in TKA where more extensive bone removal allows the use of thick tibial implants, but it is of consequence in unicompartmental prostheses when preservation of bone stock and minimal invasion are required. In fixed-bearing UKA designs, it is thought unsafe to use a polyethylene layer thinner than 6 mm [34]. However, a congruous meniscal bearing that is only 3.5 mm thick at its thinnest point wears no more rapidly than a thicker one.

In the original study based on data from Svard, there was no difference in survival between UKA with different bearing thicknesses. More recent data based on 1000 Phase 3 OUKA found that the results were substantially better with 3 mm or 4 mm bearings (94% 15 year survival) compared with 5 mm or more (75% 15 year survival) [35]. Although it is not yet clear why the difference is so marked, it confirms that wear is not an issue with the thin mobile bearings.

Volumetric wear

Penetration (linear wear plus creep) is not the only measure of wear. Another measure is the volume of debris generated (volumetric wear). Volumetric wear increases in proportion to the area of contact but, since it reduces with reduction in penetration, the beneficial effect of the low contact pressure at congruous surfaces may more than balance the adverse effect of their large contact areas. Calculations of the mean volume of wear debris produced at the articular surfaces of the Oxford bearing give a figure of about 6 mm^3/year (for bearings without impingement). The St Georg fixed-bearing implant had a measured volumetric wear rate of 17.3 mm^3/year [24]. No comparable data are available for other knee replacements, but the volumetric acetabular wear rates (assessed *in vivo*) for various designs of hip prosthesis, which also have congruous surfaces, vary from 26 to 89 mm^3/year [36]. The tissues around the hip are believed to be able to tolerate a mean of 600 mm^3 of polyethylene debris before bone resorption necessitates revision [37].

Therefore, it is unlikely that the volume of wear particles from a properly functioning meniscal bearing will cause problems. However, with the accelerated wear rate associated with impingement, it is possible that particle debris accumulated in the long term might become great enough to cause osteolysis.

There is a suspicion that it is the very small particles generated by wear at congruous surfaces that cause osteolysis and aseptic loosening. However, the study by Kendrick *et al.* [16] of 47 retrieved Oxford bearings (Fig. 2.13) showed that even those most damaged by impingement came from knees with no evidence of osteolysis. Sathasivam *et al.* [3] stated that '*there is no disadvantage with regard to particle size or type associated with large contact areas*'. The survival rates better than 90% at 20 years also imply an absence of significant osteolysis [28].

The debris generated by extra-articular impingement probably consists of larger particles. These may act as third bodies and hasten wear, as suggested by the observed correlation of impingement and increased penetration. Furthermore impingement may cause failure. The surgeon therefore needs to take all necessary precautions to ensure the bearing tracks freely and does not impinge.

Bearing fracture

Figure 2.17 shows a set of eight bearings which had fractured *in vivo*. We have reported on ten such fractured bearings on which we had data on implantation time [38]. Four others were sent to us without such information. Over 500,000 of these bearings have been implanted and these are the only instances of fractures which we have seen, seven from one practice of over 1000 cases. From the latter practice, it is estimated that the fracture rate of Phase 1 bearings was 3.2%, that of Phase 2 bearings was 0.74% and that of Phase 3 was 0.35%. The mean duration of the prosthesis *in situ* was 16.8 years (range 6.6 to 23.9). Five of the bearings had a minimum thickness of 3.5 mm, three had 4.5 mm and two had 5.5 mm at implantation. The mean age of the patients at implantation was 60.3 years (range 50 to 69) and the mean weight was 80.1 kg (range 70 to 100).

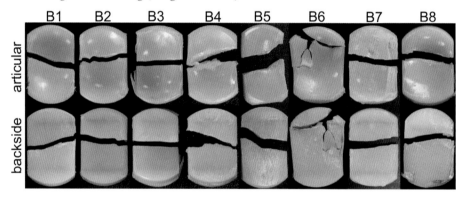

Figure 2.17 Photographs of the femoral and tibial surfaces of the fractured bearings.

All of the fractured bearings showed evidence of impingement and excessive wear (>0.05 mm per year). In most cases, the fractures appeared to be systematic, occurring on the coronal plane through or near the point of minimum thickness of the bearing. Finite element stress analysis confirmed the presence of tensile stresses on this plane needed to resist the forwards facing components of the pressure on the anterior half of the spherical upper surface of the bearing and the backwards facing components of the pressure on the posterior part of the upper surface (Fig. 2.18) [39]. Tensile stress is necessary both to initiate and propagate fatigue cracks.

The posterior metal wire used as an x-ray marker appeared to be implicated in some of the specimens and, since 1999, this has been replaced by two tantalum balls in short holes on the medial and lateral edges at the back of the bearing. However, Lim *et al.* [40] have reported an instance of a fractured Phase 3 bearing with a tantalum ball posterior marker. They remarked on evidence of impingement on the retrieved specimen.

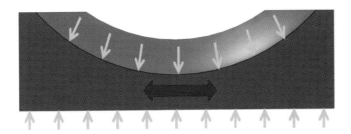

Figure 2.18. The anteriorly directed pressure at the front of the upper surface of the bearing and the posteriorly directed pressure at the back can generate the type of tensile stresses necessary to propagate fatigue cracks but they have been observed only in severely worn bearings. (This material has been reproduced from the Journal of Engineering in Medicine: Proceedings of the Institution of Mechanical Engineers Part H. 2013 Vol 227 pp 1213-23. Fracture of mobile unicompartmental knee bearings, Pegg E, Murray DW, Pandit HG, O'Connor JJ, Gill HS. Permission is granted by the Council of the Institution of Mechanical Engineers.)

We conclude that fracture occurs only after significant reduction of bearing thickness due to impingement-induced wear and that fracture can be avoided if impingement is avoided. As bearing thickness is reduced, the anteroposterior tensile stresses are increased. The most recent instrumentation, Microplasty (Chapter 7), introduces an anterior mill specifically designed to help avoid anterior impingement.

Comparison between fixed and mobile

With fixed bearing UKA, a divot appears within the surface of the tibial components almost as soon as they are used, partly as a result of creep and partly by wear, (Fig. 2.19). This tends to constrain the movement of the femoral component on the tibia. In contrast with the mobile bearing Oxford implant, Figure 2.20(a), except for the effects of friction, there is free movement of the mobile bearing both in the short and long term.

The differences between mobile and fixed have significant implications for function in the longer term. Figure 2.20(a) and (b) shows schematic diagrams of the response to an oblique load of both mobile bearing (a) and fixed bearing (b) UKA with the cruciate ligaments. With the mobile bearing implant, the femur can translate freely along the plateau, allowing one of the cruciate ligaments to stretch and to develop tensile forces to balance the component of the oblique force parallel to the tibial plateau. The interface between the implant and the tibia is not involved in this balance and the bone/implant stresses remain compressive, ideal for fixation. (More detailed descriptions of the interactions between the mobile bearing implant and the ligaments are given in Chapter 3 and the Appendix, with animations on the website www.oxfordpartialknee.com also relevant.)

After a period of usage, the divot worn in the surface of the fixed bearing implant resists anteroposterior translation of the femur on the tibia by developing shear forces parallel to the bone/implant interface (Fig. 2.20(b)), while allowing both cruciate ligaments to slacken. These shear forces tend to tilt the implant, with the development of tensile forces. The shear and tensile forces will be transmitted to the implant/bone interface and may cause loosening.

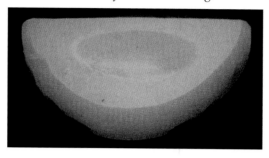

Figure 2.19 Divot in a fixed bearing UKA, unpublished photograph by Professor W Plitz, Munich.

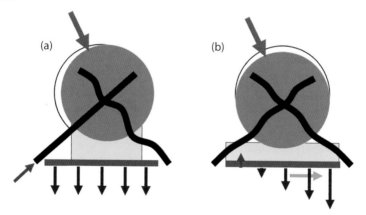

Figure 2.20 Interface reactions to an oblique load (shown in brown), mobile (a) v fixed (b). Compressive stresses at the bone/implant interface are shown in blue, tensile stresses are shown in red, shear stresses in green.

If the cruciate ligaments are not loaded normally, they may, with time, fail. Evidence that this happens comes from a study by Argenson et al. [41] which showed, at 10 years after Miller-Galante fixed bearing arthroplasty, many knees were functioning like ACL deficient knees which increases the loading in the PFJ. Studies of the OUKA show that not only at one but also 10 years post operation, the kinematics following OUKA are virtually normal, with normal bearing movement [42]. This difference may explain in part why, after the mobile bearing arthroplasty, there do not seem to be problems with the patellofemoral joint in the long term whereas, after the fixed bearing, progression of the OA into the patellofemoral joint is one of the commonest causes for failure [43].

Cementless Oxford arthroplasty

With good long term results achieved with the cemented Oxford arthroplasty, there seems little justification to develop a cementless device, particularly as cementless

TKA have not performed as well as cemented TKA [44]. There are however potential advantages. For example, many failures are caused by cementing errors, which often occur with inexperienced surgeons using the Minimally Invasive Surgical (MIS) approach. Furthermore, many of the failures in the Registers are reported as being from loosening. Some of these are likely to be true loosening but others may be the result of misinterpretation of the radiolucent lines that commonly are seen in association with a cemented tibial component. Both of these issues could potentially be addressed with cementless components.

The mechanical environment at the bone/implant interface is very different in TKA to UKA, with the forces in a TKA not being ideal for cementless fixation whereas those in UKA, particularly mobile bearing UKA, are. Despite cementless TKA not performing well [44], it is therefore well worth considering cementless mobile bearing UKA. Optimally there will be only compressive forces at the interface. With the mobile bearing OUKA, excluding the effects of friction, the forces are

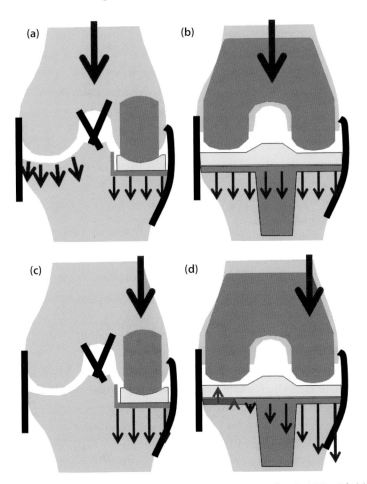

Figure 2.21 The mechanical environment at the bone/implant interface in UKA with (a) central and (c) eccentric loading and TKA with (b) central and (d) eccentric loading.

predominantly compressive.

With UKA, whether the load across the knee is central (Fig. 2.21(a)) or eccentric (Fig. 2.21(c)) there is always compressive load under the tibial component. However, following TKA, although central loading (Fig. 2.21(b)) causes compression, eccentric loading (Fig. 2.21(d)) may cause tilting and loosening of the tibia.

Anecdotal evidence that suggests that cementless components will work comes from an Italian surgeon who implanted Phase 2 Oxford components without cement. Despite having no fixation, these components functioned well. We were able to review some radiographs taken five years postoperatively. They were satisfactory, albeit with radiolucencies. This confirms that the loading on the components is predominantly compressive and that even without any formal fixation, the components function well. Therefore, with cementless fixation, one would expect a reliable result.

Potential problems with the tibia

Most of the early complications following both cemented and cementless OUKA relate to the tibia. These include early pain, tibial plateau fractures and tibial subsidence. It is perhaps not surprising that complications occur more at the tibial side than the femoral side because the bone resection significantly weakens the tibia. The resection involves both a vertical and a horizontal cut. The resected bone includes all the subchondral plate which usually provides a tension band supporting the buttress of the medial tibial condyle. Once the bone resection has been done, the stresses in the underlying bone increase substantially which in turn increases the risk of fracture as well as of bone pain.

Finite element analyses have been undertaken to study these problems. These include studies that estimated the strain in the cortical bone a few centimeters below the joint anteromedially in an area where pain commonly occurs [45], and studies estimating the strain within the bone in the region where tibial plateau fractures may occur [46]. These analyses have shown that, even with perfectly performed UKA, bone stresses anteromedially in the tibia increase by about 60% which may explain why there is anteromedial pain (Fig. 2.22). With bone remodelling, the bone may strengthen and the strains decrease which probably explains why the strains settle. In addition, following UKA, the strain within the bone at the site of a possible plateau fracture increases. Both studies have shown that errors in surgical technique are likely to increase the risk of pain or fracture (Fig. 2.23). In particular, it has been shown that vertical saw cuts that go too deep, horizontal resections that are too low, damage to the back of the keel slot or vertical saw cuts that are too medial, all increase the risk of fracture or pain. Furthermore, a cadaver study by Seeger et al. [47] has shown that the load to fracture is lower following a cementless rather than a cemented component. Although the tibia is undoubtedly weakened during its preparation, we have found that the risk of fracture or pain is very low if the surgery is undertaken carefully without any of the errors described above. Surgeons need to be aware of these risks and take care with tibial preparation.

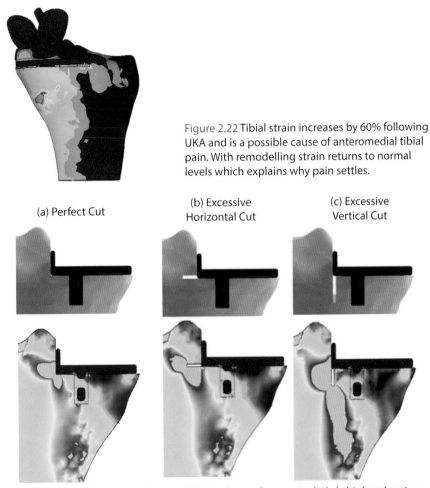

Figure 2.22 Tibial strain increases by 60% following UKA and is a possible cause of anteromedial tibial pain. With remodelling strain returns to normal levels which explains why pain settles.

(a) Perfect Cut

(b) Excessive Horizontal Cut

(c) Excessive Vertical Cut

Figure 2.23 With a perfect cut (a) the risk of tibial plateau fracture is slightly higher than in a normal knee. It is not appreciably increased by an extended horizontal cut (b). It is however high (grey) with a deep vertical cut (c).

Conclusion

We have demonstrated that the use of an unconstrained fully congruous mobile bearing in a unicompartmental knee prosthesis can minimise polyethylene wear provided that impingement of bone surfaces or cement against the polyethylene is avoided. This has remained true over the 40-year life of the prosthesis, despite several changes in the material and its processing over that time. A rare complication has been fracture of the bearing, which has been observed only when excessive wear caused by impingement occurred. The interface stresses under a mobile bearing are ideal, particularly for cementless fixation, which should help to minimise loosening. When complications occur they are frequently related to the tibia. Careful surgery is needed to avoid these problems. The theoretical basis for this, and for the surgical technique needed to minimise the risk, are discussed in Chapter 11.

References

1. Taylor WR, Heller MO, Bergmann G, Duda GN. Tibio-femoral loading during human gait and stair climbing. *J Orthop Res* 2004; **22**(3): 625-32.

2. Rostoker W, Galante JO. Contact pressure dependence of wear rates of ultra high molecular weight polyethylene. *J Biomed Mater Res* 1979; **13**(6): 957-64.

3. Sathasivam S, Walker PS, Campbell PA, Rayner K. The effect of contact area on wear in relation to fixed bearing and mobile bearing knee replacements. *J Biomed Mater Res* 2001; **58**(3): 282-90.

4. Fairbank TJ. Knee joint changes after meniscectomy. *J Bone Joint Surg Br* 1948; **30B**(4): 664-70.

5. Bullough PG, Munuera L, Murphy J, Weinstein AM. The strength of the menisci of the knee as it relates to their fine structure. *J Bone Joint Surg Br* 1970; **52**(3): 564-7.

6. Shrive NG, O'Connor JJ, Goodfellow JW. Load-bearing in the knee joint. *Clin Orthop Relat Res* 1978; (**131**): 279-87.

7. Borelli GA. *De Motu Animalium*. Heidelberg: Springer Verlag, 1989; 1680.

8. Kapandji I. The physiology of the joints. Edinburgh: Churchill Livingstone; 1970.

9. Thompson WO, Thaete FL, Fu FH, Dye SF. Tibial meniscal dynamics using three-dimensional reconstruction of magnetic resonance images. *Am J Sports Med* 1991; **19**(3): 210-5; discussion 215-6.

10. Vedi V, Williams A, Tennant SJ, Spouse E, Hunt DM, Gedroyc WM. Meniscal movement. An in-vivo study using dynamic MRI. *J Bone Joint Surg Br* 1999; **81**(1): 37-41.

11. Goodfellow J, O'Connor J. The mechanics of the knee and prosthesis design. *J Bone Joint Surg Br* 1978; **60-B**(3): 358-69.

12. Buechel FF, Pappas MJ. The New Jersey Low-Contact-Stress Knee Replacement System: biomechanical rationale and review of the first 123 cemented cases. *Arch Orthop Trauma Surg* 1986; **105**(4): 197-204.

13. Schlueter-Brust K, Kugland K, Stein G, Henckel J, Christ H, Eysel P, Bontemps G. Ten year survivorship after cemented and uncemented medial Uniglide ® unicompartmental knee arthroplasties. *Knee* 2014; **21**(5): 964-70.

14. Argenson JN, O'Connor JJ. Polyethylene wear in meniscal knee replacement. A one to nine-year retrieval analysis of the Oxford knee. *J Bone Joint Surg Br* 1992; **74**(2): 228-32.

15. Psychoyios V, Crawford RW, O'Connor JJ, Murray DW. Wear of congruent meniscal bearings in unicompartmental knee arthroplasty: a retrieval study of 16 specimens. *J Bone Joint Surg Br* 1998; **80**(6): 976-82.

16. Kendrick BJ, Longino D, Pandit H, Svard U, Gill HS, Dodd CA, Murray DW, Price AJ. Polyethylene wear in Oxford unicompartmental knee replacement: a retrieval study of 47 bearings. *J Bone Joint Surg Br* 2010; **92**(3): 367-73.

17. Price AJ, Short A, Kellett C, Beard D, Gill H, Pandit H, Dodd CA, Murray DW. Ten-year in vivo wear measurement of a fully congruent mobile bearing unicompartmental knee arthroplasty. *J Bone Joint Surg Br* 2005; **87**(11): 1493-7.

18. Kendrick BJ, Kaptein BL, Valstar ER, Gill HS, Jackson WF, Dodd CA, Price AJ, Murray DW. Cemented versus cementless Oxford unicompartmental knee arthroplasty using radiostereometric analysis: A randomised controlled trial. *Bone Joint J* 2015; **97-B**(2): 185-91.

19. Kendrick BJ, Simpson DJ, Kaptein BL, Valstar ER, Gill HS, Murray DW, Price AJ. Polyethylene wear of mobile-bearing unicompartmental knee replacement at 20 years. *J Bone Joint Surg Br* 2011; **93**(4): 470-5.

20. Murray DW, Goodfellow JW, O'Connor JJ. The Oxford medial unicompartmental arthroplasty: a ten-year survival study. *J Bone Joint Surg Br* 1998; **80**(6): 983-9.

21. Walker PS, Blunn GW, Broome DR, Perry J, Watkins A, Sathasivam S, Dewar ME, Paul JP. A knee simulating machine for performance evaluation of total knee replacements. *J Biomech* 1997; **30**(1): 83-9.

22. Scott R, Schroeder D. Correlation of knee simulator to *in-vivo* use: evaluating the Oxford Unicompartmental Knee. Transactions of the 46th Annual Meeting of the Orthopaedic Research Society; 2000; Orlando, Florida: Orthopaedic Research Society; 2000. p. 434.

23. Morra EA, Greenwald AS. Effects of walking gait on ultra-high molecular weight polyethylene damage in unicompartmental knee systems. A finite element study. *J Bone Joint Surg Am* 2003; **85-A Suppl 4**: 111-4.

24. Ashraf T, Newman JH, Desai VV, Beard D, Nevelos JE. Polyethylene wear in a non-congruous unicompartmental knee replacement: a retrieval analysis. *Knee* 2004; **11**(3): 177-81.

25. Collier MB, Engh CA, Jr., McAuley JP, Engh GA. Factors associated with the loss of thickness of polyethylene tibial bearings after knee arthroplasty. *J Bone Joint Surg Am* 2007; **89**(6): 1306-14.

26. Oral E, Christensen SD, Malhi AS, Wannomae KK, Muratoglu OK. Wear resistance and mechanical properties of highly cross-linked, ultrahigh-molecular weight polyethylene doped with vitamin E. *J Arthroplasty* 2006; **21**(4): 580-91.

27. Oral E, Neils A, Yabannavar P, Muratoglu OK. The effect of an additional phosphite stabilizer on the properties of radiation cross-linked vitamin E blends of UHMWPE. *J Orthop Res* 2014; **32**(6): 757-61.

28. Price AJ, Svard U. A second decade lifetable survival analysis of the Oxford unicompartmental knee arthroplasty. *Clin Orthop Relat Res* 2011; **469**(1): 174-9.

29. Wroblewski BM. Direction and rate of socket wear in Charnley low-friction arthroplasty. *J Bone Joint Surg Br* 1985; **67**(5): 757-61.

30. Plante-Bordeneuve P, Freeman MA. Tibial high-density polyethylene wear in conforming tibiofemoral prostheses. *J Bone Joint Surg Br* 1993; **75**(4): 630-6.

31. Hamelynck KJ, Stiehl JB, Voorhorst PE. Worldwide multicentre outcome study. In: Hamelynck KJ, Stiehl JB, eds. *LCS Mobile Bearing Arthoplasty: 25 Years of Worldwide Experience*. Berlin: Springer; 2002: 212-24.

32. Keblish PA, Briard JL. Mobile-bearing unicompartmental knee arthroplasty: a 2-center study with an 11-year (mean) follow-up. *J Arthroplasty* 2004; **19**(7 Suppl 2): 87-94.

33. Bartel DL, Bicknell VL, Wright TM. The effect of conformity, thickness, and material on stresses in ultra-high molecular weight components for total joint replacement. *J Bone Joint Surg Am* 1986; **68**(7): 1041-51.

34. Marmor L. The Modular (Marmor) knee: case report with a minimum follow-up of 2 years. *Clin Orthop Relat Res* 1976; (**120**): 86-94.

35. Pandit H, Hamilton TW, Jenkins C, Mellon SJ, Dodd CA, Murray DW. The clinical outcome of minimally invasive Phase 3 Oxford unicompartmental knee arthroplasty: a 15-year follow-up of 1000 UKAs. *Bone Joint J* 2015; **97-B**(11): 1493-500.

36. Kabo JM, Gebhard JS, Loren G, Amstutz HC. In vivo wear of polyethylene acetabular components. *J Bone Joint Surg Br* 1993; **75**(2): 254-8.

37. Hall RM, Siney P, Unsworth A, Wroblewski BM. The association between rates of wear in retrieved acetabular components and the radius of the femoral head. *Proc Inst Mech Eng H* 1998; **212**(5): 321-6.

38. Pegg E, Pandit H, Gill HS, Keys GW, Svard UG, O'Connor JJ, Murray DW. Examination of ten fractured Oxford unicompartmental knee bearings. *J Bone Joint Surg Br* 2011; **93**(12): 1610-6.

39. Pegg EC, Murray DW, Pandit HG, O'Connor JJ, Gill HS. Fracture of mobile unicompartmental knee bearings: a parametric finite element study. *Proc Inst Mech Eng H* 2013; **227**(11): 1213-23.

40. Lim HC, Shon WY, Kim SJ, Bae JH. Oxford phase III meniscal bearing fracture: case report. *Knee* 2014; **21**(1): 340-2.

41. Argenson JN, Komistek RD, Aubaniac JM, Dennis DA, Northcut EJ, Anderson DT, Agostini S. In vivo determination of knee kinematics for subjects implanted with a unicompartmental arthroplasty. *J Arthroplasty* 2002; **17**(8): 1049-54.

42. Price AJ, Rees JL, Beard DJ, Gill RH, Dodd CA, Murray DM. Sagittal plane kinematics of a mobile-bearing unicompartmental knee arthroplasty at 10 years: a comparative in vivo fluoroscopic analysis. *J Arthroplasty* 2004; **19**(5): 590-7.

43. Argenson JN, Blanc G, Aubaniac JM, Parratte S. Modern unicompartmental knee arthroplasty with cement: a concise follow-up, at a mean of twenty years, of a previous report. *J Bone Joint Surg Am* 2013; **95**(10): 905-9.

44. Ranawat CS, Meftah M, Windsor EN, Ranawat AS. Cementless fixation in total knee arthroplasty: down the boulevard of broken dreams - affirms. *J Bone Joint Surg Br* 2012; **94**(11 Suppl A): 82-4.

45. Simpson DJ, Price AJ, Gulati A, Murray DW, Gill HS. Elevated proximal tibial strains following unicompartmental knee replacement--a possible cause of pain. *Med Eng Phys* 2009; **31**(7): 752-7.

46. Pegg EC, Walter J, Mellon SJ, Pandit HG, Murray DW, D'Lima DD, Fregly BJ, Gill HS. Evaluation of factors affecting tibial bone strain after unicompartmental knee replacement. *J Orthop Res* 2013; **31**(5): 821-8.

47. Seeger JB, Haas D, Jager S, Rohner E, Tohtz S, Clarius M. Extended sagittal saw cut significantly reduces fracture load in cementless unicompartmental knee arthroplasty compared to cemented tibia plateaus: an experimental cadaver study. *Knee Surg Sports Traumatol Arthrosc* 2012; **20**(6): 1087-91.

3

Mobility and Stability of the Intact and Replaced Knee

Having demonstrated in Chapter 2 that a fully conforming mobile bearing can minimise polyethylene wear, in this chapter we show that a mobile bearing prosthesis, unconstrained in the sagittal plane, can restore natural mobility and stability.

For surgeon readers who are less interested in the theoretical background, it might be advisable to go straight to Chapter 4, Indications, or to start by reading the final section of this chapter, The Loaded Prosthetic Knee. If that proves interesting, the surgeon might attempt The Unloaded Prosthetic Knee. For the more research minded surgeon or engineer, it seems more logical to start with the Unloaded Natural Knee (the longest section of the chapter) and to read from there. The chapter may also be of interest to those surgeons embarking on the use of a bi-cruciate retaining total knee replacement.

The numerous writings on knee movement and the many methods used for its measurement and analysis over the past two centuries have been reviewed in detail by Pinskerova, Maquet and Freeman [1] and by Freeman and Pinskerova [2]. We will not attempt to repeat such reviews. We present our own evidence as to how the passive soft tissues of the human knee interact to control the passive motion of the bones and how this motion is modified in activity in the presence of muscle force, external loads and consequent tissue deformation. This provides a base with which to compare the kinematics and mechanics of the Oxford Knee in cadaver specimens and in living patients. In designing these studies, we have used as our model the example of D'Arcy Thompson:

.... ligaments and membrane, muscle and tendon, run between bone and bone; and the beauty and strength of the mechanical construction lie not in one part or another, but in the harmonious concatenation which all the parts, soft and hard, rigid and flexible, tension-bearing and pressure-bearing, make up together.

    D'Arcy Wentworth Thompson, *On Growth and Form*, 1945, Cambridge
      University Press, Macmillan Edition.

The shapes of the articular surfaces of the Oxford Knee components do not match those of either compartment of the natural joint and, even if they did, they could hardly be expected to match exactly the shapes of the surfaces of each individual patient. How is it possible for such an implant to restore normal mobility and stability, normal kinematics and mechanics?

The complex three-dimensional pattern of movement of the natural knee depends upon the following:

(1) the shapes of its articular surfaces which hold the bones apart;

(2) the design of the array of ligaments that hold the bones together;

(3) the deformation of the tissues dependent on the magnitude and direction of the forces applied by muscle contraction in response to gravity and ground reaction and other external loads.

In any particular joint, features (1) and (2) are constant and therefore the movements of the **unloaded** knee should be predictable and repeatable. However, the forces applied during activity are as infinitely variable as the uses to which the human limb is put, and the consequent patterns of movement of the **loaded** knee are also infinitely varied. Blankevoort *et al.* [3] noted that *"the basis for the understanding of the kinematics of the knee joint lies in the description of its passive motion characteristics"*. Passive motion is what the surgeon observes on the operating table with the patient under anaesthetic.

The unloaded human knee

Relative movements of the bones

The pattern of movement of the unloaded knee is highly ordered. In a study in which the movements were controlled solely by the intact ligaments and articular surfaces, 12 unloaded cadaver knee specimens were examined with the muscle tendons removed, the proximal tibia fixed with its plateau approximately horizontal and an intramedullary rod in the distal femur lying on a horizontal rod which was gently lowered and raised to control flexion and extension (Fig. 3.1) [4-6]. The only load present was the weight of the distal femur (about 5 N, 1 lb), shared between the horizontal rod and the knee specimen. An electromagnetic digitiser (Isotrack II, Polhemus Inc, Vermont, USA) was used to track all six degrees of freedom of movement of the femur relative to the tibia. The entire rig was made of plastic so as not to distort the magnetic field of the digitiser.

Figure 3.2 shows axial rotation of the femur relative to the tibia plotted against flexion angle for one specimen. External rotation of about 20° accompanied 120° of flexion but it is notable that the path followed during flexing was almost exactly reproduced during extending, with very little hysterisis. Axial rotation was uniquely coupled to flexion angle.

The graph of axial rotation from Figure 3.2 is included again in Figure 3.3 together with plots against flexion angle of the angle of abduction/adduction and the three components of translation of a single point on the femur relative to the tibia (dotted lines). Movements are plotted relative to a coordinate system with flexion/extension calculated about a medio-lateral axis parallel to a line joining the centres of curvature of the posterior femoral condyles, axial rotation about an axis perpendicular to the medio-lateral axis and fixed in the tibia according to a method

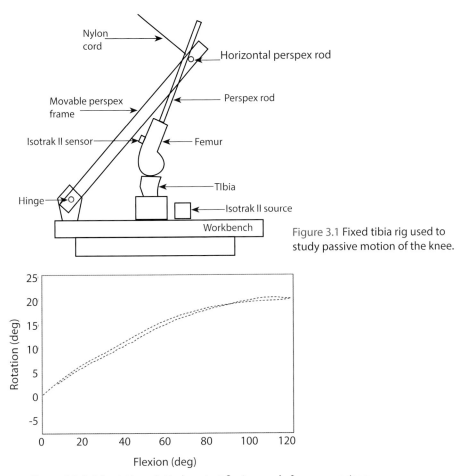

Figure 3.1 Fixed tibia rig used to study passive motion of the knee.

Figure 3.2 Axial rotation plotted against flexion angle for one specimen.

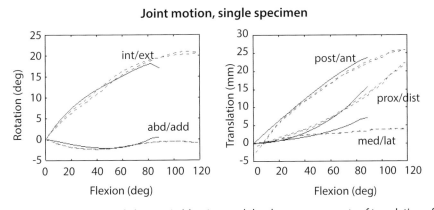

Figure 3.3 Axial rotation, abduction/adduction, and the three components of translation of a single point in the femur (the most proximal anterior point on the PCL attachment area) plotted against flexion angle for a single specimen (dotted curves). The solid lines on the graphs will be discussed later. (Adapted from Wilson DR, Feikes JD, Zavatsky AB, O'Connor JJ. The components of passive knee movement are coupled to flexion angle. *J Biomech* 2000; **33**:465-73, with permission.)

described by Yoshioka *et al.* [7], ab/adduction was calculated about a 'floating' antero-posterior axis perpendicular to both. The three components of translation were also calculated relative to these axes.

The figures show that axial rotation, abduction/adduction and the three components of translation of an arbitrarily chosen point on the femur (in this case, the most proximal point on the attachment of the PCL) were all uniquely coupled to flexion angle. In particular, for all five degrees of freedom, the path followed during flexion was almost exactly retraced during extension, with virtually no hysteresis. These curves are therefore characteristic of the unique path of passive motion followed by this specimen. Specifying the flexion angle completely determined the configuration of this knee joint, which therefore behaved like a single degree of freedom system. The solid lines in these figures will be discussed below.

Average Passive Motion (n=12)

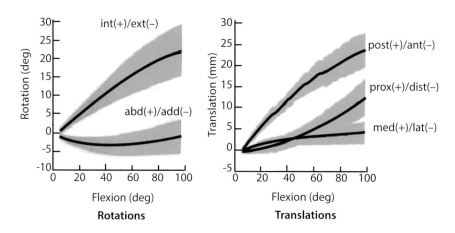

Figure 3.4 Axial rotation, abduction/adduction, and the three components of translation of a point in the femur (the most anterior point on the PCL attachment area) plotted against flexion angle for twelve specimens, the curves give mean values, the shaded areas defined by ± one standard deviation. (Reprinted from Wilson DR, Feikes JD, Zavatsky AB, O'Connor JJ. The components of passive knee movement are coupled to flexion angle. *J Biomech* 2000; 33: 465-73, Fig. 3, with permission.)

Figure 3.4 shows similar curves for 12 specimens tested in the same rig. All specimens exhibited minimal hysteresis. The results from specimen to specimen were quite repeatable and could be said to define the path of passive motion of the human knee. During passive flexion to 90°, the femur rotates externally on a fixed tibia (or the tibia rotates internally on a fixed femur) through about 22°. There is also a small amount of abduction/adduction. The components of translation vary from point to point on the femur but all are uniquely coupled to flexion angle. All specimens exhibited just one degree of freedom.

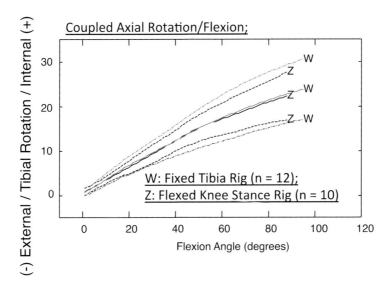

Figure 3.5 Axial rotation (mean values ± one standard deviation) plotted against flexion angle for the 12 specimens of Fig. 3.4 (marked W) and for 10 further unloaded specimens when tested in a six-degree of freedom rig simulating deep squats with the hip moving vertically above the ankle (marked Z).

Figure 3.5 shows results obtained by Zavatsky from 10 specimens tested in a rig simulating deep squats during passive motion [8–10]. The 'Z' curves are almost identical to the graphs of axial rotation of Figures 3.2, 3.3 and 3.4, demonstrating that the passive motion described by these figures is characteristic of the human knee and not of the apparatus in which the measurements are made. Such results can be achieved only if the apparatus used to hold the specimens allows them six independent degrees of freedom so that the only constraints applied to the motion of the specimens are the passive constraints of the ligaments and articular surfaces [10].

Blankevoort *et al.* [3] did not find such a unique path but defined an envelope of external/internal rotation about 40° wide obtained when the knee was flexed first with an internally rotating torque then with an externally rotating torque of 3 Nm. We show below that ordered motion is observed also in the presence of torques of value ±1 and ±2 Nm (Fig. 3.22).

The highly ordered pattern of movement suggested by Figures 3.2, 3.3 and 3.4 was not repeated in three further specimens which showed disorderly movements and wide hysteresis loops (Fig. 3.6). On subsequent dissection, two of these specimens were found to have articular surfaces eroded by disease (Figs. 3.6(a) and 3.6(b)) and the third had partial division of the MCL (Fig. 3.6(c)). For each specimen, the path followed during flexion was very different to that followed in extension, and the angle of axial rotation and the other four degrees of freedom were no longer uniquely coupled to the flexion angle. These specimens, which no longer had any preferred path, did not resist being positioned anywhere between the upper and lower curves. These results demonstrate that the ordered movement exhibited by the human knee during passive movement requires fully intact articular surfaces and fully intact ligaments.

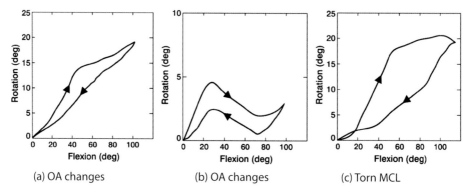

(a) OA changes   (b) OA changes   (c) Torn MCL

Figure 3.6 External femoral rotation plotted against flexion angle for three specimens: (a) and (b) had severe osteoarthritic lesions, and (c) had a partially divided MCL. (Reproduced from the DPhil Thesis of JD Feikes [4].)

Relative movements of the articular surfaces

From the point of view of prosthesis design, it is important to understand how the articular surfaces of the natural joint move on each other.

It is obvious that, during flexion, the points of contact on the femur move from the inferior surfaces of the femoral condyles to their posterior surfaces. However, the positions of the contact points on the tibial plateau are less obvious because of the presence of the menisci. Radiographic studies of the natural joint are not ideal because cartilage is radiolucent, and MRI is unreliable because the fine detail of the contacting surfaces can be trapped within one line of pixels on the VDU monitor, and can appear as straight line segments [11]. Also, MRI scanning during continuous movement is not possible. Load deforms the cartilage surfaces and the menisci, and creates areas, not points, of contact. These technical problems may account for some of the variability in descriptions of the contact regime.

After completion of the passive movement experiments [6], the positions of a number of reference points (defined by small nails or plastic plugs) on the external surface of each bone were recorded with the joint in full extension and the posterior capsule tight [4]. The specimens were then disarticulated and the electromagnetic digitiser was used to record the relative positions of over 4000 points on each of the bones, with particular attention to the articular surfaces and the areas of attachment of the ligaments and to the aforesaid reference points. It was then possible to reconstruct mathematically the relative movements of each of the digitised points during the passive movement experiments, using an algorithm developed by Veldpaus *et al.*[12].

Feikes [4] fitted surfaces mathematically through the data points from the articular surfaces of each of the posterior femoral condyles and tibial plateaux of each specimen, with a mean error of <0.5 mm (see the images of the articular surfaces in Fig. 3.13 below). She could then determine the relative movements of these surfaces during passive flexion/extension through successive steps of 5°.

Because of inevitable experimental or reconstruction error, the surface images at various positions of flexion usually appeared either to separate (Fig. 3.7(b)), or interpenetrate (Fig. 3.7(c)).

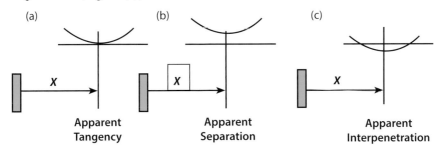

(a) (b) (c)

Apparent Tangency   Apparent Separation   Apparent Interpenetration

X : Distance of sphere centre from fixed reference

(Anterior edge of ACL tibial attachment)

Figure 3.7 Proximity method used to determine the position of the *Point of Closest Approach* of the articular surfaces, simplified in this example as a spherical femoral condyle and a flat tibial plateau. Whether the surfaces appeared to separate (b) or interpenetrate (c) due to experimental and/or reconstruction error, the position of the point of closest approach was taken to be defined by the position of the perpendicular to the flat surface through the centre of the sphere. (Reproduced from the DPhil thesis of JD Feikes [4].)

Feikes calculated the movement during flexion of a line through each of the surfaces joining their centres of curvature, defining the points of closest approach, and took that to be the movement of the contact point on each surface.

Table 3.1 gives the values of the contact point movement on the tibial plateaux from full extension to 100° flexion in the twelve intact specimens. Where Max movement exceeds Net movement at 100°, the maximum movement occurred at a flexion angle less than 100° and the contact point then moved forward with further flexion. A prosthesis designer probably should take account of the maximum rather than the net movement.

All specimens exhibited backwards movement of the contact point on the lateral tibial plateau during flexion, consistent with rolling of the femoral condyle on the tibia. One of the specimens (M) exhibited *forward* movement of the contact point on the medial plateau but all the others exhibited *backwards* rolling movement, with an overall average of 7.9 mm for the twelve specimens (SD 7.0 mm). The large variation on the medial side is reflected in the correspondingly larger standard deviation from the mean, compared with that on the lateral side.

Table 3.1 Estimated posterior movement of the tibial contact points with flexion. Negative values indicate anterior movement. Net movement corresponds to that recorded from full extension to 100° flexion while maximum (Max) movement is the maximum occurring within the range.

Specimen	Side	Medial		Lateral	
		Net (mm)	Max (mm)	Net (mm)	Max (mm)
J	L	11.4	13.1	9.2	9.2
D	R	6.3	6.3	13.1	13.1
L	L	0.7	0.7	16.5	16.5
M	R	-4.5	-7.3	9.0	9.0
X	R	7.4	7.4	18.0	18.0
I	R	3.3	3.5	24.6	24.6
E	R	1.9	1.9	22.3	22.3
G	L	19.6	19.8	12.9	14.5
F	L	9.1	9.8	10.2	10.2
B	L	18.0	18.1	15.2	15.2
A	L	8.8	10.5	11.6	11.6
H	R	12.4	12.4	13.5	13.5
Mean		**7.9**	**8.0**	**14.7**	**14.8**
SD		7.0	7.8	5.0	4.9

Table 3.1 does not tell the whole story. Goodfellow and O'Connor [13] introduced the concept of *slip ratio*, being the ratio of the distance the contact point moved on the tibial plateau divided by the distance it moved on the femoral condyle. For pure rolling without slip (as with a car wheel on the ground), the contact point would move the same distance on both surfaces and the slip ratio would equal unity. For pure sliding on the tibia, the contact point would remain stationary on the tibia while moving on the femur and the slip ratio would be zero. By this definition, it should perhaps have been better called the 'roll ratio'.

For each of the specimens, Feikes [4] calculated the slip ratio for 5° degree flexion steps from extension to 100° (Fig. 3.8). The slip ratio in the lateral compartments averaged about 0.5 while, for the medial compartments, it averaged about 0.3. In neither compartment was the mean value zero at any flexion angle so that rolling took place *continuously* and at a reasonably constant rate over the flexion range, but less so in the medial compartment. In each compartment, the femur rolls backwards while sliding forwards on the tibia during flexion, *vice versa* during extension, as described by Goodfellow and O'Connor [13] and O'Connor et al. [14] The differences in the rolling movements in the two compartments reflects the coupled effect of internal tibial rotation with passive flexion, reducing but not eliminating medial rolling, relatively increasing lateral rolling.

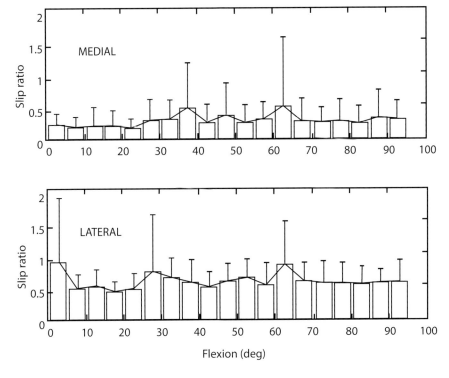

Figure 3.8. Average slip ratio plotted against flexion angle for the medial and lateral compartments of twelve cadaver specimens, plus one standard deviation.

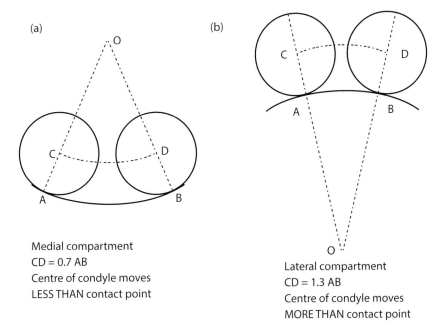

(a)

(b)

Medial compartment
CD = 0.7 AB
Centre of condyle moves
LESS THAN contact point

Lateral compartment
CD = 1.3 AB
Centre of condyle moves
MORE THAN contact point

Figure 3.9. A smaller circle moving on a larger concave (a) and larger convex (b) circle. As contact moves from **A** to **B**, the centre of the smaller circle moves from **C** to **D**.

The digitising of the tibial plateau confirmed the widely held belief that the medial tibial plateau is concave and the lateral plateau is convex, particularly in sagittal sections [15]. Figure 3.9(a) shows that when contact between a small circle (the medial femoral condyle) and a larger fixed concave circle (the medial tibial plateau) moves from *A* to *B*, the centre of the small circle moves from *C* to *D*. The ratio of these distances is about 0.68 for radii typical of the posterior surface of the medial femoral condyle (22.5 mm) and the medial tibial plateau (about 70 mm). Even without the contribution of axial rotation, the centre of the medial femoral condyle would be expected to move 5.4 mm, 32% less than the contact point (mean 7.9 mm Table 3.1). When contact between a small circle and a larger convex circle (the lateral tibial plateau) moves from *A* to *B* (Fig. 3.9(b)), the centre of the small circle moves from *C* to *D*. Thus, the centre of the lateral condyle would be expected to move about 27% more than the contact point, about 18.7 mm.

Iwaki *et al.* [16] analysed sagittal plane MRI images of (nominally) unloaded cadaver knees. The centre of a circle fitted to the image of the posterior lateral condyle moved backwards by 19 mm on a straight line fitted to the (convex) lateral plateau, almost identical to our result 18.7 mm just quoted. Two intersecting circles were fitted to the image of the medial condyle, and two intersecting straight lines to the (concave) medial plateau. They claimed that the centre of the anterior medial circle remained stationary on the anterior *'extension'* facet of the tibia during flexion from –5° to +5°; the centre of the posterior medial circle then moved backwards ± 1.5 mm on the posterior *'flexion facet'* during flexion from 5° to 120°.

However, Iwaki *et al.* [[16], caption to Fig. 6] described a discontinuity of 8 mm in the position of the medial condylar centre between 5° and 30° flexion as contact moved from the anterior facet to the posterior facet of the tibial plateau (see Fig. 2.4). They interpreted this as evidence that the posterior movement of the condyle was due to its *rocking*, not rolling, on the tibia. This apparent discontinuity could have arisen from their use of two straight lines to represent the articular surface of the medial tibial plateau, with a discontinuity of slope at their point of intersection.

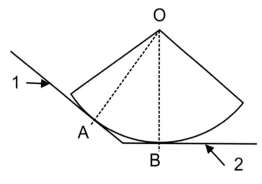

Figure 3.10. A continuous circle rolling on two intersecting straight lines, at the instant that contact transfers from *A* to *B*.

If Figure 3.10 represents a circular femoral condyle flexing clockwise on the discontinuous tibial plateau at the instant of contact transfer, it must be concluded that the cartilage on the surface of the tibia between points *A* and *B* never comes into contact with the condyle, an intuitively unsatisfactory conclusion.

We conclude that the rocking motion apparent in the Iwaki *et al.* [16] paper is an artefact created by their method of fitting discontinuous lines to the MRI images of the articular surfaces.

Ligaments

Figure 3.11 shows sketches of the fascicles of the anterior (Fig. 3.11(a)) and posterior cruciate ligament (Fig. 3.11(b)) drawn by Friederich, Muller and O'Brien [17] and augmented by Feikes [4] from her own investigations. The diagrams show clear relations between the position on the femur of the origins of individual fascicles and the position on the tibia of their insertions, a relationship we have called *fibre mapping* [18, 19]. The sketches by Mommersteeg *et al.* [20] confirmed the pattern of fibre mapping in the ACL (Fig. 3.11(c)). Feikes [4] also confirmed these observations and found similar patterns of fibre mapping for the collateral ligaments.

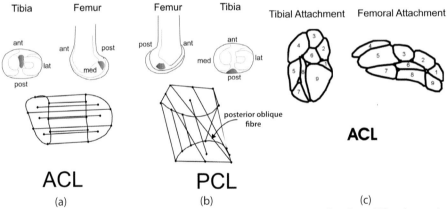

Figure 3.11 Fibre mapping of the ACL (a) and PCL (b) according to Friederich *et al.* [17] and mapping of the ACL (c) according to Mommersteeg *et al.* [20]. The sketches demonstrate clear relationships between the position of the origin of a fascicle on the femur and the position of its insertion on the tibia. (Reproduced with permission from Friederich NF, Müller W, O'Brien WR. [Clinical application of biomechanical and functional anatomical data of the knee joint.] *Orthopäde* 1992; 21:41-50 and Mommersteeg TJ, Kooloos JG, Blankevoort L, Kauer JM, Huiskes R, Roeling FQ. The fibre bundle anatomy of human cruciate ligaments, *J Anatomy* 1995;**187** Pt II: 461-71.)

Figure 3.12 reproduces sketches of fascicles of the ACL and the PCL with the knee at extension, 60° and 120° published by Friederich *et al.* [17]. These figures confirm the patterns of fibre mapping of Figure 3.11 and demonstrate how the apparent shapes of the ligaments in the sagittal plane change as their attachment areas rotate relative to each other and the points of origin and insertion of different fascicles move relative to each other. Figure 3.12 suggests that the most anterior fibre of the ACL (shown as a straight line) remains isometric during passive flexion. Other fibres are tight in extension but slacken (and are shown buckled) and then retighten again during further flexion. Friederich's sketch of the PCL suggests that a fibre within the body of the ligament, closer to the posterior edge, remains isometric during passive flexion. More anterior fibres are slack in extension (shown as buckled) but tighten as the joint is flexed. More posterior fibres are tight in extension and slacken and retighten as the joint is flexed.

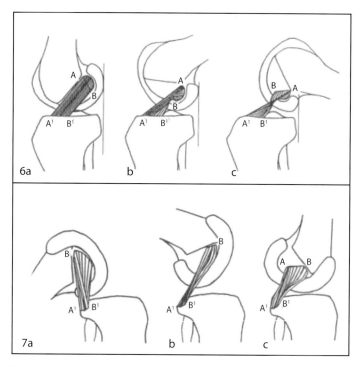

Figure 3.12. Sketches of the fascicles of the ACL and PCL in extension and flexion. (Reproduced with permission from Friederich NF, Müller W, O'Brien WR. [Clinical application of biomechanical and functional anatomical data of the knee joint]. *Orthopäde* 1992;21:41-50.)

This pattern of isometry within the ACL is well supported by independent evidence [4, 21-23]. The concept of isometry of fibres within the interior of the PCL has also been supported by independent evidence from Covey et al. [24] and Feikes [4]. Feikes used a fibre mapping of the PCL and calculated the distances apart of the points of origin and insertion of various ligament fascicles over the range of flexion. Her analysis shows that a band of fascicles within the ligament remain isometric while the distance between the points of origin and insertion of the most anterior fascicle of the PCL increases by as much as 30% as the joint flexes to 90°. Brantigan and Voshell [25] stated that "*some portion*" of the posterior cruciate ligament is "*taut in all positions of [passive] extension and flexion*".

Using the same technique, Feikes showed that anterior superficial fibres of the MCL also remain isometric during passive flexion.

Parallel spatial mechanism model of the knee

The Appendix to this book describes a three-dimensional mathematical model of passive knee flexion which is predictive of the coupling of axial rotation, ab/adduction and three components of translation of one bone relative to each other (Fig. 3.13). Indeed, the solid lines in the five graphs of Figure 3.3 were calculated from the model and fit the experimental values quite well, giving confidence in the relevance of the model and the assumptions on which it is based.

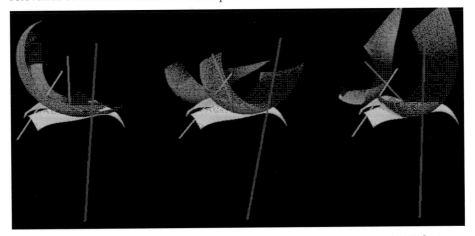

Figure 3.13. Parallel spatial mechanism model of the knee at extension, 60° and 120° flexion. The surfaces of the femoral condyles remain in continuous contact with the tibial plateaux while the isometric fibres of the ACL (red), PCL (green) and MCL (blue) rotate about their insertions on the tibia.

The formulation of the model assumes that passive motion of the knee is constrained by isometric ligament fibres in the ACL, the PCL and the MCL and by continuous contact between the articular surfaces of the medial and the lateral compartments [4, 5, 26, 27]. The mathematical formulation was based on the assumptions that, during passive motion, the ligament fibres do not stretch or shorten and that the articular surfaces in each compartment do not separate or interpenetrate. These five constraints to motion reduce the possible six degrees of freedom of the tibia relative to the femur to unity, a single degree of freedom system, and explain the coupling of five components of movement at the joint to flexion angle observed experimentally (Figs. 3.2, 3.3 and 3.4)). The model is a theory of the screw-home mechanism. Figure 3.13 and the animation of the model (see website www.oxford-partialknee.com, Animation 1) show the external rotation of the femur on a fixed tibia during flexion, internal rotation during extension. The five constraints can be satisfied during passive motion because the articular surfaces, while remaining continuously in contact, are free to roll and slide on each other and the three ligament fibres, while remaining isometric, can rotate about their points of origin and insertion on the bones. These movements can occur without tissue deformation, without stretching of ligament fibres or indentation of articular surfaces, suggesting that, during passive motion, the human knee has one degree of *unresisted* freedom.

The model reinforces the conclusions from Figure 3.6 above that intact articular surfaces and intact ligaments are necessary to achieve the ordered passive movement of the human knee. It suggests that the practice in current total knee replacement of sacrificing the cruciate ligaments and releasing the deep fibres of the MCL is unlikely to restore ordered movement. It seems improbable that additions or projections to the articular surfaces of a prosthesis (which resist interpenetration but not separation) can replace the ligamentous constraints which resist separation but not interpenetration.

Four-bar linkage model of the knee in the sagittal plane

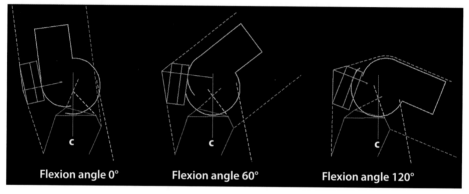

Figure 3.14 Sagittal plane model of the knee.

Figure 3.14 shows a model of the knee in the sagittal plane, at extension, 60° and 120° flexion (see website, Animation 2). The joint is represented as a four-bar linkage with the two bones and isometric fibres of the two cruciate ligaments acting as the four links. It is a model of passive flexion/extension. The articular surface of the tibia is taken to be flat, a compromise between the convex lateral tibial plateau and the concave medial plateau of the human knee. The fibres of the ACL and PCL are assumed to remain isometric during passive flexion. The instantaneous centre of the joint, through which the flexion axis passes, lies at the intersection of the two isometric fibres. Figure 3.14 shows that it moves backwards on the tibia during flexion and forwards during extension as the two ligament fibres rotate relative to each other.

The shape of the femoral condyle is calculated from the condition that, in each position, the condyle must touch the tibial plateau at the point where the perpendicular to that plateau passes through the flexion axis (the line C in each diagram) (the 'common normal theorem')[14]. When a similar calculation is performed assuming the tibial plateau to be a concave circle (the medial tibial plateau) or a convex circle (the lateral tibial plateau), the calculated shape of the corresponding condyle fits well with parasagittal sections taken through the medial or lateral condyles respectively of a human knee[14].

For these cruciate ligament fibres to remain isometric and for the surfaces to remain in contact during flexion and extension, the model femur has to roll backwards while sliding forwards on the tibia during passive flexion and *vice versa* during extension. Any other movement would require the application of load, the stretching or slackening of the fibres, the separation or indentation of the surfaces. Because the model tibial plateau has been taken to be flat, the backward excursion of the centre of curvature of the model femoral condyle during flexion is the same as that of the contact point. As Figure 3.9 above demonstrates, this is not true for concave or convex tibial plateaux.

During flexion to 140°, the isometric fibre of the model ACL rotates through 40° towards the tibia. The isometric fibre of the PCL rotates through 40° away from the tibia, as shown in Zuppinger's original sketch of the four-bar linkage model [1]. The rotation of the model PCL about its tibial insertion is similar in magnitude and direction to that shown by Nakagawa et al. [28].

The sulcus of the trochlear groove in Figure 3.14(a) is modelled as a circle anterior to the tibial facet of the femur; it appears not to be continuous with the femoral condyle because images of the trochlear flanges have been omitted (but see Figs. 3.17 and 3.18 below). The patella is modelled as a rectangle with two articular surfaces, the more posterior making contact with the trochlea in extension and at 60° [29]. By 120°, the more anterior articular surface of the patella, modelling its medial and lateral facets, makes contact with the model femoral condyle.

Apart from the assumptions about the geometry of the trochlea and the patellar surfaces, the model also assumes that the patellar tendon remains of constant length and that the line of action of the patellofemoral contact force passes through the intersection of the patellar and quadriceps tendons. (This latter condition has been used as the basis of an experimental method to measure the patellofemoral force in cadaver specimens under load [30].) As a result, during trochlear contact, the patella rolls proximally on the trochlea during passive flexion and vice versa during passive extension. Such rolling movements have been observed by Goodfellow et al. [31] (see Fig. 5.1) and discussed in Chapter 5 below in the context of patellofemoral arthritis. These authors also observed the transition to condylar contact in the flexed knee.

The magnitude of the backwards rotation of the patellar tendon during flexion agrees well with measurements on intact specimens by Buff et al. [32] and has been used as a measure of tibiofemoral movement after arthroplasty (see Fig. 3.27). Gill and O'Connor [29] showed that about two thirds of the rotation of the patellar tendon is due to the cam-like shape of the distal femur and one third due to the rolling of the femur on the tibia.

The model of Figure 3.14 also shows how straight lines representing the lines of action of the hamstrings and gastrocnemius tendons change their directions relative to the bones at the knee during flexion. The model has been used to discuss how antagonistic extensor/flexor action may be used to protect ligaments after injury or repair [33].

An animation of this model will be found as Animation 2 on the website. It shows roll-back of the femur on the tibia, the rotation of the isometric cruciate fibres about their insertions on the tibia and that the transition from trochlear patellar contact to condylar contact occurs at about 99° of flexion. The total roll-back of the model femur on the tibia over 120° is 11.5 mm, in reasonable agreement with the average movement (11.3 mm) of the contact points medially (7.9 mm) and laterally (14.7 mm) calculated by Feikes [4] from her experiments (Table 3.1 above).

Ligament fibre arrays

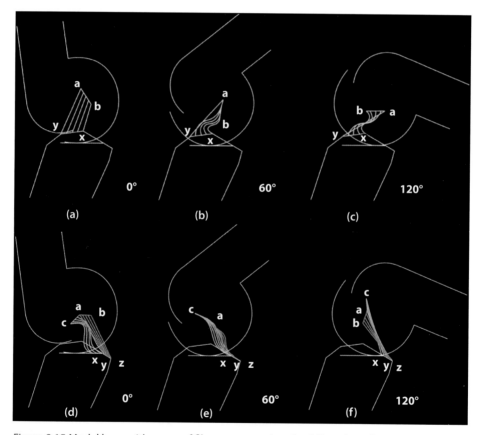

Figure 3.15 Model knee with arrays of fibres representing the ACL and two bundles of the PCL, attached to the femur along ab and cab respectively. (At 60°, the attachment point b of the PCL lies under the fibres and is not visible.)

Figure 3.15 shows an elaboration of the model with each of the cruciate ligaments represented as arrays of fibres [19, 34] (see website, Animation 3).

The fibre mapping in both ligaments is based on the anatomical studies of Friederich *et al.* [17] and Mommersteeg *et al.* [20] (Fig. 3.11). For both ligaments, the fibres marked *ay* are the isometric fibres of Figure 3.14 and the rolling and sliding movements of the femur on the tibia are the same as in the simpler model. The ACL is modelled as an array of fibres almost parallel to and passing behind the isometric fibre in extension. The PCL is shown as two bundles of fibres, one passing in front of the isometric fibres in extension and the other lying behind. In extension, all fibres of the ACL and the posterior fibres of the PCL are assumed to be just tight and are shown straight. In extension, the anterior fibres of the PCL are assumed to be slack and are shown buckled (Fig 3.15(d)).

During flexion through 120°, the femoral attachment areas *ab* and *cab* rotate through 120° relative to the tibia and points of fibre origin on the femur either approach or move away from the tibia so that most fibres either slacken or tighten. The posterior fibres of the ACL slacken (and are shown buckled) during flexion to 80°. The ACL in the human knee passes from the lateral condyle on the femur to insert medially on the tibia. Zavatsky and O'Connor [35] have shown how posterior fibres such as *bx* (Fig. 3.15), can pass under the anterior fibres and are then positioned anterior to the isometric fibre and to the flexion axis. Such fibres then begin to tighten again with further flexion. The same is true of the most posterior fibres of the PCL such as *bz* (Fig. 3.15). The anterior bundle of the PCL is slack in extension (and shown buckled) but tightens progressively as the joint flexes.

The drawings of the model cruciate ligaments in Figure 3.15 are remarkably similar to the sketches made by Friederich *et al.* [17] (Fig. 3.12 above), Brantigan and Voshell [25], and Girgis *et al.* [36]. The apparent shape changes of the model ligaments are similar to those shown by the same authors and to those derived from the RSA studies of van Dijk *et al.* [37]. The calculated patterns of model fibre slackening and tightening are similar to those reported for the ACL by Sidles *et al.* [23], Sapega *et al.* [22], and Wang and Walker [21] and to those reported for the PCL by Covey *et al.* [24].

It should be emphasised again that the fibre arrays of Figure 3.15 contain the isometric fibres shown in Figure 3.14. The drawings of the PCL look quite similar to the photographs in Nakagawa *et al.* [28] although those photographs were used by those authors as part of their argument that, quoting Strasser (1917), "*soon after the beginning of flexion the whole PCL is loose*". Our experimental and mathematical analyses support the large body of work which shows that not to be the case.

Lu and O'Connor [18] showed that the calculated values of the rotations of the model ligaments and muscle tendons about their tibial insertions agreed well with measurements on cadaver specimens by Hertzog and Read [38].

Discussion

In unloaded knees, as far as possible free from the effects of intrinsic and extrinsic loads, passive movements are controlled solely by the shapes of the articular surfaces and the design of the ligaments. The pattern of these movements is constant and repeatable as long as the surfaces and the ligaments are all intact. Flexion and extension are coupled to obligatory rotation and require backward translation of the contact areas on the tibia in flexion ('rollback'), with the medial contact area moving less than the lateral contact area. The ACL, the PCL and the MCL contain fibres which remain isometric during passive flexion/extension. All other fibres slacken and tighten as the joint flexes and extends so that ligaments can appear to be loose. All these slack fibres can be recruited to bear load in activity, as we shall shortly discuss, giving the joint its passive and dynamic laxity. The three-dimensional and two-dimensional models of the knee with its ligaments predict and explain behaviour similar to that observed experimentally in many laboratories.

The unloaded prosthetic knee

It is only in the laboratory, using a rig with six degrees of freedom and the weight of the bones counterbalanced, that it is possible to be sure of moving the knee without applying load to stretch its ligaments or indent its articular surfaces [9]. However, passive movements performed by the clinician while supporting the limb, particularly in anaesthetised subjects without muscle tone, can be similar to the unloaded state of the laboratory preparation.

In 1978, we reported that, in cadaver specimens with bicompartmental Oxford implants, forward movement of the meniscal bearings (from the rolled back position) was essential to the movement of extension and that, if bearing movement was blocked, extension was also blocked [13].

Bearing and condyle movements in four unloaded cadaver knees flexed and extended in our deep squats rig [9] after bicompartmental replacement were measured using a depth micrometer [39]. The medial bearings and condyles moved on average 12.5 mm backwards on the tibial component during flexion to 90° whereas the lateral bearings moved an average of 15.1 mm. Bearing movements of this order of magnitude are routinely observed on the operating table before closure. Bearing movements have also been measured during passive extension/flexion using fluoroscopy in nine patients with medial OUKA (a) after wound closure while they were still anaesthetised and (b) six months later in the follow-up clinic [40]. They reported a total backwards movement in the anaesthetised patients of 13 mm (SD 3 mm) during flexion to 120°, with differences between the anaesthetised and awake states only near extension (Fig. 3.16). Thus, roll-back in the replaced joint is accommodated by sliding at both the femoro-bearing and tibio-bearing interfaces. Although the total sliding distance (on both upper and lower interfaces) is greater than it would be in a fixed bearing implant, our evidence presented above in Chapter 2 demonstrates that full congruity between the components ensures minimal wear.

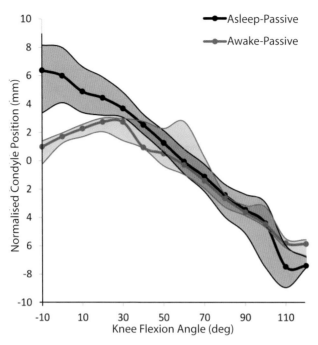

Figure 3.16. Bearing and condyle position on the tibial plateau in nine patients while anaesthetised and conscious during passive flexion/extension [40].

Bradley *et al.* [41] compared lateral radiographs of the knee in extension and in 90° flexion up to 5 years after OUKA (medial or lateral). The films were taken with the subjects lying on their side on the X-ray table with the muscles as relaxed as possible. The mean position of the bearings and condyles in flexion was 4.4 mm (range 0–13.5) posterior to their position in extension medially and 6.0 mm (range 1.6–13.0) laterally. The differences between these observations and those just described were attributed to the presence of passive muscle forces during the radiographic investigation.

Discussion

In the anaesthetised patient during passive extension/flexion, the only forces available to thrust the medial bearing forwards are the compressive forces at the articular surfaces and the tensile forces in the ligaments, both engendered by the force that the examiner applies in attempting to extend the leg or to support the flexing leg.

The movements of the bearings in the prosthetic joint, immediately after implantation and without muscle tone, were similar to the movements of the contact areas in the unloaded natural cadaveric knee (Table 3.1 above). The radiographic study at a longer follow-up time showed that bearings continue to move in the same sense for at least 5 years after implantation. However, the mean movement in that study was about half that seen intraoperatively and the spread of the data was greater; the differences were attributed to the presence of passive muscle tensions in the conscious patient. Bearing and condyle movements accommodate roll-back of the femur on the tibia during passive flexion.

The mathematical model of passive flexion of the replaced knee described in the Appendix and shown in Figure 3.17 explains the observations made on the unloaded prosthetic joint. At each flexion angle, the anteroposterior position of the femur on the tibia was determined from the condition of zero force in each ligament, a condition which required a roll-back of the model femur on the tibia of 7.5 mm over 90° of flexion. At each flexion angle, if the femur is placed anterior to this neutral position, the ACL (and MCL) are stretched and the PCL and LCL slackened (Fig. A8 in the appendix below), requiring the application of external force. If the femur is placed posterior to the neutral position, the PCL and LCL are stretched and the ACL and MCL are slackened. Thus, roll-back during passive flexion of the replaced joint is required to ensure that passive structures of the joint, articular surfaces as well as ligaments, are not loaded.

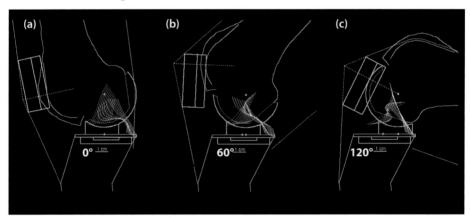

Figure 3.17. Model of the replaced knee in extension, 60° and 120° flexion, with a circular femoral component, a flat tibial component and an interposed fully conforming meniscal bearing. The model cruciate ligaments of Fig. 3.15 are also shown (see website, Animation 7).

Note that the shape changes and patterns of slackening and tightening of the ligaments in the model replaced joint are very similar to those of the model intact joint (Fig. 3.15), and those of the cadaver joint sketched by Friederich *et al.* (Fig. 3.12) [17]. For this reason, the Oxford implant can be said to be a *ligament compatible prosthesis*. Although the articular surfaces of the prosthesis are not exactly anatomical, they are sufficiently compatible with the retained ligaments to allow close restoration of natural passive motion. Calculations with the model of the replaced joint suggest that the most anterior fibres of the ACL and of the posterior bundle of the PCL remain isometric to within 0.5% during passive flexion/extension. Restoration of natural passive and dynamic laxity, and of normal kinematics and mechanics, might therefore be expected. Of course, restoration of natural laxity requires that the ligaments are restored to their natural strain patterns. This is achieved by matching the thickness of the gaps between the metal components at 110° and at 20° flexion, and filling the matched gap with a meniscal bearing of appropriate thickness, as explained in Chapters 6 and 7 below.

Note also that the model patella rolls on the anterior femur, making trochlear contact in Figures 3.17(a) and (b) and contact with the femoral component in Figure 3.17(c). This changing pattern of patellar contact is very similar to the pattern of contact in the intact knee (Figure 5.1 below). In our model, the transition from trochlear contact to component contact happens at 99° flexion, as shown in Figure 3.18. The figure shows the posterior surface of the patella (representing the central ridge) in contact with the trochlea and, simultaneously, the more anterior contact surface (representing the medial facet) in contact with the metal femoral component. The patella does not have to make contact with the hiatus between the trochlear flange and the implant and this may well be a reason for the very few revisions of the arthroplasty associated with patellar problems (Chapters 5 and 10).

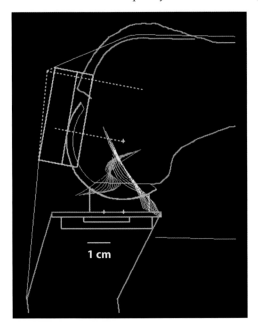

1 cm

Figure 3.18. The transition between contact of the patella with the trochlea and with the femoral component.

The loaded human knee

The unloaded knee behaves in a predictable fashion because its articular surfaces do not alter their shapes and the ligaments do not stretch during passive motion. When significant loads are applied, both these things happen. Ligaments stretch under tension and articular surfaces indent under compression, straining the constraints to movement and profoundly modifying, even reversing, the underlying patterns of movement described above.

The role of the ligaments in controlling this pattern of movement is readily demonstrated. Ligament sectioning studies [42-45] have established that the anterior cruciate ligament (ACL) is the primary constraint upon anterior tibial translation (and a secondary constraint on internal tibial rotation) and the posterior cruciate ligament (PCL) is the primary constraint on posterior tibial translation (and a secondary constraint on external tibial rotation). The collateral ligaments are the primary constraints on abduction and adduction and on internal rotation (MCL) and external rotation (LCL). This and similar evidence was not confronted by Freeman's group in dismissing the contribution of the PCL to the kinematics and mechanics of the knee, concluding that the strength of the PCL in man "*may represent an evolutionary vestige, not a contemporary necessity*", Nakagawa *et al.* [28].

The role of the articular surfaces is difficult to study because it is not possible to alter the shape of an articular facet without simultaneously making some ligament fibres slack (causing instability) or tightening others (causing limitation of movement). Therefore, unlike the ligaments, no particular movement constraint can be attributed to any particular feature of joint surface shape, *the function of the articular surfaces being mainly to keep the ligaments at their appropriate tension by resisting interpenetration.* As we shall see, prosthetic articular surfaces, if they reproduce *only* this function, can restore normal movement even if they are not shaped exactly like the natural surfaces.

Perturbation tests

We return to the study of cadaver specimens described earlier in Figures 3.1 to 3.4. During some of those tests, the specimens were held stationary at a number of positions within the flexion range and medial and lateral forces applied by the experimenter's finger-tip to the proximal end of the intramedullary rod attached to the femur. The object was to establish the extent to which the passive path of motion could be perturbed by the application of external force. Figure 3.19 shows how the tight hysteresis loops of Figures 3.2 and 3.3 were readily perturbed by the application of even such light forces but that the perturbations to motion were immediately removed and the unique passive path of motion restored when the perturbing forces were removed. The preferred path of motion is therefore dynamically stable.

The passive laxity of the joint exhibited by these perturbations arises mainly from the deformation of the ligaments and articular surfaces.

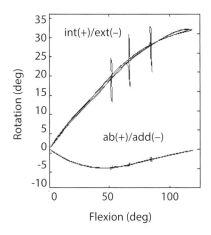

Figure 3.19 Perturbation of the passive path of motion as defined by Figs. 3.2 and 3.3 by applying and then removing medial and lateral forces to the femoral intramedullary rod at 50°, 70° and 90° flexion.

Passive anteroposterior laxity of the knee

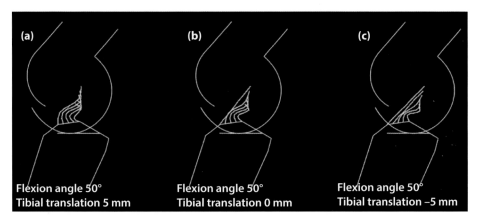

Figure 3.20 Fibres of the model ACL, with the knee at 50° flexion, (a) slacken and (c) tighten when the tibia is pulled backward and forward from the neutral unloaded position (b). Fibres shown buckled are slack, fibres shown straight are either isometric or stretched (see website, Animation 5) [34].

Figure 3.20 shows how the ACL fibres of the model knee slacken (Fig. 3.20(a)) or tighten (Fig. 3.20(c)) when the tibia is pushed backwards or pulled forward distances of 5 mm from the neutral unloaded position (Fig. 3.20(b)), in a simulation of the Lachman or Drawer test. Fig. A6(a) in the Appendix shows that backward movement of the model tibia on the femur of 5 mm is sufficient to relax the ACL completely and to stretch all fibres of the LCL, all fibres of the posterior bundle of the PCL and about half the anterior bundle. Ligament stretch leads to anterior/posterior translation of the femur on the tibia, a manifestation of passive laxity. In a further elaboration of the model, Huss et al. [47] showed that deformation of the cartilage in the model knee adds only modestly to the calculated passive laxity. The successive recruitment of ligament fibres to resist increasing load makes the ligaments increasingly resistant to elongation and increases their effective extensional stiffness. This largely explains why the effective resistance to imposed displacement of the bones, as in the drawer test, increases as the displacement increases.

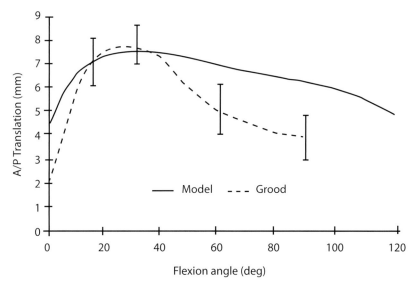

Figure 3.21 Total A/P tibial translation for applied A/P forces of 67 N plotted against flexion angle for the model knee with both cruciate and collateral ligaments intact, compared with the results of experiments by Grood and Noyes [48].

Figure 3.21 plots the total anteroposterior translation (anterior plus posterior) induced by an anteroposterior force of 67 N against flexion angle, calculated using the knee model with extensible ligaments, Zavatsky and O'Connor [46], compared with the results of measurements on human knees reported by Grood and Noyes [48]. 67 N was Grood's estimated value of the force applied by the typical examiner in performing the drawer test. The calculation predicts the value of the maximum total laxity at about 30° quite well but overestimates the measured laxity at 60° and 90°. Feikes [4] also estimated the total anteroposterior laxity using her 3-D knee model (Fig. 3.13), with similar conclusions.

Passive rotational laxity of the knee

O'Connor, Zavatsky and Gill [8] described work by Zavatsky on the path of motion when the otherwise unloaded joint was flexed and extended in the presence of either internally or externally rotating torques of 1, 2 and 3 Nm (Fig. 3.22). The applied torque rotated the knee in its own direction and, if anything, tightened further the hysteresis loops. The internally rotating torques further increased the internal tibial rotation exhibited during purely passive motion (the loop marked *0)*, while the external rotation produced near extension by the externally rotating torque tended to be cancelled out during further flexion of the joint. The curves for torques of ±3 Nm are similar to those reported by Blankevoort *et al.* [3] and described by them as the "envelopes of passive motion". Figure 3.22 shows that the paths of motion in the presence of smaller torques or none are very well defined and ordered, lying within the Blankevoort envelopes. The 0 loop is almost identical to that of Figure 3.2, though obtained in a different apparatus.

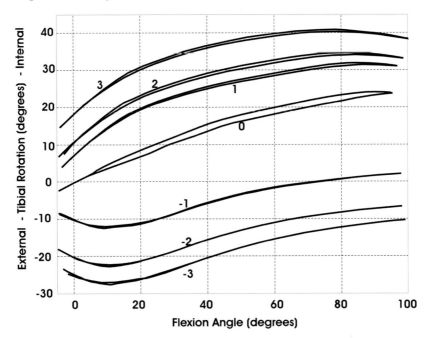

Figure 3.22 External (curves marked **-1**, **-2** and **-3**) and Internal rotation (curves marked **1**, **2** and **3**) of the tibia of a specimen knee when flexed and extended in the presence of an externally or internally rotating torque, compared to the path of passive motion of the wholly unloaded specimen (loop marked **0**).

These effects quantify the results of the perturbation tests reported in Figure 3.19 and are consistent with the reports of others, both *in vitro* [16] and *in vivo*, Hill *et al.* [49].

Quadriceps/ligament interactions, dynamic laxity

Many of the activities of daily living require action from the quadriceps muscles. We now discuss how quadriceps action alters the path of passive motion by stretching and slackening the ligaments and by indentation of the articular surfaces, giving the joint its *dynamic laxity*.

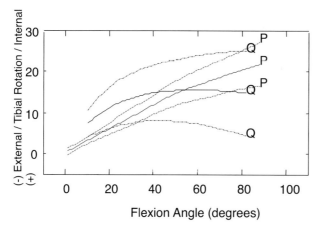

Figure 3.23 plots axial rotation of 10 cadaver specimens against flexion angle during a simulation of deep squats (mean values ± one standard deviation) and compares the path of passive motion when the specimens were flexed and extended in the absence of external load (marked **P**) with movements observed in the presence of a vertical load on the hip/ankle axis, balanced by tension in a wire sewn to the quadriceps tendon (marked **Q**).

Effect of muscle force on coupled axial rotation

Figure 3.23 demonstrates how tension in the muscle tendons changes the preferred path of motion. It compares the path recorded in ten specimens during passive deep squats (as in Fig. 3.5 above) and during deep squats in the presence of vertical load on the hip/ankle axis balanced by tension in a wire sewn to the quadriceps tendon [8]. The maximum coupled internal tibial rotation was reduced from about a mean value of 22° to about 15°, rotation occurring mainly near extension and further rotation ceasing once the knee was bent to about 50°, perhaps the reason why it is commonly called "terminal rotation". Tension in the patellar tendon near extension induces increased tibial rotation and in the flexed knee offers increasing resistance to rotation, with the patella now firmly lodged in the trochlear groove.

Isometric quadriceps contractions

Zavatsky and O'Connor [50] studied simulated isometric quadriceps action in seven cadaver specimens with the flexing effect of a force applied to the tibia parallel to the tibial plateau just balanced by extending forces applied to a wire sewn to the quadriceps tendon to give equilibrium at different flexion angles. They measured the tendon and resisting forces and the anteroposterior translation of the medial and lateral compartments of the tibia relative to the femur.

Anteroposterior translation proved to be dependent on flexion angle. When the resisting force was applied 30 cm below the tibial plateau, the tibia moved *forwards* relative to the femur at extension, 30° and 60° flexion but *backwards* at 90° and 120° (Fig. 3.24). With the resisting force at 20 cm below the plateau, motion in the same directions were observed at extension, 30°, 90°and 120° but no anteroposterior translation was observed at 60°. For both placements of the resisting force, the anterior translation was largest at 30°.

These results are consistent with measurements made *in vivo* by Jurist and Otis [51] and by Howell [52].

The results of the experiments were explained by the modelling work of Zavatsky and O'Connor [53] and Huss *et al.* [54] who used the sagittal plane knee model of Figures 3.14 and 3.15 to demonstrate that the forward pull of the patellar tendon between extension and about 65° exceeds the backwards push of the resisting force so that the tibia moves forward relative to the femur because the ACL is strained. At higher flexion angles as the patellar tendon rotates backwards about the tibial tubercle (Fig. 3.14), the backwards push of the restraining force dominates the more vertical patellar tendon force and the tibia moves backwards because the PCL is strained.

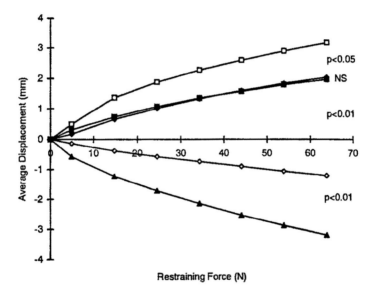

Figure 3.24 Displacement of the tibia relative to the femur during isometric quadriceps contractions plotted against the value of the resisting force at extension (■), 30° (□), 60° (◆), 90° (◇) and 120° (▲) with the resisting force placed 30 cm distal to the tibial plateau. Mean values from 7 cadaver specimens. Statistical analysis performed at the largest values of the resisting force. (Reproduced with permission from Zavatsky AB, O'Connor JJ. Anteroposterior tibial translation during simulated isometric quadriceps contractions. *The Knee. 1995;2*:85-91.)

The modelling work reveals the values of quantities which are difficult or impossible to measure, in this case the values of the forces transmitted by the cruciate ligaments.

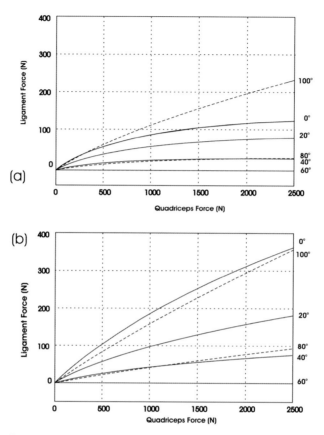

Figure 3.25 ACL forces at 0°, 20° and 40° and PCL forces (dashed lines) at 80° and 100° plotted against quadriceps force for (a) compressible and (b) incompressible cartilage when the resisting force is placed 20 cm distal to the tibial plateau. No cruciate ligament forces are required at 60°. (Reproduced with permission from Huss R A, Holstein H, O'Connor JJ. A mathematical model of forces in the knee under isometric quadriceps contractions. *Clin Biomech* 2000; **15:** 112-22.)

Figure 3.25 shows the calculated values of the ACL and PCL forces (a) taking account of the extensibility of the cruciate ligaments (Fig. 3.20) and also the indentibility of the cartilage layers. When the articular surfaces were taken to be incompressible (Fig. 3.25(b)) as in Zavatsky and O'Connor [53], the calculated values of the cruciate ligaments are larger than those from the compressible cartilage model. In both cases, the ACL is loaded up to about 60° and the PCL at higher flexion angles.

Although the calculated ACL force was largest at extension (Fig. 3.25), the calculated anterior displacement of the model tibia was largest at 20° to 30° flexion (Fig. 3.26). At extension, all ACL fibres are just tight in the unloaded state and can be recruited immediately to bear load whereas, in the flexed joint, most fibres are initially slack and have to be recruited progressively. As a result, the ACL of the flexed joint is less resistant to elongation and a smaller ACL force can produce a larger ACL extension. The calculated anteroposterior translation (Fig. 3.26) agrees well with the measurements of Zavatsky and O'Connor (Fig. 3.24) [50].

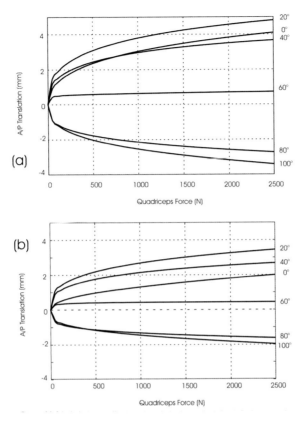

Figure 3.26 Anterior (positive) and posterior (negative) tibial displacement induced by increasing quadriceps force against a resistance placed 20 mm distal to the tibial plateau, assuming extensible ligaments and (a) compressible articular surfaces (b) assuming rigid articular surfaces. (Reproduced with permission from Huss R A, Holstein H, O'Connor JJ. A mathematical model of forces in the knee under isometric quadriceps contractions. *Clin Biomech* 2000; **15:** 112-22.)

An important lesson learnt from the mathematical models was that, as the quadriceps force was increased to 2500 N, the cruciate ligament forces (and extensions) did not increase in proportion but appeared to approach relatively small asymptotic values. Earlier studies with an inextensible ligament model predicted much higher cruciate ligament forces in association with quadriceps action. Collins and O'Connor [55] predicted large ACL forces during level walking and O'Connor et al. [56] predicted large PCL forces in flexion during deep squats. Indeed, it was this outcome which prompted the development of knee models with extensible ligaments (Fig. 3.20). The extensible-ligament knee model shows how even large muscle forces can be transmitted across the knee without involving large ACL forces. However, a study of deep squats in a group of young volunteers, taking account of ligament extensibility, found that, while peak ACL focus remained quite small, peak PCL forces reached values nearly three times body weight [57]. The ACL is protected from large forces by its own elasticity. This might help to explain the high failure rates of relatively inextensible artificial ligaments.

Movement of the contact points under load

Walker et al. [58] studied the movements of the contact points in cadaver knees in an apparatus similar to that used by Wilson et al. [6] and by Feikes [4] but with the specimen loaded by a weight hung from an intramedullary rod in the femoral shaft and resisted by tension in a wire sewn to the quadriceps tendon. Using the same methods of analysis of the measurements as Feikes (Fig. 3.7 above), they found that during the first 45° of flexion the contact points moved backwards on the tibia by 13 mm (SD 3) medially and 14 mm (SD 3) laterally, with no movement on further flexion. The patterns of movement differed in the two experiments which themselves differed only by the presence or absence of load and tissue deformation. Kurosawa et al. [59] used the same apparatus to study femoral condyle movements. During flexion to 75°, the mean movement of the centres of the medial femoral condyles was forwards 4.5 mm (SD 2.1), and then backwards 2.3 mm (SD 2.8) during flexion to 120°. The centres of the lateral condyles moved steadily backwards by a mean of 17.0 mm (SD 5.5), during flexion. The differential movements of the medial and lateral centres implied external rotation of the femur of 20.2° (SD 6).

Discussion

Even modest loads can perturb the knee from its unique path of passive motion. This occurs because the ligaments can stretch and the articular surfaces can indent under load. In activity, the ligaments serve to provide a balance between the components parallel to the tibial plateau of the muscle tendon forces and the external loads. Each activity involves its own pattern of movement and muscle force and, therefore, its own pattern of ligament forces. The detailed movements of the bones upon each other are, therefore, activity-dependent. A truly ligament compatible prosthesis should allow the soft tissues to respond in a physiological way to each different activity. The prosthesis should not resist the movements demanded by the soft tissues. It is unlikely that one could devise a prosthesis with surface shapes which alone would guide all the many possible patterns of movement of the surfaces even during the activities of daily living.

The loaded prosthetic knee

Patellar tendon angle

The patellar tendon angle (PTA) is the angle in the sagittal plane between the tendon and the long axis of the tibia. Because of its central location in the knee, it is little affected by axial rotation and gives an indirect measure of sagittal plane kinematics. The tendon rotates posteriorly during flexion, moving steadily backwards about its insertion into the tibial tubercle. The effect is predicted by the sagittal plane model of the knee during passive motion (Fig. 3.14), and by the model of passive motion of the replaced knee (Fig. 3.17). The changes in PTA with flexion arise in part due to the cam-like shape of the distal femur, with the trochlea placed anterior to the flexion axis near extension (Fig. 3.14(a)), and the closer approach of the patella to the flexion axis in deeper flexion (Fig. 3.14(c)). The PTA changes are further increased by femoral roll-back during flexion.

It was shown in cadaver studies [30] that the normal pattern of PTA was restored throughout the range of flexion after medial OUKA with both cruciates preserved. After TKA with an unconstrained fixed-bearing prosthesis (implanted after division of the ACL), anterior subluxation of the femur caused an increase in the PTA in high flexion, i.e. loss of the normal rollback. When a posterior stabilised TKA was implanted after division of both cruciates, the PTA became normal in flexion as the cam of the prosthesis artificially restored natural rollback.

Price *et al.* [60] used dynamic fluoroscopy to measure the PTA in the knees of five patients at 1 year after OUKA and five patients at 10 years during a step-up exercise. The measurements were compared with the knees of five patients who had undergone TKA and five normal volunteers (Fig. 3.27). The graphs show no significant difference in the pattern of tendon rotation between the control knees and those with OUKA. In contrast, the sagittal plane mechanics after TKA were significantly disturbed.

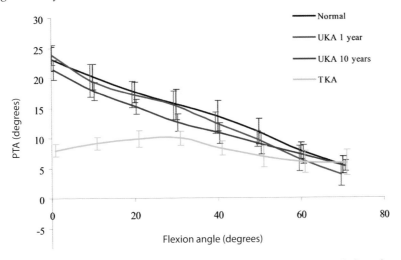

Figure 3.27 Patellar tendon angle recorded during a step-up exercise and plotted against flexion angle for groups of 5 normal volunteers, 5 patients one year and 5 patients 10 years after medial OUKA, and 5 patients one year after PCL-retaining TKA [60]. (Reproduced with permission from Price AJ, Rees JL, Beard DJ, Gill RH, Dodd CA, Murray DM. Sagittal plane kinematics of a mobile-bearing unicompartmental knee arthroplasty at 10 years: a comparative in vivo fluoroscopic analysis. *J Arthroplasty* 2004; **19**(5): 590-7.)

Bearing movement in activity

Pegg *et al.* [40] described measurements of bearing and condyle movement fluoroscopically during active extension/flexion and during step-up after OUKA. These two exercises were chosen because the quadriceps force would be expected to be largest in extension during active extension/flexion and largest in flexion during step up.

Movements in activity were very different from those measured passively (Fig. 3.16). During active extension/flexion with the femur stationary and horizontal (Fig. 3.28), the bearing lay posterior to its position in passive extension/flexion up to about 30° and anterior to that position with further flexion. Figure A9 and the website's Animation 9 show the model replaced knee during active extension/flexion. At full extension, the anteriorly directed model patellar tendon pulls the tibia anterior to the femur and stretches the ACL, allowing the model tibia to move anteriorly relative to the femur and the bearing to move backwards on the tibial plateau. As the knee flexes, the quadriceps and ACL forces diminish, reducing the difference between the active and passive position of the bearing. At larger flexion angles, the quadriceps force is further reduced and the patellar tendon is directed more posteriorly so that stretch of the PCL allows the bearing to move anterior to its position during passive movement, by about 4 mm in the fully flexed knee. The cross-over between these events occurred at about 30° in the patients (Fig. 3.28(a)) and at about 60°, according to the model calculations (Fig. 3.29(a)). The model assumed the presence only of agonistic quadriceps action and the differences between the bearing position during passive and active flexion/extension at larger flexion angles in the model was much smaller than in the patients. However, the patients could also have used antagonistic hamstrings action to control movements at the knee. In the flexed knee, the presence of hamstrings forces can greatly increase the level of force in the PCL [57], resulting in the observed significant anterior movement of the condyle in flexion.

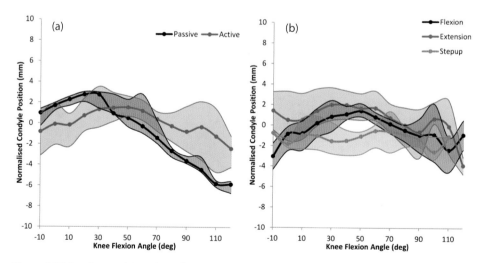

Figure 3.28 Bearing position plotted against flexion angle (a) during passive and active extension/flexion and (b) during active extension, active flexion and step-up.

Leg-Lift Experiment: Posterior Bearing Movement During Active Extension/Flexion

The bearing position at 90° flexion is taken as reference; the bearing movement during extension is anterior to this position

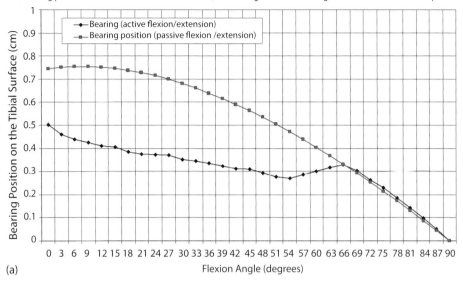

(a)

Length of Anterior Fibre of ACL During Active Extension/Flexion

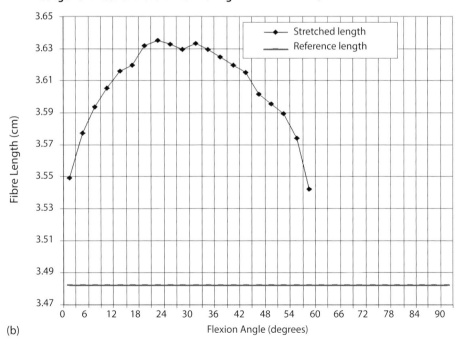

(b)

Figure 3.29 (a) Calculated position of the model bearing on the tibia during passive and active flexion/extension. (b) Length of the most anterior fibre of the model ACL during passive and active flexion/extension. The reference length is the isometric length of the fibre during unloaded passive motion. (Reproduced from O'Connor J, Imran A. Bearing Movement after Oxford Unicompartmental Knee Arthroplasty: A Mathematical Model. *Orthopedics|www.ORTHOSuperSite.com. 2007;30(5):42-45* (Supplement).)

The model calculations showed that the differences between the anterior translation of the tibia between passive motion and active extension are maximum at about 30° (Fig. 3.29(a)) where the extension of the ACL is also maximum (Fig. 3.29(b)).

There were significant differences between bearing position in the patients during active flexion/extension and during step up (Fig. 3.28(b)), particularly in mid-range. Whereas the bearing appeared to move forward and then backward as the knee was actively flexed, during step-up it appeared to remain essentially stationary on the tibia over most of the flexion range. The differences between the two activities doubtless arise from differing patterns of muscle activity and corresponding differences in the patterns of ligament stretch.

Gait analysis

Jefferson and Whittle [61] assessed a group of medial OUKA patients in the gait laboratory. Seven parameters of their normal level walking gait (speed, cadence, stride length, sagittal plane and coronal plane angles, and sagittal plane and abduction moments) were compared with those of a group of age- and sex-matched volunteers with no locomotor problems. All seven parameters of the patients' gait were restored to the normal range. This is probably the most convincing demonstration that the use of a ligament compatible unicompartmental prosthesis leads to a restoration of normal function.

Wiik et al. [62] compared the downhill walking gait pattern in 19 UKA and 14 TKA patients who were well matched demographically and with high Oxford knee scores (OKS) for their operation type at a minimum 1 year after their operation. They also compared this data with 19 healthy young subjects used as controls. Downhill gait analysis was carried out on an instrumented treadmill that was ramped at the rear to produce a declination of 7°. All subjects after a period of habituation were tested for preferred and top downhill walking speed with associated ground reaction and temporo-spatial measurements. The UKA group walked downhill 15% faster than the TKA group (1.75 ± 0.14 vs 1.52 ± 0.13 m/s, $p < 0.0001$) despite having the same cadence (134.9 ± 8.0 vs 133.9 ± 9.6 steps/min). This 15% difference in speed appeared largely due to a 15% increase in stride length (173 ± 14 vs 150 ± 17 cm, $p = 0.0007$) and normal weight acceptance, both of which were similar to the controls.

Discussion

Since there is no single pattern of knee movement under load, it is difficult to ensure that comparisons before and after surgery are valid. The pattern of forces can only be adequately regulated to produce repeatable patterns of movement with very simple defined activities, such as straight leg raise, step-up, level walking etc.

The evidence of cadaver studies and the modelling is that the anatomical features of the joint (the shapes of its articular surfaces and the design of its ligaments) define the envelope within which the bones are moved by the very large extrinsic and intrinsic forces. These forces can either reinforce or reverse the pattern of contact in the unloaded joint, depending on how the ligaments are stretched in activity, implying that the detailed shapes of the articular surfaces allow rather than control the site of their contact areas. If the main function of the natural surface shapes is to maintain the ligaments at their appropriate tensions, any other pair of surfaces that can fulfil that one function might be able to restore normal movements if all the ligaments are intact.

The evidence of the PTA, bearing movement and gait laboratory studies is that a spherical femoral condyle articulating on a flat tibial plateau can replace the natural surfaces of the medial compartment. It is stressed that, in this regard, the meniscal bearing design of the OUKA implant is not different from fixed-bearing UKA implants, most of which employ a flat, or nearly flat, tibial plateau which allows the femoral condyle the same freedoms of anteroposterior translation as the OUKA enjoys. This is borne out by the studies of Parratte *et al.*[63]. We know of no evidence, and there is no theoretical reason, for the biomechanics and kinematics of the two designs of implant to differ *as long as the tibial component of the fixed-bearing implant remains flat*. However, if, because of the effects of wear, the flat form of the polyethylene becomes concave, the translational movements of the femoral condyle may become constrained (see Figs. 2.19 and 2.20). If stability can be restored to normal during OUKA with the Oxford instrumentation (Chapters 6 and 7 below), it is likely to remain so because of the minimal wear of the meniscal bearing.

Mathematical models

Explanations for many of the above observations have been deduced from analysis of the mathematical models of the knee. The two- and three-dimensional models are further discussed in the Appendix, and animations of the models are available at www.oxfordpartialknee.com.

References

1. Pinskerova V, Maquet P, Freeman MA. Writings on the knee between 1836 and 1917. *J Bone Joint Surg Br* 2000; **82**(8): 1100-2.

2. Freeman MA, Pinskerova V. The movement of the normal tibio-femoral joint. *J Biomech* 2005; **38**(2): 197-208.

3. Blankevoort L, Huiskes R, de Lange A. The envelope of passive knee joint motion. *J Biomech* 1988; **21**(9): 705-20.

4. Feikes JD. The mobility and stability of the human knee joint [DPhil]. Oxford: University of Oxford; 1999.

5. Wilson DR. Three-dimensional kinematics of the knee [DPhil]. Oxford University of Oxford; 1995.

6. Wilson DR, Feikes JD, Zavatsky AB, O'Connor JJ. The components of passive knee movement are coupled to flexion angle. *J Biomech* 2000; **33**(4): 465-73.

7. Yoshioka Y, Siu DW, Scudamore RA, Cooke TD. Tibial anatomy and functional axes. *J Orthop Res* 1989; **7**(1): 132-7.

8. O'Connor JJ, Zavatsky AB, Gill HS. Stability of the knee. In: Pedowitz RA, O'Connor JJ, Akeson WH, eds. *Daniel's Knee Injuries: Ligament and Cartilage, Structure, Function, Injury and Repair*. Philadelphia: Lippincott Williams & Wilkins; 2003.

9. Biden E, O'Connor JJ. Experimental methods used to evaluate knee ligament function. In: Daniel D, Akeson WH, O'Connor J, eds. *Knee ligaments: Structure, Function, Injury and Repair*. New York: Raven Press; 1990.

10. Zavatsky AB. A kinematic-freedom analysis of a flexed-knee-stance testing rig. *J Biomech* 1997; **30**(3): 277-80.

11. Monk AP, Choji K, O'Connor JJ, Goodfellow JW, Murray DW. The shape of the distal femur: a geometrical study using MRI. *Bone Joint J* 2014; **96-B**(12): 1623-30.

12. Veldpaus FE, Woltring HJ, Dortmans LJ. A least-squares algorithm for the equiform transformation from spatial marker co-ordinates. *J Biomech* 1988; **21**(1): 45-54.

13. Goodfellow J, O'Connor J. The mechanics of the knee and prosthesis design. *J Bone Joint Surg Br* 1978; **60-B**(3): 358-69.

14. O'Connor JJ, Shercliff TL, Biden E, Goodfellow JW. The geometry of the knee in the sagittal plane. *Proc Inst Mech Eng H* 1989; **203**(4): 223-33.

15. Kapandji I. The physiology of the joints. Edinburgh: Churchill Livingstone; 1970.

16. Iwaki H, Pinskerova V, Freeman MA. Tibiofemoral movement 1: the shapes and relative movements of the femur and tibia in the unloaded cadaver knee. *J Bone Joint Surg Br* 2000; **82**(8): 1189-95.

17. Friedrich NF, Muller W, O'Brien WR. Klinishe Anwendung biomechanischer und funktionell anatomisher Daten am Kniegelenk. [Clinical application of biomechanic and functional anatomical findings of the knee joint]. *Orthopade (Springer Verlag)* 1992; **21**: 41-50.

18. Lu TW, O'Connor JJ. Lines of action and moment arms of the major force-bearing structures crossing the human knee joint: comparison between theory and experiment. *J Anat* 1996; **189 (Pt 3)**: 575-85.

19. Zavatsky AB, O'Connor JJ. A model of human knee ligaments in the sagittal plane. Part 1: Response to passive flexion. *Proc Inst Mech Eng H* 1992; **206**(3): 125-34.

20. Mommersteeg TJ, Kooloos JG, Blankevoort L, Kauer JM, Huiskes R, Roeling FQ. The fibre bundle anatomy of human cruciate ligaments. *J Anat* 1995; **187 (Pt 2)**: 461-71.

21. Wang C, Walker PS. The effects of flexion and rotation on the length patterns of the ligaments of the knee. *J Biomech* 1973; **6**: 587-96.

22. Sapega AA, Moyer RA, Schneck C, Komalahiranya N. Testing for isometry during reconstruction of the anterior cruciate ligament. Anatomical and biomechanical considerations. *J Bone Joint Surg Am* 1990; **72**(2): 259-67.

23. Sidles JA, Larson RV, Garbini JL, Downey DJ, Matsen FA 3rd. Ligament length relationships in the moving knee. *J Orthop Res* 1988; **6**(4): 593-610.

24. Covey DC, Sapega AA, Sherman GM. Testing for isometry during reconstruction of the posterior cruciate ligament. Anatomic and biomechanical considerations. *Am J Sports Med* 1996; **24**(6): 740-6.

25. Brantigan OC, Voshell AF. The mechanics of the ligaments and menisci of the knee joint. *J Bone Joint Surg [Am]* 1941; **23**(1): 44-66.

26. Wilson DR, Feikes JD, O'Connor JJ. Ligaments and articular contact guide passive knee flexion. *J Biomech* 1998; **31**(12): 1127-36.

27. Feikes JD, O'Connor JJ, Zavatsky AB. A constraint-based approach to modelling the mobility of the human knee joint. *J Biomech* 2003; **36**(1): 125-9.

28. Nakagawa S, Johal P, Pinskerova V, Komatsu T, Sosna A, Williams A, Freeman MA. The posterior cruciate ligament during flexion of the normal knee. *J Bone Joint Surg Br* 2004; **86**(3): 450-6.

29. Gill HS, O'Connor JJ. Biarticulating two-dimensional computer model of the human patellofemoral joint. *Clin Biomech (Bristol, Avon)* 1996; **11**(2): 81-9.

30. Miller RK, Goodfellow JW, Murray DW, O'Connor JJ. In vitro measurement of patellofemoral force after three types of knee replacement. *J Bone Joint Surg Br* 1998; **80**(5): 900-6.

31. Goodfellow J, Hungerford DS, Zindel M. Patello-femoral joint mechanics and pathology. 1. Functional anatomy of the patello-femoral joint. *J Bone Joint Surg Br* 1976; **58**(3): 287-90.

32. Buff HU, Jones LC, Hungerford DS. Experimental determination of forces transmitted through the patello-femoral joint. *J Biomech* 1988; **21**(1): 17-23.

33. O'Connor JJ. Can muscle co-contraction protect knee ligaments after injury or repair? *J Bone Joint Surg Br* 1993; **75**(1): 41-8.

34. Lu TW, O'Connor JJ. Fibre recruitment and shape changes of knee ligaments during motion: as revealed by a computer graphics-based model. *Proc Inst Mech Eng H* 1996; **210**(2): 71-9.

35. Zavatsky AB, O'Connor JJ. Three-dimensional geometrical models of human knee ligaments. *Proc Instn Mech Engrs*, Part H 1994; **208**: 229-240.

36. Girgis FG, Marshall JL, Monajem A. The cruciate ligaments of the knee joint. Anatomical, functional and experimental analysis. *Clin Orthop Relat Res* 1975; (**106**): 216-31.

37. van Dijk R, Huiskes R, Selvik G. Roentgen stereophotogrammetric methods for the evaluation of the three dimensional kinematic behaviour and cruciate ligament length patterns of the human knee joint. *J Biomech* 1979; **12**(9): 727-31.

38. Herzog W, Read LJ. Lines of action and moment arms of the major force-carrying structures crossing the human knee joint. *J Anat* 1993; **182 (Pt 2)**: 213-30.

39. Goodfellow JW, O'Connor J. Clinical results of the Oxford knee: surface arthroplasty of the tibiofemoral joint with a meniscal bearing prosthesis. *Clin Orthop Relat Res* 1986; **205**:21-42.

40. Pegg EC, Bare J, Gill HS, Pandit H, O'Connor JJ, Murray DW, Price AJ. Influence of consciousness, muscle action, and exercise on medial condyle translation after unicompartmental knee arthroplasty. *Knee* 2015; **22**(6): 646-652 .

41. Bradley J, Goodfellow JW, O'Connor JJ. A radiographic study of bearing movement in unicompartmental Oxford knee replacements. *J Bone Joint Surg Br* 1987; **69**(4): 598-601.

42. Butler DL, Noyes FR, Grood ES. Ligamentous restraints to anterior-posterior drawer in the human knee. A biomechanical study. *J Bone Joint Surg Am* 1980; **62**(2): 259-70.

43. Grood ES, Noyes FR, Butler DL, Suntay WJ. Ligamentous and capsular restraints preventing straight medial and lateral laxity in intact human cadaver knees. *J Bone Joint Surg Am* 1981; **63**(8): 1257-69.

44. Piziali RL, Seering WP, Nagel DA, Schurman DJ. The function of the primary ligaments of the knee in anterior-posterior and medial-lateral motions. *J Biomech* 1980; **13**(9): 777-84.

45. Seering WP, Piziali RL, Nagel DA, Schurman DJ. The function of the primary ligaments of the knee in varus-valgus and axial rotation. *J Biomech* 1980; **13**(9): 785-94.

46. Zavatsky AB, O'Connor JJ. A model of human knee ligaments in the sagittal plane. Part 2: Fibre recruitment under load. *Proc Inst Mech Eng H* 1992; **206**(3): 135-45.

47. Huss RA, Holstein H, O'Connor JJ. The effect of cartilage deformation on the laxity of the knee joint. *Proc Inst Mech Eng H* 1999; **213**(1): 19-32.

48. Grood ES, Noyes FR. Diagnosis of knee injuries: Biomechanical precepts. In: Feagin JA, ed. *The Crucial Ligaments: Diagnosis and treatment of ligamentous injuries about the knee.* New York: Churchill Livingstone; 1988.

49. Hill PF, Vedi V, Williams A, Iwaki H, Pinskerova V, Freeman MA. Tibiofemoral movement 2: the loaded and unloaded living knee studied by MRI. *J Bone Joint Surg Br* 2000; **82**(8): 1196-8.

50. Zavatsky AB, O'Connor JJ. Anteroposterior tibial translation during simulated isometric quadriceps contractions. *Knee* 1995; **2**(2): 85-91.

51. Jurist KA, Otis JC. Anteroposterior tibiofemoral displacements during isometric extension efforts. The roles of external load and knee flexion angle. *Am J Sports Med* 1985; **13**(4): 254-8.

52. Howell SM. Anterior tibial translation during a maximum quadriceps contraction: is it clinically significant? *Am J Sports Med* 1990; **18**(6): 573-8.

53. Zavatsky AB, O'Connor JJ. Ligament forces at the knee during isometric quadriceps contractions. *Proc Inst Mech Eng H* 1993; **207**(1): 7-18.

54. Huss RA, Holstein H, O'Connor JJ. A mathematical model of forces in the knee under isometric quadriceps contractions. *Clin Biomech (Bristol, Avon)* 2000; **15**(2): 112-22.

55. Collins JJ, O'Connor JJ. Muscle-ligament interactions at the knee during walking. *Proc Inst Mech Eng H* 1991; **205**(1): 11-8.

56. O'Connor JJ, Biden E, Bradley J, Fitzpatrick D, Young S, Kershaw C, Danial DM, Goodfellow JW. The muscle stabilised knee. In: Daniel D, Akeson WH, O'Connor JJ, eds. *Knee Ligaments: Structure, Function, Injury and Repair.* New York: Raven Press; 1990.

57. Toutoungi DE, Lu TW, Leardini A, Catani F, O'Connor JJ. Cruciate ligament forces in the human knee during rehabilitation exercises. *Clin Biomech (Bristol, Avon)* 2000; **15**(3): 176-87.

58. Walker PS, Rovick JS, Robertson DD. The effects of knee brace hinge design and placement on joint mechanics. *J Biomech* 1988; **21**(11): 965-74.

59. Kurosawa H, Walker PS, Abe S, Garg A, Hunter T. Geometry and motion of the knee for implant and orthotic design. *J Biomech* 1985; **18**(7): 487-99.

60. Price AJ, Rees JL, Beard DJ, Gill RH, Dodd CA, Murray DM. Sagittal plane kinematics of a mobile-bearing unicompartmental knee arthroplasty at 10 years: a comparative in vivo fluoroscopic analysis. *J Arthroplasty* 2004; **19**(5): 590-7.

61. Jefferson RJ, Whittle MW. Biomechanical assessment of unicompartmental knee arthroplasty, total condylar arthroplasty and tibial osteotomy. *Clin Biomech (Bristol, Avon)* 1989; **4**(4): 232-42.

62. Wiik AV, Aqil A, Tankard S, Amis AA, Cobb JP. Downhill walking gait pattern discriminates between types of knee arthroplasty: improved physiological knee functionality in UKA versus TKA. *Knee Surg Sports Traumatol Arthrosc* 2015; **23**(6): 1748-55.

63. Parratte S, Pauly V, Aubaniac JM, Argenson JN. No long-term difference between fixed and mobile medial unicompartmental arthroplasty. *Clin Orthop Relat Res* 2012; **470**(1): 61-8.

4

Indications: Anteromedial Osteoarthritis

Total knee arthroplasty is an effective treatment for most types of arthritis of the knee and requires little of the joint's anatomy to be intact for a successful outcome. On the other hand, unicompartmental arthroplasty can only succeed if the rest of the knee is functionally intact before surgery. We will discuss, first, the pathology of osteoarthritis (OA) of the knee and then how to ascertain, before operating, that the ligaments are all functionally normal and the retained articular surfaces capable of resuming their weight-bearing role.

History

The components of the OUKA prosthesis were first used (from 1976 to 1984) as a bi-compartmental knee replacement (Fig. 4.1). The patients had severe OA or rheumatoid arthritis and since, at that time, there were no proven alternative treatments, there were no specific indications. The first step towards defining a role for the implant was taken when the results of these operations were reviewed and it was found that the anatomical state of the anterior cruciate ligament (ACL) at the time of surgery was an important determinant of the long-term outcome [1]. In 1992, we reported a six-fold difference in the 7-year cumulative survival of the prosthesis between knees with or without a functioning ACL at the time of surgery, irrespective of the primary disease and of all the other variables measured [2]. This was the first publication to offer statistical evidence of the importance of that ligament in the kinematics of unconstrained resurfacing implants. During the same period we had, incidentally, observed that in osteoarthritic knees with an intact ACL, articular surface damage was usually limited to the medial compartment, with the rest of the

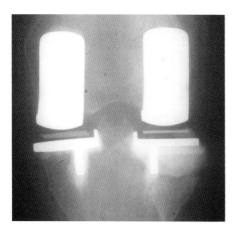

Figure 4.1 Bicompartmental Oxford Knee replacement (Phase 1, 1976-84).

joint remaining healthy. Taken together, the two observations suggested that these cases would be appropriate for treatment with the meniscal prosthesis and, since 1982, the implant has been mainly used for medial replacement in OA knees with an intact ACL [3].

Subsequently, we published a more detailed study of the pattern of cartilage damage in arthritis, correlating the preoperative clinical and radiological signs with the intraoperative findings during unicompartmental surgery [4]. In that paper we introduced the term 'anteromedial osteoarthritis' to describe the subgroup of varus knees in which both cruciate ligaments and the MCL are functionally normal, and in which the cartilage and bone erosions on the tibial plateau are in the anterior and central parts of the medial compartment with a corresponding lesion on the inferior medial femoral condyle.

We now believe that anteromedial OA is the most common indication for UKA and is present in about half the patients needing knee replacement. The condition can be recognised by a consistent association between the clinical and radiological signs and the pathological lesions that cause them.

Anteromedial osteoarthritis (Figures 4.2 & 4.3)

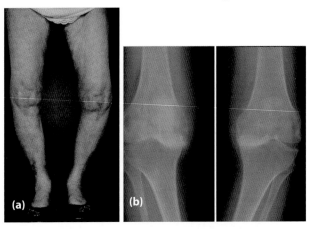

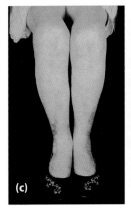

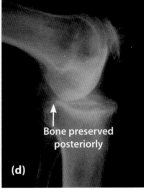

Figure 4.2 (a)–(d) The patient illustrated had unusually severe bilateral anteromedial OA. Standing, (a) she has marked varus deformities and the radiographs (b) show deep erosions of both medial tibial plateaux. Sitting, (c) the varus corrects. The radiograph (d) shows that this is because in flexion the medial condyles roll out of the anteromedial erosions on to the intact articular surfaces posteriorly.

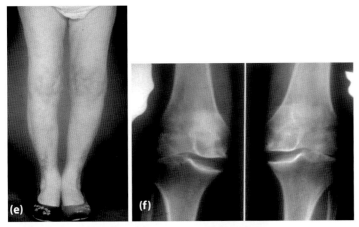

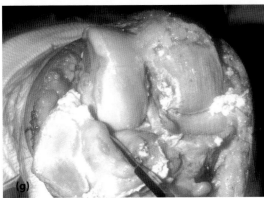

Figure 4.2 (e) –(i) Because the varus corrected every time the knees were flexed, structural shortening of the medial collateral ligament could not occur. Therefore, with the knees flexed a little, the patient could correct the varus with her own muscles (e). On the radiographs (f), the varus is corrected by applied valgus force. The intraoperative picture (g) shows the anatomical features of anteromedial OA. Note the intact ACL.

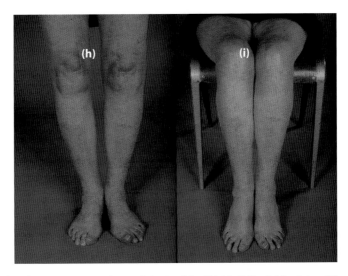

(Reproduced with permission and copyright © of the British Editorial Society of Bone and Joint Surgery [White SH, Ludkowski PF, Goodfellow JW. Anteromedial osteoarthritis of the knee. *J Bone Joint Surg [Br]* 1991; **73-B**: 582–6].) (h) & (i) show clinical photographs of the same patient with well functioning knees 23 years after her bilateral Oxford medial knee replacements. The patient died in 2013, aged 100 years.

Principal physical signs

1. Pain in the knee is present on standing and is severe when walking. It is relieved by sitting.

2. With the knee (as near as possible) fully extended, the leg is in varus (5–15°) and the deformity cannot be corrected.

3. With the knee flexed 20° or more, the varus can be corrected.

4. With the knee flexed to 90°, the varus corrects spontaneously.

Principal anatomical features

At surgery, knees with the above mentioned physical signs regularly demonstrate the following anatomical features, some of which are visible in the intraoperative photograph shown in Figure 4.2(g) and all of which are illustrated in the diagrams in Figure 4.3.

1. Both cruciate ligaments are functionally normal, though the ACL may have suffered some damage and may have longitudinal splits.

2. The cartilage on the tibia is eroded, and eburnated bone is exposed, anteriorly and/or centrally on the medial plateau. An area of full-thickness cartilage is always preserved at the back of the plateau (Fig. 4.3(a)).

3. The cartilage on the inferior articular surface of the medial femoral condyle is eroded, and eburnated bone is exposed. The posterior surface of the condyle retains its full-thickness cartilage (Fig. 4.3(a)).

4. The weight bearing articular cartilage of the lateral compartment, although often fibrillated, preserves its full thickness (Fig. 4.3(b)). In many cases, a full thickness ulcer can be present on the medial border of the lateral femoral condyle (see Fig 5.4) [5].

5. The medial collateral ligament (MCL) is of normal length (Figs. 4.3(d–f)).

6. The posterior capsule is shortened (Fig. 4.3(a)).

Correlations

The observed sites of articular surface damage, together with the intact status of the cruciate ligaments and the MCL, explain the symptoms and physical signs.

1. The cruciate ligaments maintain the normal pattern of 'rollback' of the femur on the tibia in the sagittal plane (see Chapter 3) and thereby preserve the distinction between the damaged contact areas in extension (the anterior tibial plateau and the inferior surface of the medial femoral condyle) (Figs. 4.3(a) and (b)) and the intact contact areas in flexion (the posterior tibial plateau and the posterior surface of the femoral condyle) (Figs. 4.3(c) and (d)). The short posterior capsule causes the flexion deformity (Fig. 4.3(a)).

2. The varus deformity of the extended leg, (and the pain felt on standing and walking), are caused by loss of cartilage and bone from the contact areas in extension (Figs. 4.3(a) and 4.3(b)).

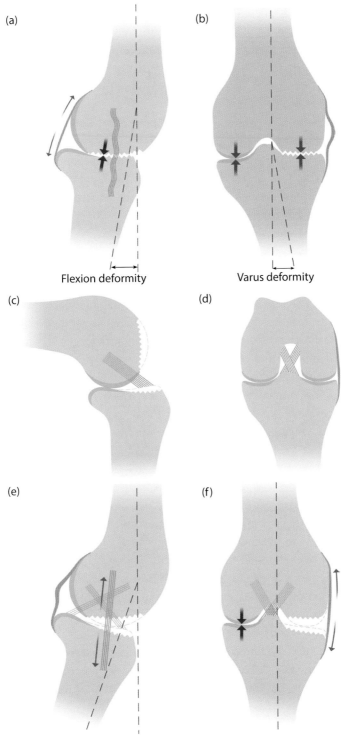

Figure 4.3 Diagramatic explanation of the physical signs of anteromedial OA in the right knee (see text).

The *angle* of varus depends on the amount of material lost. To expose bone on both surfaces, the total thickness of cartilage lost is about 5 mm, causing about 5° of varus. At least this degree of deformity is usual on presentation because pain seldom becomes severe until there is bone-on-bone contact during weight bearing. Thereafter, each millimetre of bone eroded increases the deformity by about 1°.

3. The varus deformity corrects spontaneously at 90° as the articular cartilage is intact in the areas of contact in flexion (Figs. 4.3(c) and (d)). Therefore the MCL is drawn out to its normal length every time the patient bends the knee (Fig. 4.3(d)), and structural shortening of the ligament does not occur. Thus an intact ACL ensures an MCL of normal length, as demonstrated by manual correction of the varus (Fig. 4.3(f)) when the posterior capsule is relaxed (Fig. 4.3(e)) with the knee flexed.

Progression to posteromedial osteoarthritis

The association of an intact ACL with the focal pattern of cartilage erosions described above is striking. White et al. [4] described 46 medial tibial plateaux excised sequentially from a series of OA knees treated by OUKA, all of them with an intact ACL and with cartilage erosions exposing bone (Ahlback stages 2, 3, and 4) [6]. The erosions were *all* anterior and central (Fig. 4.4). They rarely extended to the posterior quarter of the plateau and *never* reached the posterior joint margin.

Harman et al. [7] examined the tibial plateaux excised from 143 osteoarthritic knees during operations for TKA. They found that wear in ACL-deficient varus knees was located a mean 4 mm more posterior on the medial plateau than wear in ACL-intact knees ($p < 0.05$). The ACL-deficient knees also exhibited more severe varus deformity. The authors stated: '... *it is evident that anterior cruciate ligament integrity is a dominant factor affecting the location of tibiofemoral contact and the resulting cartilage wear patterns in patients with osteoarthritis*'. Similar findings were reported by Mullaji et al. [8]. The authors assessed tibial articular cartilage wear intraoperatively in 100 consecutive patients with varus OA. They noted that the posterior half of the medial tibial plateau was more commonly involved in ACL deficiency with predominant anteromedial wear in ACL-intact knees. Moschella et al. [9] reached very similar conclusions from their examination of 70 excised medial plateaux from varus osteoarthritic knees, the lesion in ACL intact knees lying centrally and medially on the medial plateau.

The site and extent of the tibial erosions can be determined reliably from lateral radiographs (see Fig. 4.11) [4]. Based on this, Keyes et al. [10] studied the preoperative lateral radiographs of 50 OA knees in which the state of the ACL had been recorded at surgery (25 ACL deficient and 25 ACL intact). Using four blinded observers, they found 95% correlation between preservation of the posterior part of the medial tibial plateau on the radiograph and an intact ACL at surgery, and 100% correlation of erosion of the posterior plateau on the radiograph with an absent or badly damaged ACL.

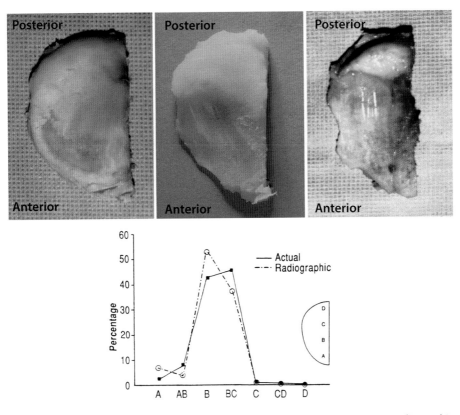

Figure 4.4 Typical tibial plateau lesions of anteromedial OA. The graph compares radiographic data with data from 46 intraoperative specimens. (The graph is reproduced with permission and copyright © of the British Editorial Society of Bone and Joint Surgery [White SH, Ludkowski PF, Goodfellow JW. Anteromedial osteoarthritis of the knee. *J Bone Joint Surg* [Br] 1991; 73-B: 582–6].)

These correlations show that, as long as the ACL remains intact, the tibiofemoral contact areas in flexion remain distinct from the areas of contact in extension. Progressive loss of bone causes the varus deformity in extension to increase but, while the ACL continues to function, the deformity corrects spontaneously in flexion and structural shortening of the MCL does not occur.

Failure of the ACL may be the event that causes the transition from anteromedial OA to the posteromedial form of the disease, with posterior subluxation of the femur and structural shortening of the MCL. Deschamps and Lapeyre [11] observed that absence of the ACL in an osteoarthritic knee was associated with posterior subluxation of the femur on the tibia in extension. Figure 4.5 demonstrates how this subluxation results in abrasion of the cartilage at the back of the tibial plateau by the exposed bone on the inferior surface of the femoral condyle. Thereafter, in flexion, the cartilage on the posterior surface of the femoral condyle is also destroyed by abrasion on the tibial plateau, now devoid of cartilage. The varus deformity is then present in flexion as well as in extension, and the MCL can shorten structurally.

(a)   (b)

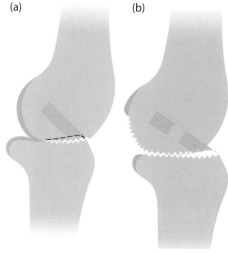

Figure 4.5 (a) The intact ACL holds the femur forward on the tibia in extension. (b) Rupture (or stretching) of the ACL allows posterior subluxation of the femur on the tibia and secondary damage to the posterior articular surface of the tibial plateau. Thereafter, the cartilage on the posterior surface of the femur is damaged when the femur flexes.

The sequence described above does not require us to assume any 'spread' of the original disease to adjacent intact cartilage. Failure of the ACL alone is enough to explain how the original lesions in the 'extension areas' of the medial compartment could cause secondary physical damage to the cartilage of its 'flexion areas' and start a process that results in a subluxed knee with progressive bone loss posteromedially and fixed varus deformity.

How and why does the ACL rupture?

How?

The stages of deterioration of the ACL observed intraoperatively in OA knees suggest the following sequence, which we have used to grade the damage:
1. Normal
2. Loss of synovial covering, usually starting distally
3. Longitudinal splits in the substance of the exposed ligament
4. Friable and fragmented with stretching and loss of strength of the collagen bundles
5. Absent or ruptured.

Why?

Among the knee's ligaments, the ACL is peculiarly at risk because of two anatomical features.
1. Its intra-articular course puts it at risk of nutritional insufficiency from chronic synovitis of any type. For instance, the ACL is frequently damaged by chronic rheumatoid synovitis. The importance of the ligament's synovial investment is also suggested by the observation that the ACL is always healthy in knees in which the *ligamentum mucosum* is intact (Dr RD Scott,

personal communication). Experimental stripping of the synovium from rabbit ACL causes a succession of changes very like those seen in human OA joints, culminating in structural disintegration of the ligament [12].

2. The ligament is at risk of physical damage from osteophytes at the margins of the condyles. In knees with anteromedial OA, osteophytes are almost always present on the lateral side, and sometimes on both sides of the intercondylar notch, and the lower part of the ligament may be damaged by them as the knee approaches full extension (Fig. 4.6).

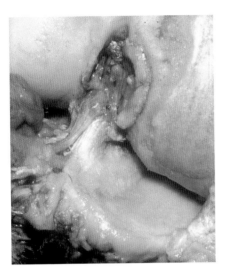

Figure 4.6 Intraoperative picture of an ACL that is partly denuded of synovium, has longitudinal splits and is surrounded by osteophytes. Chronic synovitis and osteophytosis, which are both common in antereomedial OA, probably represent the response throughout the joint cavity to material shed into it from the cartilage erosions in the medial compartment.

Summary of pathology

The primary pathological lesions of anteromedial OA are focal erosions of the cartilage on the inferior surface of the medial femoral condyle and on the anterior and central parts of the medial tibial plateau, areas that make contact with one another in extension.

Chronic synovitis and marginal osteophytosis are secondary pathological changes. The articular cartilage of the lateral compartment is functionally intact. The cruciate and collateral ligaments are of normal length.

While the ACL remains effective, the orderly flexion–extension movements of the femur on the tibia in the sagittal plane are preserved, maintaining the separation of the flexion areas from the extension areas. Progressive loss of bone causes increasing varus deformity in extension but not in flexion.

Failure of the ACL allows posterior subluxation of the femur on the tibia and offers a sufficient explanation for the progression from anteromedial arthritis to posteromedial disease, with an associated fixed varus deformity.

If this is the natural history, resurfacing the medial compartment *while the ACL is still intact* may cure the symptoms and recover the normal kinematics and mechanics of the joint. If the osteophytes have been removed, and cartilage debris is no longer shed into the joint cavity, later failure of the ACL and spread of the disease to the other compartments may be avoided.

These are the theoretical reasons for employing unicompartmental arthroplasty as the treatment for anteromedial OA.

Preoperative assessment

Preoperative assessment aims to determine, as precisely as possible, whether a particular knee has anteromedial OA.

Clinical examination

Pain

Pain is usually felt near the medial joint line but it may be anterior, posterior, and even on the lateral side of the knee. Its localisation is not a reliable sign. Pain is felt on standing and walking, but is usually absent while sitting (when the intact articular surfaces at the back of the medial compartment are in contact) and when lying down (when the damaged surfaces are unloaded).

Severity of pain, limitation of walking distance and compromised quality of life are the factors that decide the need for operation. The criteria are similar to those used to justify TKA.

Physical signs

The principal physical signs were briefly described in the previous section.

1. Varus deformity of the leg is best seen when the patient is standing. Varus is seldom less than 5° on presentation and rarely more than 15°. A 'lateral thrust' of the knee is often seen on walking and is not a contraindication. As already noted, the intra-articular varus deformity corrects spontaneously when the patient is seated with the knee flexed to 90° (Figs. 4.3(c) and (d)), and it can be manually corrected, by applying a valgus force, with the knee flexed 20° or more to relax the posterior capsule (Figs. 4.3(e) and (f)).
2. Usually the knee will not fully extend. If the ACL remains intact and functional, the fixed flexion deformity is rarely more than 15°.
3. Flexion range is usually limited but is rarely less than 110°. Flexion less than 110° is a relative contraindication to OUKA because of the difficulty it presents at surgery. However, more flexion can usually be achieved under anaesthesia than in the clinic, particularly if the limitation is due to severe pain rather than stiffness of the joint.
4. Moderate synovial swelling and joint effusion are common, and there is often tenderness to palpation over the medial joint line.

It should be noted that the 'pivot shift', the drawer test, and other manoeuvres designed to assess the cruciate ligaments after trauma are of much less value in the arthritic knee. Erroneous conclusions may result from false instability, due to intact ligaments being rendered slack by loss of articular cartilage height, or from false stability, due to interpenetration of the damaged articular surfaces, or the presence of large osteophytes, which mask ligament insufficiency. These tests are not used in preoperative decision-making.

Radiography

Radiography is the most useful adjunct to physical signs in demonstrating the suitability of a knee for OUKA.

Anteroposterior radiographs

Anteroposterior radiographs, taken in the standard way with the patient weight-bearing on the extended leg, can demonstrate loss of articular cartilage medially by showing that the condyles articulate 'bone-on-bone' (Ahlback stage 2 or more) [6]. However, in some cases in which there is full-thickness cartilage loss, this method fails to reveal it. A better projection for this purpose is a Rosenberg view with the patient standing with the knee 45° flexed, with the X-ray beam appropriately tilted, to be parallel to the tibial plateau. A varus-stressed film is more reliable than either of these methods (Fig. 4.7).

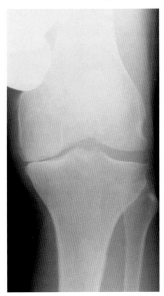

Figure 4.7 Varus stressed radiograph of anteromedial OA.

Valgus-stressed radiographs

Valgus-stressed radiographs are used to ensure that there is a normal thickness of articular cartilage in the lateral compartment and to demonstrate that the intra-articular varus deformity is correctable (i.e. the MCL is not shortened). We have found no other method of investigation to be so satisfactory in confirming these two key requirements for successful unicompartmental arthroplasty [13].

When the patient stands on a knee with a varus deformity, body weight tends to distract the lateral joint surfaces [14, 15]. Therefore, to measure the thickness of the lateral compartment cartilage, the lateral condyles must be firmly apposed to one another by applying a valgus force to the otherwise unloaded limb.

Technique (Fig. 4.8)

The patient lies supine on the X-ray couch with a support under the knee to flex it 20°. The X-ray beam is aligned 10° from the vertical (to allow for the average posterior inclination of the tibial plateau so it is parallel to the joint surfaces). The surgeon (wearing protective gloves and apron) applies a firm valgus couple of forces through the knee, while ensuring that the leg is in neutral rotation. Alternatively, a device can be used by a radiographer to apply stress. The radiographs should be examined to ensure they are of adequate quality. The radiograph should show the joint surfaces end on and the patella should be approximately central. If the quality is poor they should be repeated.

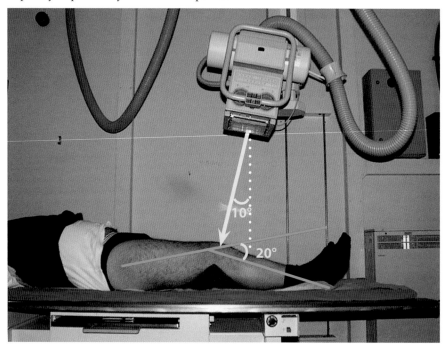

Figure 4.8 Technique of varus/valgus stress radiography.

Interpretation (Fig. 4.9)

1. The radiolucent joint space between the subchondral plates of the lateral compartment should measure not less than 4 mm, the sum of the thickness of two layers of normal cartilage (Fig. 4.9(b)). A gap of less than 4 mm implies thinning of the cartilage and its impending failure. It is a contraindication to UKA.

ACL damage

Direct examination of the ACL may cause a change of mind. ACL deterioration is gradual (as is the posterior extension of the tibial erosion), and it is sometimes difficult to determine the point at which the ACL has ceased to function adequately.

To increase the precision of the indications, we analysed retrospectively 820 OUKAs in which the state of the ACL had been recorded intraoperatively and graded as normal, synovial damage or longitudinal splits [18].

More marked macroscopic ACL damage was significantly associated with increasing age, male gender and a more extensive anteromedial tibial defect. At ten years, no difference in functional outcome or activity level was found between groups. However, compared to those with macroscopically normal ACL at ten years, a significantly greater improvement from baseline OKS and AKSS-Objective score was seen in patients with macroscopically ACL abnormalities. At fifteen years, no difference in implant survival, or failure mechanism, was detected between groups.

We therefore conclude that the macroscopic status of the ACL does not affect long term functional outcomes or implant survival providing the ACL is functionally intact.

In summary we have found that loss of synovial lining or longitudinal splits in the substance of the ligament are not contraindications. Knees in which the ligament is ruptured or its substance is demonstrably weak (friable and fragmented ACL) are unsuitable for OUKA.

A practical way to show that a ligament is 'demonstrably weak' is to insert a small tendon hook around the ACL and pull forcibly on it. If this test does not rupture the ACL, it is safe to proceed to OUKA; if it does, TKA is required.

Lateral compartment damage

Even through the small incision now used for OUKA, it is possible to see most of the articular surface of the lateral femoral condyle. Surface flaking and chondromalacia are very common and have been shown not to be significant. Occasionally, there is a medial ulcer on the lateral condyle. This can be ignored (see Chapter 5). Rarely, a full-thickness defect in the central weight-bearing cartilage is discovered. We treat this as a contraindication (although we have no evidence to support this practice).

Summary of indications

The main indication for OUKA is significant symptoms and anteromedial osteoarthritis defined as follows:

Physical signs
1. Pain severe enough to justify joint replacement.

Radiographic signs
2. Full-thickness cartilage loss with eburnated bone-on-bone contact in the medial compartment (Ahlback stage 2, 3, or 4) [6].

3. Full-thickness cartilage preserved in the lateral compartment, demonstrated on a valgus stress radiograph.
4. Intact medial articular surface at the back of the tibial plateau and of the femoral condyle, best seen on a lateral radiograph.
5. Intra articular varus deformity manually correctable (in 20° flexion), best seen on a valgus stress radiograph.

Intraoperative signs

6. Full-thickness cartilage preserved in the lateral compartment, demonstrated on a valgus stress radiograph.
7. Presence of an intact ACL (ignoring synovial damage and longitudinal splits).
8. Satisfactory appearance of the central weight-bearing articular cartilage of the lateral compartment.

Apart from the severity of the pain, all the indications that a knee is suitable for OUKA are anatomical; plain radiography and stressed films are the best ways to demonstrate them.

Many surgeons find it difficult to obtain good quality stress radiographs and therefore do not use them for assessing patients. This is not ideal as stress radiographs are the best way to assess patients and the only reliable way to assess the thickness of the lateral cartilage and the correctability of the deformity. We believe they should be used by all surgeons starting to implant the OUKA. However, many experienced surgeons believe, that if there is bone-on-bone medial OA with a functionally intact ACL and the central weight bearing area of the lateral femoral condyle is in good condition, it is acceptable to do an OUKA. Although this may be correct, we have no long term data to support it.

Discussion of indications

In this section, some of the criteria listed above are discussed in more detail.

Flexion deformity

There may be several contributory causes for the (usually small) flexion deformity commonly seen in knees with anteromedial OA.

1. The posterior capsule is structurally shortened, perhaps from the effect of chronic synovitis and/or the patient's prolonged reluctance to straighten the painful knee.
2. Osteophytes at the posterior margin of the medial femoral condyle can 'tent' the posterior capsular ligament.
3. Osteophytes at the top of the intercondylar notch of the femur can impinge, near full extension, on an osteophyte arising from the tibia in front of the attachment of the ACL.

It seems likely that there is always some structural shortening of the posterior capsule because removal of the osteophytes at surgery, although it often improves the deformity, does not immediately restore full extension. However, unlike TKA, unicompartmental replacement is followed in the postoperative period by spontaneous improvement of extension, probably from stretching of the shortened posterior capsule.

Weale *et al.* [19] reported that 28 knees with a mean preoperative flexion deformity of 8° (SD 8) reduced to a mean of 1° (SD 2) 1–2 years after OUKA (*p*< 0.001). At 10+ years, the mean deformity was not significantly changed (3° (SD 4)).

Provided that anterior and posterior osteophytes are removed, some correction will occur during the operation and improvement will continue in the succeeding year so that a preoperative flexion deformity of as much as 15° is considered acceptable. In fact, it is unusual to encounter as great a deformity as this in an OA knee with an intact ACL. However, in avascular necrosis (AVN or SONK), with severe collapse of the femoral condyle, greater degrees of flexion deformity are encountered and have been found to correct spontaneously after OUKA [20, 21].

Why does flexion deformity correct spontaneously after UKA and not after TKA?

In TKA, 'balancing the ligaments' in flexion means equalising the lengths of the MCL and the lateral collateral ligament (LCL) to create a quadrilateral flexion gap (Fig. 4.14(d)). This is achieved by lengthening the MCL (Fig 4.14(e)), which leaves the flexion gap wider than before and the posterior capsule relatively too short. Therefore, spontaneous correction of residual flexion deformity after TKA would require the posterior capsule to stretch beyond its physiological length.

In UKA, the cruciate mechanism and the MCL are both preserved intact and the flexion gap is the same after the operation as before, so that the posterior capsule is required only to stretch back to its physiological length for the flexion deformity to correct. Alteration of the interstriational angle of the lattice-like structure of the posterior capsule provides a mechanism whereby it could shorten, and lengthen again, but only within the limit set by the physiological lengths of its constituent fibres (Fig. 4.15).

(a)   (b)

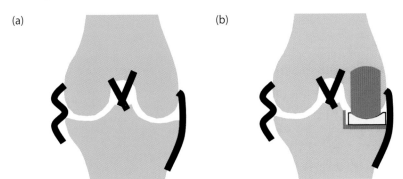

Figure 4.14 (a) In the normal knee above 20° flexion fibres within the MCL, ACL & PCL are tight and the LCL is slack. (b) During OUKA, no ligaments are released so postoperatively the MCL, ACL & PCL are tight and the LCL is slack. There is no distraction of the joint.

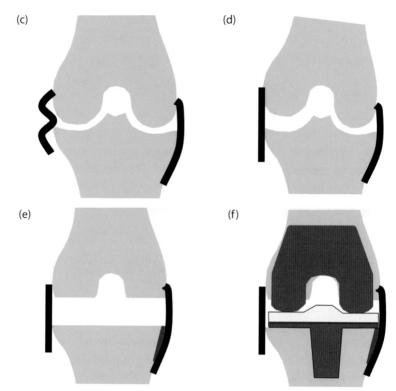

Figure 4.14 (c) During TKA, the ACL is removed and the PCL is defunctioned. (d) For the knee to be balanced, both LCL & MCL have to be tight so the lateral side is distracted. (e) Following bone cuts, a rectangular gap usually can only be achieved with a medial release (f) so when the TKA is implanted the joint is distracted.

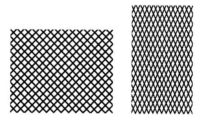

Figure 4.15 The posterior capsule's ability to shorten, and lengthen again, may be explained by the lattice-like arrangement of its collagen bundles.

Full-thickness cartilage in the lateral compartment

The full thickness of the cartilage is taken to be evidence that it is adequate to sustain load even if its surface is fibrillated and has superficial erosions.

Fibrillation and chondromalacia are almost always present in parts of the lateral (and patellofemoral) compartments of knees with anteromedial OA, probably because of the chronic synovitis present throughout the joint cavity and the abnormal loading regime experienced by the cartilage as a result of the varus deformity. It is because surface changes have proved largely irrelevant in predicting long-term outcome that arthroscopy does not appear among the necessary preoperative investigations listed above. Indeed it can overestimate the surface damage and confuse the issue.

However, thinning of the articular cartilage in the lateral compartment is taken to be a sign of its impending failure to support load and is a contraindication to UKA. Therefore, accurate measurement of cartilage thickness is important. We have tried ultrasound imaging and MRI, but have found these methods less reliable than the valgus-stressed plain radiograph (which has the added advantage of showing, at the same time, whether the varus is correctable).

The justification for the advice given above rests mainly on several published 10-year survival studies for OUKA performed using these criteria. In one study, there was no radiological evidence of deterioration during that time. Table 4.1 compares the appearance of the lateral compartment on radiographs taken immediately postoperatively with its appearance 10+ years later (mean interval 11.4 years) [19]. The films were all taken under fluoroscopic control and therefore were strictly comparable. The intra-observer error was small ($K = 0.64$) for the Ahlback classification and moderate ($K = 0.44$) for the Altman grading [6, 22]. One lateral compartment in 23 knees examined showed definite progression of arthritis, but only on the Altman classification. Statistical analysis of the scores revealed no significant deterioration with time.

Table 4.1 Radiological evaluation of the lateral tibiofemoral compartment 10+ years after OUKA compared with its status at one year. Each pair or radiographs were assessed twice

Condition	Ahlback classification		Altman classification	
	Assessment 1	Assessment 2	Assessment 1	Assessment 2
Definitely worse	0	0	1	1
Possibly worse	7	3	5	6
Same	14	19	14	13
Possibly better	2	1	3	3
Definitely better	0	0	0	0

(The table is reproduced with permission and copyright © of the British Editorial Society of Bone and Joint Surgery [Weale AE, Murray DW, Crawford R, Psychoyios V, Bonomo A, Howell G, O'Connor J, Goodfellow JW. Does arthritis progress in the retained compartments after 'Oxford' medial unicompartmental arthroplasty? *J Bone Joint Surg [Br]* 1999; **81-B**: 783–9].)

Nevertheless, failure of the lateral compartment has been a cause for revision of OUKA (see Chapter 10). The question as to whether the failure rate from this cause could be diminished by employing different, or more stringent, preoperative criteria than those advised above will only be answered by further prospective long-term studies. This matter is discussed in Chapter 10 where it is concluded that many lateral compartment failures result from overloading of the cartilage by inadvertent overcorrection into valgus, not from spontaneous degeneration with time.

Correctable varus deformity

Why do we not include full-length leg films in our preoperative radiological assessment?

Tibiofemoral varus may be due to intra-articular deformity (genu varum) (Fig. 4.16(b)), extra-articular deformity (tibia vara) (Fig. 4.16(d)), or a combination of both (Fig. 4.16(e)).

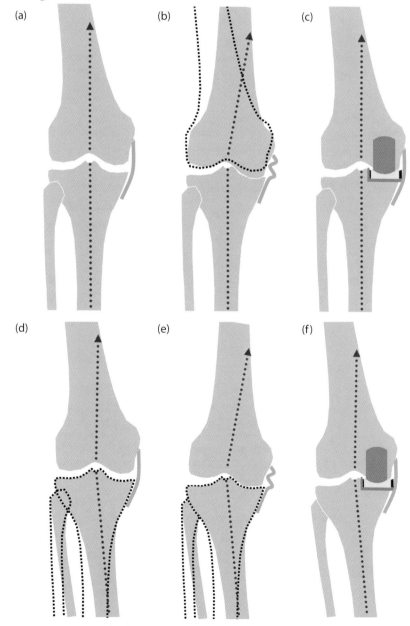

Figure 4.16 Diagrams of the knee, with femoral and tibial axes (a) showing the effect of the intra-articular deformity (genu varum) (b) and the correction achieved by OUKA (c). (d, e, and f) show the same occurring in the presence of an extra articular deformity (tibia vara).

1. The genu varum of anteromedial OA is caused by collapse of the medial compartment from loss of its cartilage and subchondral bone. The MCL is not shortened and so varus is completely correctable preoperatively, and completely corrected by OUKA. If the tibiofemoral angle was normal before the onset of arthritis (Fig. 4.16(a)), it will be returned to normal by the operation (Fig. 4.16(c)).

2. Tibia vara is a bone deformity, usually between the tibial plateau and the shaft (Fig. 4.16(d)), and is commonly developmental.

3. Not uncommonly, anteromedial OA develops in a limb with pre-existing extra-articular tibia vara, resulting in an increase in the tibiofemoral varus (Fig. 4.16(e)). This is more commonly seen in Asian patients. In these cases, OUKA corrects the intra-articular genu varum but the tibia vara persists (Fig. 4.16(f)), so that the tibiofemoral angle remains in some degree of varus. (Much less commonly, genu varum develops in a limb with extra-articular *valgus*, which is commonly in the femur. In this case, OUKA corrects the genu varum and restores whatever degree of tibiofemoral valgus was present before the arthritis developed. This is seen almost exclusively in female patients.)

Therefore the term 'fully correctable' refers only to the intra-articular component of alignment deformity. The valgus-stressed radiograph predicts full correction of the intra-articular deformity by demonstrating at least 4 mm separation of the medial femoral condyle from the tibial plateau, i.e. the MCL is not shortened (see Fig. 4.9).

Measurement of the tibiofemoral shaft angle does not distinguish between intra-articular and extra-articular deformity and therefore is not helpful.

Emerson *et al.* [23] compared the effects on postoperative leg alignment of employing either a fixed-bearing UKA (Brigham) or an OUKA (Phase 2). They measured alignment on 3-foot anteroposterior radiographs taken with the patient standing. The technique of Kennedy and White [24] was used to determine the location in the knee through which the mechanical axis passed, and the conventions of the Knee Society were used to measure the angle of alignment. The average preoperative alignment of the two groups was similar, 1.7° and 1.8° varus. After OUKA the average alignment was 5.5° valgus, and after the fixed-bearing UKA it was 2.6° valgus. The variability of alignment after OUKA was less. Figure 4.17 shows that after OUKA the mechanical axis of the limb usually passed through the intercondylar area of the knee. The authors suggested that the greater degree of valgus achieved by the OUKA might explain the late failures from lateral compartment arthritis that they experienced. However, in a more recent study, Emerson *et al.* [25] found that following Phase 3 OUKA, fewer patients were in valgus, suggesting perhaps with Phase 3 the incidence of OA progression might be less than with Phase 2. Furthermore the study demonstrated that, following OUKA, the leg alignment was similar to that of the other knee which suggests that predisease alignment was restored.

Hernigou and Deschamps [26] showed that, after medial UKA, 'severe undercorrection' (i.e. hip–knee–ankle angle <170°) caused increased polyethylene wear in the fixed-bearing implants they used; and overcorrection into valgus (>180°) was associated with an increased risk of lateral compartment arthritis. However, their method of measurement could not distinguish between intra- and extra-articular deformity. Intra-articular overcorrection, implying as it does a damaged MCL, has been associated with lateral compartment arthritis after OUKA. However, failure of a meniscal bearing from wear-through has not been recorded, although some limbs have residual extra-articular varus.

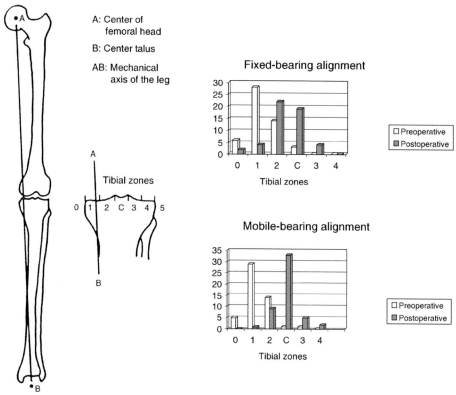

Figure 4.17 The mechanical axis of the leg is shown with the tibial surface divided into zones. The zone location of the mechanical axis for the fixed- and mobile-bearing knee implants taken with 3-foot radiographs obtained with the patient standing are shown in graphical form. The tibial zones are according to Kennedy and White [24]. (Reproduced with permission of Lippincott Williams & Wilkins from Emerson RH Jr., Hansborough T, Reitman RD, Rosenfeldt W, Higgins LL. Comparison of a mobile with a fixed-bearing unicompartmental knee implant. *Clin Orthop* 2002; **404**: 62–70.)

We believe that no attempt should ever be made to correct an extra-articular varus malalignment intra-articularly, for example by MCL release. On the contrary, that ligament's fibres should all be carefully preserved, and 'overstuffing' of the medial compartment with a bearing that is too thick should be avoided. We have found no differences in clinical outcome between those with varus and normal alignment at the end of the operation [27].

References

1. Goodfellow JW, O'Connor J. Clinical results of the Oxford knee. Surface arthroplasty of the tibiofemoral joint with a meniscal bearing prosthesis. *Clin Orthop Relat Res* 1986; (**205**): 21-42.

2. Goodfellow J, O'Connor J. The anterior cruciate ligament in knee arthroplasty. A risk-factor with unconstrained meniscal prostheses. *Clin Orthop Relat Res* 1992; (**276**): 245-52.

3. Goodfellow JW, Tibrewal SB, Sherman KP, O'Connor JJ. Unicompartmental Oxford Meniscal knee arthroplasty. *J Arthroplasty* 1987; **2**(1): 1-9.

4. White SH, Ludkowski PF, Goodfellow JW. Anteromedial osteoarthritis of the knee. *J Bone Joint Surg Br* 1991; **73**(4): 582-6.

5. Kendrick BJ, Rout R, Bottomley NJ, Pandit H, Gill HS, Price AJ, Dodd CA, Murray DW. The implications of damage to the lateral femoral condyle on medial unicompartmental knee replacement. *J Bone Joint Surg Br* 2010; **92**(3): 374-9.

6. Ahlback S. Osteoarthrosis of the knee. A radiographic investigation. *Acta Radiol Diagn (Stockh)* 1968: Suppl 277:7-72.

7. Harman MK, Markovich GD, Banks SA, Hodge WA. Wear patterns on tibial plateaus from varus and valgus osteoarthritic knees. *Clin Orthop Relat Res* 1998; (**352**): 149-58.

8. Mullaji AB, Marawar SV, Luthra M. Tibial articular cartilage wear in varus osteoarthritic knees: correlation with anterior cruciate ligament integrity and severity of deformity. *J Arthroplasty* 2008; **23**(1): 128-35.

9. Moschella D, Blasi A, Leardini A, Ensini A, Catani F. Wear patterns on tibial plateau from varus osteoarthritic knees. *Clin Biomech (Bristol, Avon)* 2006; **21**(2): 152-8.

10. Keyes GW, Carr AJ, Miller RK, Goodfellow JW. The radiographic classification of medial gonarthrosis. Correlation with operation methods in 200 knees. *Acta Orthop Scand* 1992; **63**(5): 497-501.

11. Deschamps G, Lapeyre B. [Rupture of the anterior cruciate ligament: a frequently unrecognized cause of failure of unicompartmental knee prostheses. Apropos of a series of 79 Lotus prostheses with a follow-up of more than 5 years]. *Rev Chir Orthop Reparatrice Appar Mot* 1987; **73**(7): 544-51.

12. Robinson D, Halperin N, Nevo Z. Devascularization of the anterior cruciate ligament by synovial stripping in rabbits. An experimental model. *Acta Orthop Scand* 1992; **63**(5): 502-6.

13. Gibson PH, Goodfellow JW. Stress radiography in degenerative arthritis of the knee. *J Bone Joint Surg Br* 1986; **68**(4): 608-9.

14. Thomas RH, Resnick D, Alazraki NP, Daniel D, Greenfield R. Compartmental evaluation of osteoarthritis of the knee. A comparative study of available diagnostic modalities. *Radiology* 1975; **116**(3): 585-94.

15. Dacre JE, Cushnaghan J, Jack MJ, Kirwan JR, Dieppe PA. Knee X-rays: Should we take them lying down? *Br J Rheumatol* 1991; **30**(Abstr Suppl 1): 3.

16. Jacobsen K. Gonylaxometry. Stress radiographic measurement of passive stability in the knee joints of normal subjects and patients with ligament injuries. Accuracy and range of application. *Acta Orthop Scand Suppl* 1981; **194**: 1-263.

17. Sharpe I, Tyrrell PN, White SH. Magnetic resonance imaging assessment for unicompartmental knee replacement: a limited role. *Knee* 2001; **8**(3): 213-8.

18. Hamilton TW, Pistritto C, Jenkins C, Mellon SJ, Dodd CA, Pandit H, Murray DW. Unicompartmental knee replacement: does the macroscopic status of the anterior cruciate ligament affect outcome? *Knee* 2016; **23**(3): 506-510.

19. Weale AE, Murray DW, Crawford R, Psychoyios V, Bonomo A, Howell G, O'Connor J, Goodfellow JW. Does arthritis progress in the retained compartments after 'Oxford' medial unicompartmental arthroplasty? A clinical and radiological study with a minimum ten-year follow-up. *J Bone Joint Surg Br* 1999; **81**(5): 783-9.

20. Langdown AJ, Pandit H, Price AJ, Dodd CA, Murray DW, Svard UC, Gibbons CL. Oxford medial unicompartmental arthroplasty for focal spontaneous osteonecrosis of the knee. *Acta Orthop* 2005; **76**(5): 688-92.

21. Marmor L. Unicompartmental arthroplasty for osteonecrosis of the knee joint. *Clin Orthop Relat Res* 1993; (**294**): 247-53.

22. Altman RD, Fries JF, Bloch DA, Carstens J, Cooke, T, Genant H, Gofton P, Groth H, Mcshane DJ, Murphy WA, Sharp JT, Spitz P, Williams CA, Wolfe F.. Radiographic assessment of progression in osteoarthritis. *Arthritis Rheum* 1987; **30**(11): 1214-25.

23. Emerson RH, Jr., Hansborough T, Reitman RD, Rosenfeldt W, Higgins LL. Comparison of a mobile with a fixed-bearing unicompartmental knee implant. *Clin Orthop Relat Res* 2002; (**404**): 62-70.

24. Kennedy WR, White RP. Unicompartmental arthroplasty of the knee. Postoperative alignment and its influence on overall results. *Clin Orthop Relat Res* 1987; (**221**): 278-85.

25. Emerson RH Jr, Higgins LL. Unicompartmental knee arthroplasty with the Oxford prosthesis in patients with medial compartment arthritis. *J Bone Joint Sur Am*. 2008 Jan; **90**(1):118-22.

26. Hernigou P, Deschamps G. Alignment influences wear in the knee after medial unicompartmental arthroplasty. *Clin Orthop Relat Res* 2004; (**423**): 161-5.

27. Gulati A, Pandit H, Jenkins C, Chau R, Dodd CA, Murray DW. The effect of leg alignment on the outcome of unicompartmental knee replacement. *J Bone Joint Surg Br* 2009; **91**(4): 469-74.

5

Contraindications in Anteromedial Osteoarthritis

While it is important to ensure that all the necessary indications are met [1], it is also important not to apply unnecessary contraindications. Some published lists of supposed contraindications have achieved wide acceptance without having much evidence to support them. We have recently argued with evidence that many of the suggested contraindications are unnecessary [2].

The suggested contraindications for UKA are based on Kozinn & Scott's 1989 publication which stated that patients who weigh more than 82 kg, were younger than 60 years, undertook heavy labour, had exposed bone in the PFJ or chondrocalcinosis were not ideal candidates for UKA [3]. We wanted to establish whether these potential contraindications should apply to candidates for OUKA. In order to do this, the outcome of patients with these potential contraindications was compared with that of patients without the contraindications in a prospective series of 1000 OUKAs [3]. The outcome was assessed using the Oxford Knee Score, American Knee Society Score, Tegner activity score, revision rate and survival. The clinical outcome of patients with each of the potential contraindications was similar to, or better than, those without each contraindication. Overall, 678 UKA (68%) were performed in patients who had at least one potential contraindication and only 322 (32%) in patients deemed to be ideal for UKA. The 10-year survival was 97% (95% CI 93.4 to 100) for those with potential contraindications and 93.6% (95% CI 87.2 to 100) in the 'ideal' patients. This difference was maintained at 15 years as well. The 15-year survival was 94% (95% CI 88 to 100) for those with potential contraindications and 90% (95% CI 78 to 100) in the 'ideal' patients.

Each of these contraindications, and others, are discussed in detail in this chapter.

Patellofemoral arthritis

Almost all authors have included 'patellofemoral arthritis' in the list of contraindications to unicompartmental arthroplasty and it may strike the reader as strange that we have not yet mentioned it in the discussion of AMOA, because, intuitively, associated patellofemoral joint OA must influence the outcome of UKA.

In anteromedial OA, the patellofemoral compartment very commonly exhibits chondromalacia, fibrillation, and cartilage erosions that sometimes expose bone. These lesions are mainly on the medial longitudinal (or 'odd') and medial facets of the patella and the equivalent surfaces of the femoral trochlea (see Fig. 4.2(g)), but they are also seen astride the median ridge of the patella and in the groove of the trochlea. They are much less common on the lateral facets. Marginal osteophytes are often seen on the preoperative radiographs and even more commonly when the joint is open to inspection.

The presence of any of these lesions has frequently been taken to contraindicate unicompartmental replacement. However, there are some evidence-based arguments for believing that this is unnecessary.

Table 5.1 Patellofemoral state versus postoperative pain (a) at rest and (b) during activity. Each entry in a table gives the number of knees with PFJ state at surgery as defined by the column and the report of pain at last follow-up as defined by the row. Each table is also a graph on which is plotted the linear regression line (shown dashed) that fits the data with minimum squared error. Both lines are nearly horizontal showing that the outcome was independent of the preoperative state.

Patellofemoral state (a) — Pain at rest

Pain at rest	1	2	3	4	5	Total
1	9	21	14	12	3	59
2	3	4	4	4	0	15
3	2	1	0	2	1	6
4	0	2	0	0	0	2
Total	14	28	18	18	4	82

Patellofemoral state (b) — Pain in activity

Pain in activity	1	2	3	4	5	Total
1	11	22	13	10	3	59
2	2	2	4	6	1	15
3	2	2	3	1	0	8
4	0	2	0	0	0	2
Total	15	28	20	17	4	84

Patellofemoral state: 1 = good; 2 = moderate; 3 = poor; 4 = grossly disorganized; 5 = previous patellectomy.

Pain: 1 = none; 2 = mild; 3 = moderate; 4 = severe.

We first reached this opinion in 1986 [4] based on a study of 125 bicompartmental Oxford arthroplasties performed for OA (n = 74) or rheumatoid arthritis (n = 51). In these procedures only the tibiofemoral articular surfaces were replaced; the patella and the trochlea were retained. The state of the patella's articular surface was recorded intra-operatively. At postoperative review (mean follow-up 49 months), no correlation was found between the intraoperative state of the patellofemoral joint and the patients' postoperative complaints of pain (Table 5.1).

Despite the mixture of diagnoses in this study (and its questionable relevance to unicompartmental replacement), at that time it provided the only scientific evidence on which to base our practice. Accordingly, ever since that publication, we have continued to ignore the state of the patellofemoral joint, whether assessed clinically, radiographically or intraoperatively, when deciding between OUKA and TKA. Subsequently, Carr *et al.* [5] found no correlation between the perioperative state of the PFJ and the patients' postoperative complaints of pain at a mean 44 months after surgery in a series of 121 knees treated for anteromedial OA by

OUKA. Despite the degeneration of the PFJ in these patients (and in those of surgeons to whom we have given similar recommendations), patellofemoral problems have rarely been the cause of failure after OUKA [6]. In all the published series of OUKA with 10-year or longer results that we are aware of, including nearly 10,000 patients, there was not one revised for PFJ problems. The 2004 report from the Swedish Knee Arthroplasty Register gave causes for the 50 revisions from a total of 699 OUKAs, only one of which was for PFJ problems [7].

In 28 knees, the state of the PFJ was assessed on radiographs taken 1–2 years after OUKA and was compared with films taken 10+ years later. No significant difference between them was found [8]. (This study was based on anteroposterior and lateral radiographs of the patellofemoral joint because 'skyline' views were not available.)

Beard *et al.* [9] have reported on 100 consecutive OUKA cases for anteromedial OA. In all these cases, the location of preoperative pain (anterior, medial, lateral, generalised) was independently determined and the radiological status of the patellofemoral joint was defined using Altman systems [10]. There was no relationship between the presence of the pre-operative anterior knee pain (AKP) and the state of the PFJ. Also pre-operative AKP settled in every case and did not compromise the outcome. We therefore do not consider AKP to be a contraindication.

In this study [9], arthritis, however severe, seen on the medial side of the PFJ on the skyline view did not compromise the outcome, so we ignore medial PFJ OA. However, although the numbers were small, there was some evidence to suggest that severe lateral PFJ OA does compromise the outcome. Therefore in the rare cases (less than 1% of patients) when there is severe lateral PFJ OA with bone loss, grooving and subluxation, we would now recommend a TKA.

In a further study of 824 knees in 793 patients, the state of the PFJ peri-operatively was correlated with the clinical outcome [11]. There was exposed bone in the trochlea in 15%, on the medial side of the patella in 9%, and on the lateral side in 4%. Exposed bone did not compromise the outcome. Therefore we do not consider exposed bone seen in the PFJ to be a contraindication.

Berend *et al.* [12] correlated the pre-operative state of the PFJ assessed radiographically with the six year survival in 626 OUKA. 61% of the cases had a normal PFJ and a survival of 94%; 39% had an abnormal PFJ with a 98% survival; and 15% had significant PFJ damage and a 97% survival. There was no statistically significant difference in survival between the groups.

Discussion

Although we cannot offer a full explanation for the (apparent) enigma that the pre-operative state of the patellofemoral joint has so little long-term predictive power, there are considerations that make it less inexplicable than at first sight.

First, similar lesions to those seen radiographically and intraoperatively in anteromedial OA are common in the joints of most middle-aged and elderly people and, presumably, must be compatible with adequate function. Owre [13] found flaking and fissuring of some part of the patellar cartilage at necropsy in all but one of 16 subjects aged 60–80 years. Wiles *et al.* [14] recorded that nearly all adult patellofemoral joints showed some pathological changes. The medial border of the medial facet was the most frequent site, and severe degeneration was associated with marginal osteophytes. Outerbridge [15] reported the state of the patellar cartilage during 101 open meniscectomies. He found 'surface fissuring and fragmentation' with increasing frequency at each decade in up to 12 of 15 subjects aged 50–69 years. Emery and Meachim [16] gave a detailed description of the topography of surface degeneration at necropsy. They found fibrillation in almost every knee they examined. In young subjects, degeneration was limited to the articular margins and the medial longitudinal facet of the patella, but in middle-aged subjects fibrillation was seen elsewhere on the patella surface. At these sites it became progressively more common and more severe with increasing age, frequently exposing subchondral bone. The cartilage lesions and marginal osteophytes referred to above were all chance findings at necropsy or at arthrotomy performed for reasons not associated with the patellofemoral joint. Therefore the lesions can be assumed to be generally compatible with adequate patellofemoral function. They are likely to be at least as common in the joints of candidates for unicompartmental replacement as they are in the rest of the middle-aged and elderly population, and to have as little significance.

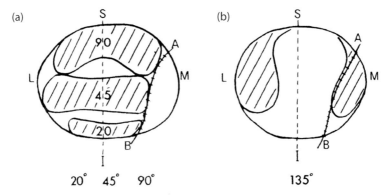

Figure 5.1 Diagrammatic representation of contact areas on the patella in varying degrees of flexion. (Reproduced with permission and copyright © of the British Editorial Society of Bone and Joint Surgery [Goodfellow JW, Hungerford DS, Zindel M. Patellofemoral joint mechanics and pathology. 1. Functional anatomy of the patellofemoral joint. *J Bone Joint Surg [Br]* 1976; **58-B**: 287–90].)

Secondly, lesions on the medial margin of the patella may have no secondary effect on the rest of the knee joint. There are two unusual features of the medial longitudinal, or 'odd', facet. It is the *only* part of the patella's surface that articulates with the medial femoral condyle in full flexion (Fig. 5.1(b)) [17]. In anteromedial OA, the inferior surface of that condyle is devoid of cartilage, and so it is almost inevitable that the odd facet will be secondarily damaged. However, the odd facet *only* articulates with the femoral condyle, and never with the medial trochlear facet

(Fig. 5.1(a)); therefore a lesion on the odd facet has no potential to cause secondary damage to the rest of the patellofemoral joint. After OUKA, the odd facet articulates in full flexion only on the metal prosthetic condyle (Figs. 3.17(c) & 3.18). Therefore its circumstances are similar to those of the retained patella after TKA.

Thirdly, preoperative genu varum tends to overload the medial patellofemoral facets, the most commonly damaged surfaces [18]. Also, osteophytes at the anterior margin of the erosion on the medial femoral condyle can impinge on the medial facet of the patella in flexion. After OUKA, the intra-articular varus deformity is corrected, tending to unload the medial facet, and the osteophytes are excised during the operation.

It is striking that, after OUKA, problems with the PFJ are very rare [11] whereas after fixed bearing UKA they are relatively common, particularly in the second decade. For example, Argenson et al. [19] in a series of 160 Miller-Galante UKA with 20 year survival of 74% found that PFJ progression was such an issue in the second decade that they concluded PFJ cartilage loss should be a contraindication to UKA.

In fixed bearing UKA, long term problems with the PFJ may be the result of deteriorating kinematics or impingement. With fixed bearing UKA, the femur tends to wear a 'divot' in the polyethylene which affects the kinematics [20] (see Chapter 2, Fig. 2.19). Argenson et al. [21] studied the gait of 17 subjects after Miller-Galante medial arthroplasty at 5 – 10 years and demonstrated that about one third of the knees functioned similar to PCL-retaining TKA, as if the ACL was absent. This would dramatically increase the PFJ contact forces [18].

In fixed bearing UKA, the femoral component must be mounted on the femur so that its anterior margin is flush with the retained cartilage of the trochlear facet. If this is not achieved, the patella has to negotiate a ridge as it moves distally on the femur. Hernigou and Deschamps [22] demonstrated that, if such a femoral component is implanted too far anteriorly, the patella can sustain severe damage from impingement in flexion. The technical error may only be revealed by skyline radiographs taken in 90° flexion (Fig. 5.2) and may have been overlooked in the past, with late failure from patellofemoral pain being wrongly attributed to spontaneous progression of degeneration in the patellofemoral joint. Impingement may explain the high incidence of patellofemoral deterioration reported by Berger et al. [23]. Of 49 knees treated by UKA (Miller–Galante) and followed for 10 – 13 years, seven (14%) had radiographic evidence of progressive medial facet patellofemoral joint-space loss. Two of these knees had already been revised (at 7 and 10 years postoperatively) for anterior knee pain attributed to the patellofemoral joint. Of the remaining five, four (one lateral arthroplasty) demonstrated 'severe patellofemoral joint-space loss secondary to impingement with the femoral component'. These deteriorations occurred despite use of the strict preoperative selection criteria of Kozinn and Scott [2] which include '… only mild radiographic signs of deterioration of the patellofemoral joint' (Outerbridge grades 1 and 2) and absence of preoperative patellofemoral symptoms.

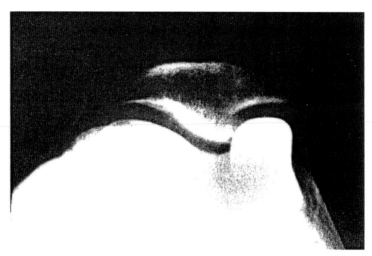

Figure 5.2 Radiograph, taken 15 years after medial arthroplasty with a polyradial fixed-bearing implant, demonstrating severe erosive changes due to impingement of the femoral component on the patella. (Reprinted with permission from The Journal of Bone and Joint Surgery, Inc [Hernigou P, Deschamps G. Patellar Impingement Following Unicompartmental Arthroplasty. J Bone Joint Surg [Am] 2002; **84-A**: 1132–7].)

Unlike polyradial components, the spherical femoral component of the OUKA does not reach the medial trochlear facet of the femur (see Chapter 3, Fig. 3.18 and Appendix, Fig. A10). Therefore, accurate alignment of its surface with that of the articular cartilage is not required as its anterior edge is always buried a few millimetres below the patellofemoral joint line. Furthermore, with the mobile UKA, the kinematics of the knee continues to be normal in the long term so the mechanics of the PFJ will remain normal [24].

Hernigou and Deschamps [22] also observed progressive OA of the patella in the second postoperative decade, quite separately from impingement. Joint-space narrowing was most commonly seen in the lateral patellofemoral compartment (Fig. 5.3). It was associated with significant symptoms, and was predicted by lack of joint congruency on the preoperative skyline radiographs. However, the symptoms from this type of degeneration were less severe than those arising from impingement and therefore no revision operation had been performed.

Conclusion

The studies referred to above support the conclusion that the presence of peripheral osteophytes, chondromalacia, fibrillation, and even full-thickness cartilage loss in the patellofemoral compartment need not significantly prejudice the function of the knees of older people. The presence of such lesions in the joints of candidates for UKA is to be expected, and the rarity of revision of OUKA from patellofemoral symptoms suggests that they can be ignored.

We therefore continue to recommend that, in a patient with AMOA, when deciding whether to do an OUKA, the state of the PFJ should be ignored. In particular anterior knee pain, full thickness cartilage loss, or PFJ arthritis seen on skyline radiographs should be ignored. However, we now usually exclude knees in which the lateral side of the patellofemoral joint exhibits bone loss with eburnation and longitudinal grooving, although very few such cases (<1%) have been encountered and we do not have evidence to support this practice.

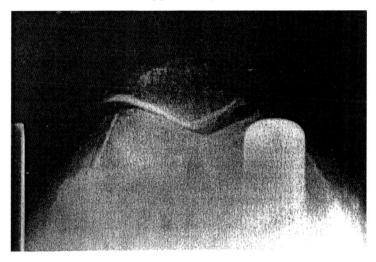

Figure 5.3 Radiograph, taken 16 years postoperatively, demonstrating osteoarthritis of the lateral part of the patellofemoral joint. Reprinted with permission from The Journal of Bone and Joint Surgery, Inc [Hernigou P, Deschamps G. Patellar Impingement Following Unicompartmental Arthroplasty. *J Bone Joint Surg [Am]* 2002; **84-A**: 1132–7].

Lateral side

Degenerative lateral meniscus

The presence of degenerative tears of the lateral meniscus has been regarded as a contraindication to UKA by some authors [25]. Arthroscopy has not been used as a routine preoperative investigation in any published series of OUKA and, as the state of the meniscus cannot be assessed adequately through the small incision now employed, we do not have data on its predictive significance. Nevertheless, as mentioned above, the most common cause for revision of OUKA (Phase 2) was arthritis of the lateral compartment, and it is possible that a more stringent approach than we have adopted would diminish the failure rate from that cause. However, necropsy studies have shown that degenerative lesions are common in both menisci in middle-aged and older people, and so they must usually be compatible with adequate function of the joint [26]. Ritter *et al.* [25] found the lateral meniscus to be 'degenerative or absent' in 69% of varus arthritic knees treated by joint replacement. Therefore, paying attention to the state of the lateral meniscus would deny the advantages of UKA to very many patients in the hope of diminishing the 1.7% 10-year cumulative revision rate (CRR) from lateral compartment failure.

Symptomatic lateral meniscal tears do rarely occur after OUKA and can be treated satisfactorily by arthroscopic meniscectomy. We do not know if these are related to the state of the lateral meniscus at the time of surgery.

Articular surface damage

Damage to the articular surface of the lateral compartment is considered to be a contraindication to UKA. We recommend that the lateral side should be assessed with a valgus stress radiograph. If this shows full thickness cartilage then we will ignore any damage to the lateral side seen at operation. The only exception to this, which is very rare, is that if a full-thickness defect in the central weight-bearing cartilage is seen, we would treat this as a contraindication (although we have no evidence to support this practice).

In about 30% of cases, there is articular cartilage damage seen on the medial side of the lateral femoral condyle [27]. This is often a circumscribed area of cartilage erosion, which can be up to 1 cm wide and 3 cm long, with eburnated bone exposed in its floor (Fig 5.4). This erosion is a consequence of the varus alignment causing the medial side of lateral femoral condyle to impinge on the tibial eminence. (Fig. 5.5(a)). Following surgery, when the varus is corrected, impingement no longer occurs (Fig. 5.5(b)). We have found that there is no difference in outcome between patients with and without articular cartilage damage on the medial side of the lateral condyle; we do not , therefore, consider it to be a contraindication to OUKA.

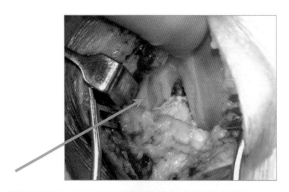

Figure 5.4 Intra-operative picture of right knee with patella retracted laterally showing the full thickness ulcer on the medial side of the lateral femoral condyle.

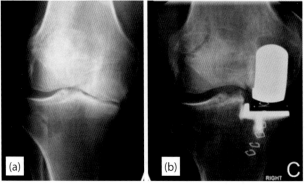

Figure 5.5 (a) Pre-op radiographs showing tibial spine impinging on the lateral condyle. (b) Post-op radiograph showing no impingement.

Age

Old age has been proposed as a relative contraindication [28]. However, in a study based on NJR data [29], we found that elderly patients had particularly good results with UKA. With increasing age, not only did the implant survival increase but also outcome scores and satisfaction improved. Furthermore, the lower morbidity and mortality and quicker recovery of UKA recommend it in the elderly, particularly the unfit elderly. It is therefore surprising that surgeons tend not to do UKA in the elderly: UKA compromises nearly 20% of knee replacements performed in patients in their 50s, but only 5% in octogenarians. This may be because surgeons believe that TKA is the best solution in the elderly, as it is highly unlikely that a revision will be required. However, the same applies to UKA in the elderly, because of the high UKA survival rates and limited life expectancy in this group. We therefore believe that all elderly patients with AMOA who need knee replacement should be treated with a UKA. Furthermore, in the elderly, particularly the unfit elderly, if the indications are borderline we would still do a UKA.

Youth is a recognised contraindication for fixed-bearing prostheses, some of which have proved susceptible to late failure from polyethylene wear, particularly in young active patients [30]. The linear wear rate of polyethylene in congruent mobile bearings is an order of magnitude lower than in fixed bearings [31, 32], and failure from wear-through of an Oxford implant has rarely been reported. So, in theory, youth need not be a contraindication for the OUKA.

Youth relative to the average age for joint replacement has been shown in many studies, including the Swedish Knee Arthroplasty Register and the NJR, to increase the risk for revision for both UKA and TKA [7]. Therefore, it is not a good criterion for deciding between the two treatments. If, because of relative youth, the patient is likely to outlive the prosthesis, UKA may still be preferred because it is easier to revise than TKA.

The detailed analysis in the study based on NJR data found that, with decreasing age, not only did the survival rate decrease markedly but also the outcome scores worsened [29]. However, in two large prospective series of the OUKA, this effect was not seen. In a combined study based on series from Goodfellow [33] and Svard [34], there were 564 knees of which 52 were less than 60 years of age at the time of surgery [35]. The survival rates of those below and above 60 were not significantly different (91%, CI 12.4 and 96%, CI 3.2 respectively), whereas the clinical scores were significantly better in those less than 60 (HSS 94% CI 3 compared to 86% CI 2). In a series of 1000 Phase 3 knees [3], of which 245 were aged less than 60, there was no significant difference between the survival rates (10-year survival <60 97.3% [CI 91 to 100%]; >60 95.1% [CI 91 to 99%], p=0.63) and the functional outcome was significantly better in those less than 60 (AKSS Function 87.8 [SD 20.2]) to those older than 60 (AKSS Function 82.1 [SD 18.8]). In contrast, Kuipers et al.[36] found that young age (<60) had a 2.2-fold increased risk of early revision with the same prosthesis. In order to determine the outcome in patients under 50 at the time of surgery, data from seven series were combined [37]. In 107 patients, with mean age 47, the seven year survival was 98% when there were 24 patients at risk.

It is interesting that in some series reported by experienced surgeons, very good results are achieved in younger patients, whereas in the national registries the results are poor in this group. One reason for this may be that some surgeons, who are relatively inexperienced with UKA, mainly use UKA in young patients with early arthritis who may not have bone-on-bone as they know that these patients tend not to do well with TKA. However these patients often do not do well with UKA [38, 39]. In contrast, we try to use the OUKA only if there is osteoarthritis with bone-on-bone OA even in young patients. In this condition the results tend to be good.

We therefore believe that age need not be a factor in choosing between OUKA and TKA. If the indications for OUKA are fulfilled, with bone-on-bone arthritis, we prefer it at all ages.

Activity level

In a series of 1000 medial OUKA followed up to 15 years, we assessed the postoperative activity level using the Tegner Score [3]. Patients with higher levels of activity, not surprisingly, had higher OKS [40]. However, contrary to accepted wisdom, there was a significant reduction in revision rate associated with increased activity (Fig. 5.6). In general, impact activity is not recommended after joint replacement. This level of activity would be 5 or more on the Tegner scale (5 being 'jogging on uneven ground' or 'heavy labour'). We found that the 115 patients with a Tegner score of five or more had an OKS of 45 and 12-year survival of 97.3%, whereas the 885 with Tegner 4 or less had OKS of 39.9 and 12-year survival of 94.0%. It is not clear why the survival improves with increased activity. It may be that the bone and cartilage are stronger in more active patients so failures due to loosening or disease progression are less likely to occur. Also with the mobile bearing, failure due to wear should not occur. Whatever the reason it is clear that, after OUKA, activity should be encouraged not discouraged. Furthermore, provided the patients have significant symptoms, high levels of activity or expectations of achieving high levels of activity should not be considered to be a contraindication to OUKA.

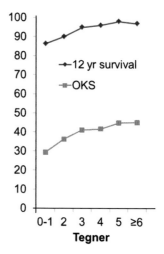

Figure 5.6 The effect of activity level (as scored by maximum postoperative Tegner Score) on the 12-year survival rate and OKS.

Weight

Although obesity has often been considered to be a contraindication to fixed bearing UKA, we have never considered it to be a contraindication for OUKA. Studies of retrieved meniscal bearings have revealed no association between patient weight and linear wear rate [41].

We studied the effect of BMI on outcome in a two centre series of 2467 patients followed up to 12 years. It was found that there was no significant difference in survival with patients of different BMI [41]. In fact in the 80 super-obese patients with BMI >45, there were no failures. The final OKS did decrease with increasing BMI. However, because the preoperative OKS decreased with increasing BMI, the improvement in OKS actually increased with increasing BMI. We therefore do not consider high BMI to be a contraindication. Indeed, in patients with high BMI, we prefer to implant the OUKA rather than a TKA because the surgery is much simpler. The instrumentation works from the front and the extensor mechanism only needs to be subluxed laterally and not everted or dislocated as in TKA.

Chondrocalcinosis

Because chondrocalcinosis can be taken as evidence of 'inflammatory arthritis', preoperative radiographic calcification in the menisci and the articular cartilage, or calcified deposits seen at arthrotomy, have been deemed to be contraindications to unicompartmental replacement [42]. Two studies have looked at the influence of chondrocalcinosis on the outcome of OUKA. In the first study [43] of 96 patients with Phase 1 or Phase 2 OUKA there were 20 knees with histologically proven chondrocalcinosis (HCCK). There was no difference in clinical outcome or 10-year survival between those with or without chondrocalcinosis. In the second study [44] using Phase 3 OUKA, 88 patients with radiographically diagnosed chondrocalcinosis (RCCK) and 67 with histological chondrocalcinosis were matched to control patients without chondrocalcinosis. RCCK was not associated with any difference in outcome score or survival, whereas HCCK was associated with significantly greater improvement in OKS but a lower survival. It is difficult to know how to interpret the data relating to HCCK and further study is needed. However, when assessing patients for OUKA, the diagnosis of chondrocalcinosis is made radiographically, based on the appearance of calcification seen in the menisci or articular cartilage. As RCCK is not associated with a worse outcome we do not consider the presence of chondrocalcinosis to be a contraindication.

What proportion of patients with osteoarthritic knees needing surgery is suitable for OUKA?

The proportion of osteoarthritic knees deemed suitable for medial unicompartmental arthroplasty depends on the selection criteria. Early in our experience, using the indications given above, we found that about a quarter of knees with OA severe enough to need joint replacement were suitable for OUKA. Now we find that about half of the knees are suitable, presumably because patients are presenting with less severe arthritis. The criteria are evidence-based in that they have been employed with little variation since the 1980s and are attested by a number of long term survival studies of several independent cohorts [34]. In addition we have reviewed 1000 cases with 15 year follow up and found that two thirds have a Kozinn and Scott [2] contraindication yet there is no difference in outcome or survival between those with and without the contraindications. This confirms that the Kozinn and Scott contraindications do not apply to the OUKA.

In contrast, Stern et al. [45] applied the often quoted criteria of Kozinn and Scott [2] to knees with OA severe enough to warrant joint replacement and found only 6% suitable for UKA.

Ritter et al. [25] examined retrospectively the preoperative and intraoperative records of 4021 osteoarthritic varus knees treated by TKA to determine how many of them would have been 'ideal candidates' for UKA. They first applied anatomical criteria, i.e. '… *a normal ACL, a normal lateral meniscus, no more than mild osteophytes in the patellofemoral and/or lateral compartment, no more than grade 2 chondromalacia in the patellofemoral compartment and no more than grade 1 chondromalacia in the lateral compartment*'. Only 6% met these criteria. They then applied clinical criteria attributed to Kozinn and Scott [2], i.e. patients should be more than 60 years old and weigh less than 82 kg, the flexion contracture should be less than 5°, and varus deformity less than 10°. This reduced the number to 2% of the original cohort.

If, in fact, UKA were useful in as few patients as these studies suggest, few surgeons would ever see enough suitable patients to become adept in its use. However, the detailed data provided by Ritter et al. [25] reveal that the criteria that they applied retrospectively and those that we have used prospectively are so dissimilar that the 15-fold difference between our practice and their prediction is readily explained.

Strikingly, they found that 45% of their cohort of knees had a normal ACL and an undefined percentage would have had an ACL that was functionally normal although slightly damaged; both of which are appropriate for an OUKA. However, this large group was diminished to 6.1% because of the presence of lateral compartment chondromalacia (74%), a degenerative lateral meniscus (69%), patellofemoral chondromalacia (55%), lateral compartment osteophytes (33%), or patellofemoral osteophytes (30%), all of which can occur in middle-aged people with no knee complaints and none of which has played a part in our selection process. The clinical criteria (overweight (53%), more than 5° flexion deformity (32%), age (12%)) that further reduced the number of suitable knees to 2.2% have also all been ignored in our practice.

The contraindications criticised above were elaborated by surgeons whose experience was with fixed-bearing prostheses. Their criteria have been widely accepted and few knees outside these narrow limits may have been treated by UKA. Consequently, there is little evidence other than ours to contradict them. However, our experience has been with a meniscal-bearing prosthesis implanted (since 1987) by a fully instrumented method. The proportion of suitable cases may not be the same for fixed-bearing devices that are susceptible to medium-term polyethylene wear and patella problems and, until recently, have been implanted with little instrumental assistance.

Summary

Patient selection is simple when it is considered in the light of positive indications for OUKA rather than its contraindications. If a patient has only anteromedial OA and symptoms severe enough to justify the surgery and associated risks, we would do an OUKA and there are no contraindications. AMOA is clearly defined and to make this diagnosis a patient should be shown to have medial osteoarthritis with bone-on-bone, a functionally intact ACL and MCL and full thickness cartilage laterally.

For completeness, the following list brings together all the contraindications, most of which have already been discussed or implied.

General

All the general contraindications recognised in the practice of joint replacement surgery apply to unicompartmental replacement and are not rehearsed exhaustively here. Among them, OUKA (like TKA) is likely to fail in limbs with sensory and/or motor neurological impairment.

The use of a tourniquet during the operation, almost a necessity for OUKA (Phase 3) performed through a small incision, is dangerous in limbs with vascular insufficiency. It may also be dangerous to apply tourniquets to both lower limbs, and for this reason we seldom perform bilateral OUKA in one session, preferring to stage the procedures with an interval of not less than 6 weeks.

Particular

Unicompartmental arthroplasty is contraindicated in the inflammatory forms of arthritis because they are diseases of the synovium and therefore cannot be limited to one compartment.

We have already noted the anatomical contraindications listed below:

➤ absent or severely damaged ACL (or PCL or MCL)

➤ failure to demonstrate eburnated bone-on-bone contact in the medial compartment

➤ intra-articular varus not fully correctable

➤ mediolateral subluxation, not corrected on valgus-stressed films

➤ flexion deformity >15°, which is suggestive of ACL deficiency

➤ flexion range <100° (under anaesthesia)

➤ erosion of central cartilage in the lateral compartment

➤ bone loss with eburnation and grooving in the lateral part of the patello-femoral joint

➤ previous valgus tibial osteotomy (see Chapter 8).

References

1. Pandit H, Jenkins C, Gill HS, Barker K, Dodd CA, Murray DW. Minimally invasive Oxford phase 3 unicompartmental knee replacement: results of 1000 cases. *J Bone Joint Surg Br* 2011; **93**(2): 198-204.

2. Pandit H, Jenkins C, Gill HS, Smith G, Price AJ, Dodd CA, Murray DW. Unnecessary contraindications for mobile-bearing unicompartmental knee replacement. *J Bone Joint Surg Br* 2011; **93**(5): 622-8.

3. Kozinn SC, Scott R. Unicondylar knee arthroplasty. *J Bone Joint Surg Am* 1989; **71**(1): 145-50.

4. Goodfellow JW, O'Connor J. Clinical results of the Oxford knee. Surface arthroplasty of the tibiofemoral joint with a meniscal bearing prosthesis. *Clin Orthop Relat Res* 1986; (**205**): 21-42.

5. Carr A, Keyes G, Miller R, O'Connor J, Goodfellow J. Medial unicompartmental arthroplasty. A survival study of the Oxford meniscal knee. *Clin Orthop Relat Res* 1993; (**295**): 205-13.

6. Price AJ, Svard U. A second decade lifetable survival analysis of the Oxford unicompartmental knee arthroplasty. *Clin Orthop Relat Res* 2011; 469(1): 174-9.

7. Lidgren L, Knutson K, Robertsson O. Swedish Knee Arthroplasty Register: Annual Report 2004. Lund, 2004.

8. Weale AE, Murray DW, Crawford R, Psychoyios V, Bonomo A, Howell G, O'Connor J, Goodfellow JW. Does arthritis progress in the retained compartments after 'Oxford' medial unicompartmental arthroplasty? A clinical and radiological study with a minimum ten-year follow-up. *J Bone Joint Surg Br* 1999; **81**(5): 783-9.

9. Beard DJ, Pandit H, Ostlere S, Jenkins C, Dodd CA, Murray DW. Pre-operative clinical and radiological assessment of the patellofemoral joint in unicompartmental knee replacement and its influence on outcome. *J Bone Joint Surg Br* 2007; **89**(12): 1602-7.

10. Altman RD, Fries JF, Bloch DA, Carstens J, Cooke TD, Genant H, Gofton P, Groth H, McShane DJ, Murphy WA, Sharp JT, Spitz P, Williams C A, Wolfe F. Radiographic assessment of progression in osteoarthritis. *Arthritis Rheum* 1987; **30**(11): 1214-25.

11. Beard DJ, Pandit H, Gill HS, Hollinghurst D, Dodd CA, Murray DW. The influence of the presence and severity of pre-existing patellofemoral degenerative changes on the outcome of the Oxford medial unicompartmental knee replacement. *J Bone Joint Surg Br* 2007; **89**(12): 1597-601.

12. Berend KR, Lombardi AV, Morris MJ, Hurst JM. Does preoperative patellofemoral joint state affect medial unicompartmental arthoplasty survival? (P204). AAOS. San Diego, USA; 2011.

13. Owre A. Chondromalacia patellae. *Acta Chirurg Scand* 1936; **Supple 41**.

14. Wiles P, Andrews PS, Devas MB. Chondromalacia of the patella. *J Bone Joint Surg Br* 1956; **38-B**(1): 95-113.

15. Outerbridge RE. The etiology of chondromalacia patellae. *J Bone Joint Surg Br* 1961; **43-B**: 752-7.

16. Emery IH, Meachim G. Surface morphology and topography of patello-femoral cartilage fibrillation in Liverpool necropsies. *J Anat* 1973; **116**(Pt 1): 103-20.

17. Goodfellow J, Hungerford DS, Zindel M. Patello-femoral joint mechanics and pathology. 1. Functional anatomy of the patello-femoral joint. *J Bone Joint Surg Br* 1976; **58**(3): 287-90.

18. Miller RK, Goodfellow JW, Murray DW, O'Connor JJ. *In vitro* measurement of patellofemoral force after three types of knee replacement. *J Bone Joint Surg Br* 1998; **80**(5): 900-6.

19. Argenson JN, Blanc G, Aubaniac JM, Parratte S. Modern unicompartmental knee arthroplasty with cement: a concise follow-up, at a mean of twenty years, of a previous report. *J Bone Joint Surg Am* 2013; **95**(10): 905-9.

20. Ashraf T, Newman JH, Desai VV, Beard D, Nevelos JE. Polyethylene wear in a non-congruous unicompartmental knee replacement: a retrieval analysis. *Knee* 2004; **11**(3): 177-81.

21. Argenson JN, Komistek RD, Aubaniac JM, Dennis DA, Northcut EJ, Anderson DT, Agostini S. *In vivo* determination of knee kinematics for subjects implanted with a unicompartmental arthroplasty. *J Arthroplasty* 2002; **17**(8): 1049-54.

22. Hernigou P, Deschamps G. Patellar impingement following unicompartmental arthroplasty. *J Bone Joint Surg Am* 2002; **84-A**(7): 1132-7.

23. Berger RA, Meneghini RM, Jacobs JJ, Sheinkop MB, Della Valle CJ, Rosenberg AG, Galante JO. Results of unicompartmental knee arthroplasty at a minimum of ten years of follow-up. *J Bone Joint Surg Am* 2005; **87**(5): 999-1006.

24. Price AJ, Rees JL, Beard DJ, Gill RH, Dodd CA, Murray DM. Sagittal plane kinematics of a mobile-bearing unicompartmental knee arthroplasty at 10 years: a comparative *in vivo* fluoroscopic analysis. *J Arthroplasty* 2004; **19**(5): 590-7.

25. Ritter MA, Faris PM, Thong AE, Davis KE, Meding JB, Berend ME. Intra-operative findings in varus osteoarthritis of the knee. An analysis of pre-operative alignment in potential candidates for unicompartmental arthroplasty. *J Bone Joint Surg Br* 2004; **86**(1): 43-7.

26. Noble J, Hamblen DL. The pathology of the degenerate meniscus lesion. *J Bone Joint Surg Br* 1975; **57**(2): 180-6.

27. Kendrick BJ, Rout R, Bottomley NJ, Pandit H, Gill HS, Price AJ, Dodd CA, Murray DW. The implications of damage to the lateral femoral condyle on medial unicompartmental knee replacement. *J Bone Joint Surg Br* 2010; **92**(3): 374-9.

28. Sisto DJ, Blazina ME, Heskiaoff D, Hirsh LC. Unicompartment arthroplasty for osteoarthrosis of the knee. *Clin Orthop Relat Res* 1993; (**286**): 149-53.

29. Liddle AD, Judge A, Pandit H, Murray DW. Determinants of revision and functional outcome following unicompartmental knee replacement. *Osteoarthritis and Cartilage*. 2014 Sep; **9**(22): 1241-1250

30. Witvoet J, Peyrache MD, Nizard R. [Single-compartment «Lotus» type knee prosthesis in the treatment of lateralized gonarthrosis: results in 135 cases with a mean follow-up of 4.6 years]. *Rev Chir Orthop Reparatrice Appar Mot* 1993; **79**(7): 565-76.

31. Argenson JN, O'Connor JJ. Polyethylene wear in meniscal knee replacement. A one to nine-year retrieval analysis of the Oxford knee. *J Bone Joint Surg Br* 1992; **74**(2): 228-32.

32. Psychoyios V, Crawford RW, O'Connor JJ, Murray DW. Wear of congruent meniscal bearings in unicompartmental knee arthroplasty: a retrieval study of 16 specimens. *J Bone Joint Surg Br* 1998; **80**(6): 976-82.

33. Murray DW, Goodfellow JW, O'Connor JJ. The Oxford medial unicompartmental arthroplasty: a ten-year survival study. *J Bone Joint Surg Br* 1998; **80**(6): 983-9.

34. Svard UC, Price AJ. Oxford medial unicompartmental knee arthroplasty. A survival analysis of an independent series. *J Bone Joint Surg Br* 2001; **83**(2): 191-4.

35. Price AJ, Dodd CA, Svard UG, Murray DW. Oxford medial unicompartmental knee arthroplasty in patients younger and older than 60 years of age. *J Bone Joint Surg Br* 2005; **87**(11): 1488-92.

36. Kuipers BM, Kollen BJ, Bots PC, Burger BJ, van Raay JJ, Tulp NJ, Verheyen CC. Factors associated with reduced early survival in the Oxford phase III medial unicompartment knee replacement. *Knee* 2010; **17**(1): 48-52.

37. Price A J, Longino D, Svard U, Kim KT, Weber P, Fiddian N, Shakespeare D, Keys G, Beard D, Pandit H, Dodd CAF, Murray DW. Seven year survival analysis of mobile bearing UKA in patients 50 years of age or less. *J Bone Joint Surg [Br]* Proceedings 2010; 92-B (Supp III): 412-12.

38. Pandit H, Gulati A, Jenkins C, Barker K, Price AJ, Dodd CA, Murray DW. Unicompartmental knee replacement for patients with partial thickness cartilage loss in the affected compartment. *Knee* 2011; **18**(3): 168-71.

39. Niinimaki TT, Murray DW, Partanen J, Pajala A, Leppilahti JI. Unicompartmental knee arthroplasties implanted for osteoarthritis with partial loss of joint space have high re-operation rates. *Knee* 2011; **18**(6): 432-5.

40. Ali A, Pandit H, Liddle AD, Jenkins C, Mellon SJ, Dodd CA, Murray DW. Does activity affect the outcome of the Oxford unicompartmental knee replacement? British Association for Surgery of the Knee Annual Meeting. Telford; 2015.

41. Murray DW, Pandit H, Weston-Simons JS, Jenkins C, Gill HS, Lombardi AV, Dodd CA, Berend KR. Does body mass index affect the outcome of unicompartmental knee replacement? *Knee* 2013; **20**(6): 461-5.

42. Kozinn SC, Marx C, Scott RD. Unicompartmental knee arthroplasty. A 4.5-6-year follow-up study with a metal-backed tibial component. *J Arthroplasty* 1989; **4 Suppl**: S1-10.

43. Woods D, Wallace D, Woods C, McLardy-Smith P, Carr AJ, Murray DW, Martin J, Gunther T. Chondrocalcinosis and medial unicompartmental knee arthroplasty. *Knee* 1995; **2**: 117-19.

44. Kumar V, Pandit HG, Liddle AD, Borror W, Jenkins C, Mellon SJ, Hamilton TW, Athanasou N, Dodd CA, Murray DW. Comparison of outcomes after UKA in patients with and without chondrocalcinosis: a matched cohort study. *Knee Surg Sports Traumatol Arthrosc* 2015.

45. Stern SH, Becker MW, Insall JN. Unicondylar knee arthroplasty. An evaluation of selection criteria. *Clin Orthop Relat Res* 1993; **(286)**: 143-8.

6

Principles of the Oxford Operation

This chapter is intended to be read in parallel with the description of the operative technique (Chapter 7). That chapter is concerned with 'how' to do the operation; this chapter provides the rationale—'why' the various steps of the procedure are necessary. It may help also to watch the videos of the operation which can be found at www.oxfordpartialknee.com.

Although the surgeon operates exclusively on the bones, carefully avoiding any interference with the ligaments, the operation is essentially about 'soft tissue balance'. The aim is to implant the prosthetic surfaces so that the ligaments are at their resting tensions throughout the range of passive movement. This should restore both normal alignment, normal mobility and normal stability.

In what follows, we will often refer to the 'gap' between the medial femoral and tibial condyles, meaning the space between them created by distraction of their surfaces. With the muscles relaxed, the width of this gap can be used as a measure of the lengths of the ligaments spanning it.

The ligaments

The normal intact knee

In full extension, most of the fibres of the ligaments of the normal knee and the posterior capsule are just tight (i.e. at their resting unstretched lengths), and neither the medial nor the lateral joint surfaces can be separated without applying force to stretch the ligaments. With the knee flexed (beyond about 20°) all the fibres of the posterior capsule and the LCL slacken, and distraction of the articular surfaces produces a gap in either compartment. These 'physiological' gaps are limited by the compliance of the other three ligaments that span the joint (the MCL and the cruciates), some of whose fibres maintain their resting tension and remain isometric throughout the range of passive flexion (see Chapter 3 and Appendix).

The effect of increasing flexion on the width of these gaps is different in the two compartments.

In the **lateral compartment,** the gap produced by distraction increases with increasing flexion to about 7 mm at 90° (mean 6.7 ± 1.9 mm) (Fig. 6.1(b)) [1].

In the **medial compartment,** the width of the gap does not alter significantly throughout the range of passive flexion, measuring about 2 mm at 90° (mean 2.1 mm ±1.1 mm) (Fig. 6.1(c)).

Since the LCL and the posterior capsule are demonstrably slack in the flexed knee, the constant width of the medial gap at all angles of flexion (except full extension) implies that the MCL and the cruciates exert a net isometric effect on that compartment throughout that range of movement. After medial unicompartmental replacement, both the stability of the knee and the entrapment of the free bearing depend upon reproducing this isometric mechanism. (The difference between the compliance of the two compartments in flexion explains why bearing dislocation is a problem laterally.)

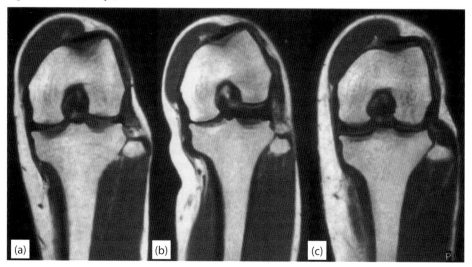

(a)   (b)   (c)

Figure 6.1 Representative MR scans of the left knee in (a) a neutral position, (b) under passive varus stress, and (c) under passive valgus stress. (Reproduced with permission and copyright © of the British Editorial Society of Bone and Joint Surgery [Tokuhara Y, Kadoya Y, Nakagawa S, Kobayashi S and Takaoka K. The flexion gap in normal knees. An MRI study. *J Bone Joint Surg [Br]* 2004; **86-B**: 1133–6].)

The knee with anteromedial osteoarthritis

In anteromedial OA, the MCL and the cruciate ligaments are intact and have the same mechanical effects as in the normal joint. However, the posterior capsule tends to be shortened and there is an associated fixed flexion deformity. The effect of this is to close down the medial compartment gap *before full extension is reached* (Figs. 6.2(a) and 6.2(b)). For this reason, we assess the gap with the knee flexed at 20° to ensure that the posterior capsule is slack (Fig. 6.2(c)). (In anteromedial OA with an intact ACL, the flexion deformity tends to be less than 15°, so 20° flexion should always achieve this.)

In all positions of flexion greater than 20°, the medial condyles can be distracted the same distance as in the normal knee because the gap is limited by the normal MCL and cruciates. Therefore, distraction in flexion above 20° (Fig. 6.2(c)) restores normal alignment of the leg (Fig. 6.2(d)). The medial gap appears wider than normal only because cartilage and bone have been lost from the joint surfaces.

Balancing the ligaments in TKA and OUKA

In TKA, the term 'ligament balancing' usually implies elongation of the MCL by medial release to match the length of the LCL so that, at 90° flexion, the medial and lateral gaps are equal (the flexion gap is quadrilateral, Fig. 4.14(e)). As Figures 1.10 and 6.1(b) demonstrate, this is not the physiological state.

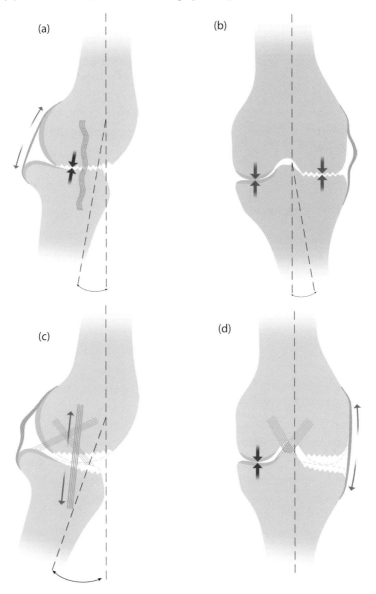

Figure 6.2 (a) With the knee extended, as far as possible, the shortened posterior capsule closes down the medial gap before full extension is reached, causing a flexion deformity, and (b) a varus deformity that is not correctable although the MCL is slack (c). At 20° flexion, however, the posterior capsule is slack and (d) an applied valgus force can distract the damaged medial articular surfaces. Because the MCL is of normal length, this corrects the varus deformity.

In OUKA, medial release should never be undertaken. The MCL is of normal length in anteromedial OA; mobility and stability of the joint, alignment of the leg, and entrapment of the bearing all depend upon its integrity. *Balancing the ligaments means adjusting the position of the femoral component relative to the femur (by removing bone) so that the medial distraction gap is the same in flexion and extension.*

In other words the 'flexion gap' and 'extension gap' should be equal. As explained above, the extension gap is measured in 20° flexion because the posterior capsule is slack. The flexion gap is measured at 90° to this, at 110° knee flexion. The instrumentation is designed to adjust the extension gap without changing the flexion gap. The flexion gap is established first, then the extension gap is adjusted to match it by milling bone from the inferior femoral condyle.

Because the lateral collateral ligament plays no part in the balancing of ligaments in OUKA, it is not represented on any of the explanatory diagrams.

The joint level

The prosthetic joint level

The prosthetic joint level is shown in the construct in Figure 6.3. It is at the interface between the femoral component and the polyethylene bearing, the level at which flexion–extension occurs. The operation aims to remove enough bone from the femoral and tibial condyles to create a flexion gap that the constructed implant will just fill. The thickness of the posterior facet of the femoral component varies with its radius from 5.50 mm (extra small) to 7.45 mm (extra large). The thickness of the tibial component is 3 mm which is constant throughout the range of sizes. The thinnest bearing usually considered safe to use (3 mm) has 3.5 mm of polyethelene at its thinnest point. We do however recommend a 4 mm bearing for all but small and extra small femoral components.

In this respect, the thickness of bone removed from the tibia is not critical. If more is removed than the minimum required, the widths of the flexion and extension gaps are increased equally, and their 'balance' does not alter. A thicker bearing will be needed to restore stability, but this will affect neither the joint level nor, therefore, the kinematics of the replaced compartment (Fig. 6.3(c)).

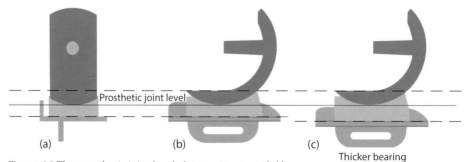

(a)　　　　　(b)　　　　　(c)

Thicker bearing

Figure 6.3 The prosthetic joint level, the continuous solid line.

The anatomical joint level

For the MCL and cruciate ligaments to resume their isometric function, the prosthesis should be implanted so that its prosthetic joint level coincides, throughout the range of movement, with the old anatomical joint level, i.e. the articular surface of the femoral condyle before it was modified by disease. The relative thicknesses of bone removed from the posterior and the inferior surfaces of the femur is critical because this determines the relative widths of the flexion/extension gaps.

In anteromedial OA, the posterior articular surface of the condyle is preserved (Fig. 6.4(a)). If a layer of cartilage and bone the same thickness as the metal implant is excised from the back of the condyle, the prosthetic and the anatomical joint levels will coincide (Fig. 6.4(b)). This establishes the width of the flexion gap which will not subsequently be changed.

The position of the anatomical joint level anteriorly is lost because all the cartilage, plus an unknown quantity of bone, has been eroded from the inferior surface of the femoral condyle. However, its site can be deduced because the ligaments that once matched it are still intact. As these ligaments are isometric throughout the joint range, the prosthetic joint level will be at the anatomical joint level when the extension gap is the same as the flexion gap (already established). The non-articular surfaces of the femoral component are designed so that removing bone from the inferior surface of the femoral condyle widens the extension gap without altering the flexion gap (Fig. 6.4(b)).

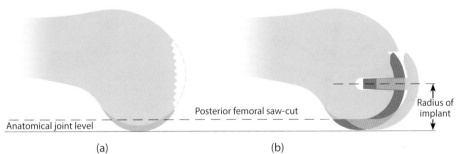

(a)   (b)

Figure 6.4 The anatomical joint level posteriorly, the continuous solid line.

Effect of using a spherical femoral component

The natural medial femoral condyle is polyradial; its inferior articular surface has a radius of curvature greater than its posterior radius. The prosthetic condyle is circular in the sagittal plane, and so the most anterior part of its articular surface cannot coincide with the old anatomical joint level but is proximal to it. This does not affect the gap measurements described above since the natural condyle is virtually circular between the points of contact at which the extension gap (20°) and flexion gap (110°) are measured and also in higher flexion [2] (see Fig. 2.9).

The rationale of balancing the ligaments assumes that, if the prosthetic and the anatomical joint levels coincide at these two points, they will also coincide at all intervening contact points and in higher flexion, maintaining the ligaments at constant tension throughout that range. This approximation will be closest if a femoral component with a radius similar to that of the posterior natural condyle has been chosen.

How the instruments work

We will first describe how the instruments are used to position the component and to balance the ligaments. Reference to the videos may be found helpful.

The tibial component

The extramedullary tibial saw guide is used to direct the transverse saw cut. The saw guide is positioned at the correct height using a system of femoral sizing spoons and G-clamps that reference off the posterior femur with the knee in flexion (Fig. 6.5). It ensures that the appropriate amount of bone is resected from the tibia.

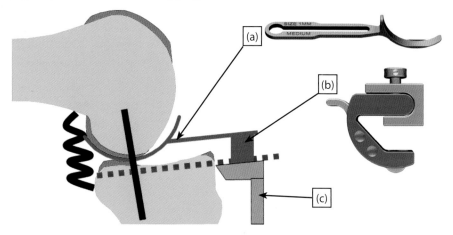

Figure 6.5 Level of tibial saw-cut and of its guiding surface (a) femoral sizing spoon, (b) Oxford G-clamp, (c) EM guide.

The level of the transverse tibial saw cut

We commonly use a 4 mm thick bearing except for small patients, in whom we would use a 3. However, as the operation is easier with a 4 bearing, we would recommend that, when starting, surgeons should aim for a 4. In order to make a space for a 4 mm thick bearing and a tibial component 3 mm thick, the tibial saw cut should be made about 7 mm below the posterior femoral articular surface with the ligament just tight. This will ensure that when the femoral component is appropriately positioned, with its articular surface where the original articular surface was, a 4 bearing will have the appropriate tightness.

To guide the height of the horizontal cut we use a stylus, otherwise known as a spoon (Fig. 6.5(a)), which is linked to the extramedullary tibial saw guide using a G-clamp, (Fig. 6.5(b)). The spoons come in five different sizes, extra small, small, medium, large, and extra large, to match the sizes of the femoral component. We use medium for most patients, small for small women and large for large men. The spoons can be used to confirm the size of femoral component. When inserted, the front of a spoon of appropriate size should be about where the original surface of the condyle was, 3 to 5 mm in front of the eburnated bone (see Fig. 7.8).

Spoons also come in different thicknesses, 1 mm, 2 mm, 3 mm, which are used to ensure that the ligaments are just tight (Fig. 6.6). Usually the 1 spoon is appropriate as it just tightens the ligaments. However, occasionally with a very deep tibial defect or with lax ligaments, a 2 or 3 spoon is necessary. When a thicker spoon is inserted, less tibia is removed so the ligaments will be just tight when the bearing is inserted.

3 and 4 mm G-clamps are available; the 3 should be selected for a 3 bearing and the 4 for a 4 bearing. With the 4 G-clamp, 1 mm more bone is removed than with a 3 mm G-clamp, allowing a 1 mm thicker bearing to be inserted.

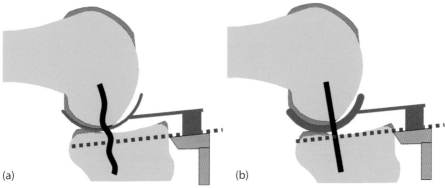

(a)   (b)

Figure 6.6 A spoon of correct thickness (a or b) is selected to just tighten the MCL. With a thicker spoon less tibia is removed.

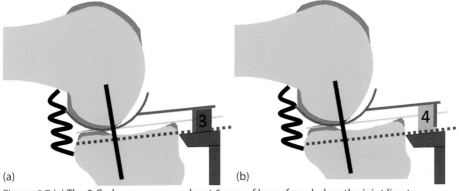

(a)   (b)

Figure 6.7 (a) The 3 G-clamp removes about 6 mm of bone from below the joint line to accommodate a 3 mm bearing and a 3 mm thick tibial plateau and (b) the 4 G-clamp removes one more millimetre of bone to accommodate a 4 mm bearing.

Varus–valgus inclination

In the frontal plane, the extramedullary tibial guide aims to place the tibial plateau at about 90° to the tibial axis. In UKA, the alignment of the limb (tibiofemoral angle) is independent of the alignment of the plateau. Therefore, any minor angular inaccuracies do not have the same significance as in TKA. Furthermore, the ball-and-socket configuration of the femoromeniscal articulation of the OUKA accommodates a small amount of angulation of the plateau relative to the femoral component without loss of congruence. We have found that ±5° malalignment of the tibial component does not compromise the outcome [3].

Posteroinferior inclination

The natural medial tibial plateau is inclined backwards and downwards in the sagittal plane at a mean angle of 7°, but with a wide range of 0°–15°. As the knee flexes and extends relative to the tibial crest, the femoral condyle moves backwards and forwards on the plateau so alteration of the slope will effect the ligament balance in flexion and extension. We have always implanted the tibial plateau at the mean inclination, irrespective of the knee's anatomy, and a 7° angle is built into the tibial saw guide. Because the 20° and 110° gaps are measured relative to the cut surface of the tibia, the effects of altering the tibial slope are automatically taken into account when the gaps are balanced.

Mediolateral position

The mediolateral position of the tibial plateau is defined by the vertical saw cut. With the G-clamp and spoon removed and with the knee flexed, the cut is made into the intercondylar eminence, just medial to the apex of the medial tibial spine and is directed towards the ipsilateral Anterior Superior Iliac Spine (ASIS). The direction of the cut will then be in the flexion–extension plane of the knee, the approximate direction of the anteroposterior movements of the mobile bearing. The cut is advanced until the saw blade rests on the guiding surface of the tibial saw guide. When the vertical cut is completed, the transverse cut is carried out, to release the medial tibial plateau.

Choice of plateau size

The tibial component should cover as much of the cut surface as possible to maximise the area available for the transmission of load, and hence minimise the risk of complications such as pain, loosening, or fracture. It is particularly important that the tibial component lies on the posterior and medial cortices [4].

It *must* reach as far as the medial cortex; therefore the implant is chosen from the range of sizes by its *width*. The plateau can overhang medially by up to 2 mm without risk of soft tissue irritation. (More overhang than this is unnecessary as the next smaller size component is 2 mm smaller.) Some overhang is preferable to underhang which will lead to incomplete coverage.

The tibial component *must* be placed as far back as possible so that it reaches to the posterior cortex. Full coverage is needed at this site because the bearing slides to, and beyond, the posterior edge of the plateau in flexion. In addition, very high loads may be transmitted across the flexed knee, and so the posterior part of the tibial implant needs to be supported by the posterior tibial cortex. Comparing the sawn plateau with tibial templates of the opposite side guides choice of the optimum component.

The parametric range of sizes cannot always provide a component that satisfies these two criteria *and also* reaches to the anterior cortex, so that often a small area of the cut surface is uncovered anterolaterally. However if the component is 3 mm or more from the anterior cortex the vertical cut should be repeated 2 mm further lateral so a larger size component can be used. (A larger component will be 2 mm wider and 3 mm longer.)

Femoral component

The femoral drill guide

The femoral drill guide, femoral saw guide, and concave spherical mill are all available in five sizes to match the diameters of the five sizes of femoral component. With the knee flexed, the drill guide is inserted with its upper foot touching the intact cartilage on the posterior surface of the medial femoral condyle and its face touching the eburnated bone on the inferior surface of the condyle (Fig. 6.8(a)). The correct alignment of the drill guide is achieved by linking it to an intramedullary rod. A drill (with a fixed collar) passes through the guide to make a hole in the bone. The axis of the hole is the same distance from the foot of the instrument as the radius of the chosen femoral component, and the depth of the hole is the same as the length of the shafts of the spigots.

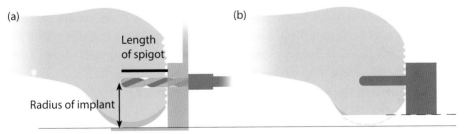

Figure 6.8 Level of posterior femoral saw-cut.

Femoral saw guide

The guide is positioned in the drill hole and directs the saw to remove from the femoral condyle a slice of bone and cartilage the same thickness as the metal of the posterior part of the femoral implant. This restores the level of the joint line in flexion (see Fig. 6.4).

The concave spherical mill (Fig. 6.9)

The mill is used to remove bone incrementally from the inferior surface of the femoral condyle, simultaneously shaping the bone to match the inner surface of the femoral implant. The mill rotates about a spigot inserted into the drill hole already made in the condyle.

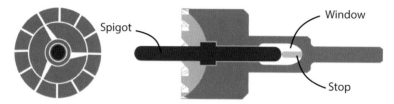

Figure 6.9 Concave spherical mill used to mill the inferior surface of the condyle. Milling is complete when the shaft of the spigot is seen, through the window, to touch the stop.

The spigots (Fig. 6.9) are provided in a range numbered 0 to 7 depending on the thickness of the collar that acts as a stop to the mill. As the thickness of the collar decreases in 1 mm steps from spigot 0 to spigot 7, the amount of bone removed increases similarly.

The lengths of the shafts on both sides of the collar are the same, and are constant throughout the range, so each spigot can be used either way around. The depth of the drill hole in the condyle is the same as the length of the shafts (see Fig. 6.8(a)), and so the spigots register at two sites, the worn surface of the condyle and the bottom of the drill hole (Fig. 6.10(a)).

The 0 spigot (the one with the thickest collar) is always used first (Fig. 6.10(b)). The mill then shapes the surface of the bone (Fig. 6.10(c)) so that a trial femoral component can be inserted (Fig. 6.10(d)). This establishes (as the spigot's number suggests) a zero point from which subsequent measurements are made. Because the contour of the arthritic condyle has been flattened by loss of bone and cartilage, the bone removed is peripheral and mostly anterior; no bone is removed centrally (Figs. 6.10(b) and 6.10(c)). After milling with the zero spigot, the articular surface of the trial femoral component lies about 4 mm distal to the eburnated surface of the bone (Fig. 6.10(d)) so that the extension gap is smaller than the flexion gap, an essential requirement for the next step.

First gap measurement (Fig. 6.11, p.130)

With the tibial template and the trial femoral component in place (Fig. 6.11(a)), the flexion gap (with the knee flexed to about 110°) is measured with a gap gauge (say, 4 mm). The joint is then extended (to 20° flexion) and the extension gap is measured (say, 1 mm). The difference between the flexion gap and the extension gap (4 mm − 1 mm = 3 mm) gives the thickness of bone to be milled from the inferior surface of the femur to make the gaps equal. The 3 spigot (with a collar 3 mm thinner than the 0 spigot) is inserted into the drill hole and the second milling is completed, having removed 3 mm of bone (Figs. 6.11(b) and 6.11(c)).

Spigot registers at two points

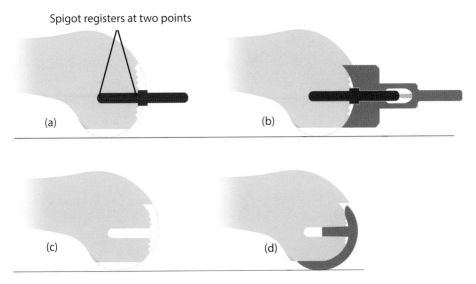

(a)

(b)

(c)

(d)

Figure 6.10 First milling.

Second gap measurement

The tibial template and the trial femoral component are reinserted and the gaps are again measured; they are usually found to be the same (Fig. 6.11(d)).

Occasionally, the second measurement shows that the extension gap remains narrower than the flexion gap, and that more bone must be milled away to achieve balance. To remove a further 1 mm, the 4 spigot (with a collar 1 mm thinner than the 3 spigot) is inserted and a third milling is performed. As Figure 6.11(c) shows, the small ring of bone under the collar of the spigot escapes the second milling and has to be removed to allow the femoral component to seat. This robs the spigot of one of its points of reference (Fig 6.10(a)). However, if a third milling has to be undertaken, the spigots continue to function as before by registering off the bottom of the drill hole. Figure 6.12 shows that, in this case, the temptation to hammer the spigot into the hole until the collar touches the bone must be resisted.

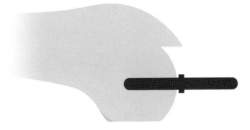

Figure 6.12 Third milling.

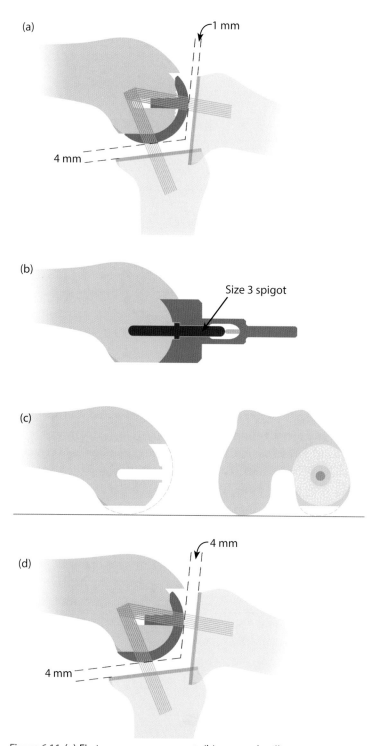

Figure 6.11 (a) First gap measurement; (b), second milling (c) resultant bone shape; (d) second gap measurement.

The bearing

The mobile bearing passively follows the track of the femoral condyle as it moves anteroposteriorly and mediolaterally relative to the plateau. The limits of these movements are set by the lengths of the ligaments, and, within these limits, the freedom of the bearing to translate in all directions should be unrestricted. If the bearing is unrestrained, loads are transmitted across the joint as a combination of compressive force (perpendicular to the articular surface) and tensile forces in the soft tissues. Shear stresses at the bone–implant interfaces are thereby minimised. If bearing movement is resisted (by impingement against bone, cement, or the lateral wall of the tibial component), shear and tensile stresses may develop at the femoral and/or tibial interfaces and could cause loosening of the fixed components, dislocation of the bearing and perhaps pain (see Fig. 2.20).

The largest translational movements of the femoral condyle relative to the tibia are in the anteroposterior direction. The flat plateau of the tibial component, having no anterior or posterior rim, offers no limits to movement of the bearing in these directions, nor do the soft tissues interfere. In flexion, when the bearing moves posteriorly, the posterior capsule is relaxed; in extension, when the bearing moves forward, so does the anterior capsule. In a normally functioning OUKA, the excursion of the bearing regularly brings its posterior margin beyond the posterior edge of the tibial plateau in flexion, and anteromedial overhang is common in full extension. Despite these movements of the bearing, the centre of pressure always lies within the middle third of the tibial implant, maintaining the bone/implant interface in compression.

In a knee with normally tensioned ligaments, the femoral condyle has very little freedom to translate mediolaterally, and the bearing needs equivalently little freedom to follow it. However, the bearing should not be jammed against the lateral wall of the tibial component.

Rotation and entrapment

As well as the translational movements described above, the femoral condyle rotates axially relative to the tibial plateau. Obligatory internal rotation of the femur, of about 20° (see Figs. 3.2 and 3.3(a)), occurs during passive extension, and a range of forced internal/external rotation is available in all flexed positions due to tissue deformation, increasing with increasing flexion (see Fig. 3.22). Axial rotation of the femur relative to the tibia is accomplished by means of spinning movements at the femoromeniscal interface and anteroposterior translational movements at the meniscotibial interface. Since the femoromeniscal interface of the prosthesis is a ball-in-socket and the meniscotibial interface is flat-on-flat, spinning movements can occur at both surfaces of the bearing. One of these levels of rotation is superfluous, and so spin can be limited at the lower interface, by the tibial wall, without limiting the joint's freedom to rotate. The design takes advantage of this to maximise entrapment of the bearing.

The prototype bearing (1976 to 1978) was circular in plan and the amount of entrapment, i.e. the height of the socket wall above its deepest point, was the same all round (Fig. 6.13(a)). However, dislocation proved more likely to occur anteriorly or posteriorly than sideways and it was desirable to have more entrapment at the front and the back of the socket than at the sides [5]. Furthermore, with the circular design, entrapment can only be increased by decreasing the radius of the femoral component or increasing the width of the bearing, and the latter would make the bearing too wide for the tibial plateau. The solution was to make the bearing quadrilateral in plan, with its longer axis in the anteroposterior direction (Fig. 6.13(b)). This allowed the anterior and posterior lips of the socket to be higher (increasing anteroposterior entrapment without affecting mediolateral entrapment).

Since it is difficult to stretch the ligaments more than 3 mm, the posterior wall of the socket cannot provide greater entrapment than that (or the bearing cannot be inserted). Therefore the centre of the socket was moved towards the back of the quadrilateral, diminishing the height of the posterior lip to about 3 mm and raising the anterior lip to about 5 mm (Fig. 6.13(c)). This is the general form that the medial bearing has had ever since the Phase 1 implant was introduced in 1978.

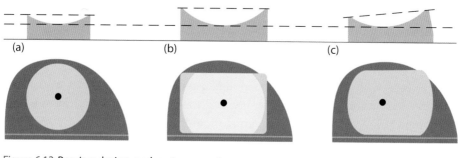

(a) (b) (c)

Figure 6.13 Bearing design and entrapment.

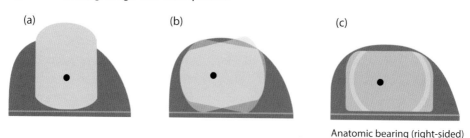

(a) (b) (c)

Anatomic bearing (right-sided)

Figure 6.14 Limiting rotation of the bearing.

Obviously, this mechanism can only work if the bearing maintains its anteroposterior alignment. If it spins through 90°, the socket will present reduced resistance to anterior or posterior dislocation (Fig. 6.14(a)). Figure 6.14(b) shows how its quadrilateral shape limits spin of the bearing if the centre of the socket (about which spin occurs) is close enough to the lateral wall of the tibial implant. This is achieved by positioning the femoral component appropriately. Unlimited spin is still allowed at the meniscofemoral interface and the fundamental requirement, that the bearing be free to translate in all directions, is still satisfied.

In order to minimise further the risk of bearing rotation, 'anatomic' bearings (right- and left-sided) with an extended lateral edge were introduced in 2002/3 (Fig. 6.14(c)). Also, the anteromedial corner has been rounded off to minimise bearing overhang in extension and the potential for soft tissue irritation.

The femoral component

Mediolateral position

The mediolateral position of the femoral component controls the mediolateral position of the bearing on the tibia. The main 6 mm hole for the peg of the femoral component should be placed centrally in the femoral condyle (Fig. 6.11(c)). If the femoral component is positioned in this manner and the vertical tibial cut is made just medial to the apex of the spine, the bearing should be close to, but not jammed against, the wall. A common mistake is for the vertical saw to slide down the tibial spine and the cut is made too far medially. If this is the case, the bearing can jam against the vertical wall. To prevent this, a trial reduction of the tibial template and the trial femoral component with a trial bearing should be made, prior to preparing the slot for the keel of the tibial component. If the bearing is found to jam against the wall, the vertical saw cut should be moved 2 mm further laterally. Occasionally, due to the femoral component being sited too far medial relative to the tibial component, the bearing is some distance from the wall. The risk here is that the bearing would rotate and dislocate. This is now unlikely to occur because of the asymmetric design of the bearing and therefore should be accepted. The only exception is if the vertical tibial cut has in error been made lateral to the medial spine in which case the tibial component should be moved medially a millimetre or two.

Rotation and 'attitude'

The articular surface of the femoral component is a segment of a sphere (with its centre at the tip of its peg). The position of a complete spherical surface does not alter when it rotates around its centre and so, in some sense, the rotational alignment of the femoral implant is an irrelevance. Figure 6.15 shows, for instance, that rotational alignment of the femoral component about the axis of its peg does not alter the position of the bearing in the flexed knee. Nevertheless, because the femoral component is an incomplete sphere, its 'attitude' is altered by rotation in any of the three planes. The attitude of the component affects (1) the availability of its limited articular surfaces and (2) its appearance on radiographs. However, because the contact area is so large (about 6 cm^2), some malalignment of the component is unlikely to compromise the contact area. We have found that ±10° malalignment does not compromise the outcome [5].

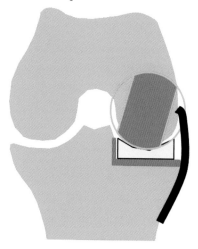

Figure 6.15 Femoral component attitude: rotation about the axis of its peg (knee flexed to 110°). We consider angular alignment up to 10° acceptable.

The alignment of the femoral component is controlled by the femoral drill guide, which is linked to an intramedullary rod (see Fig. 7.15). The linkage is such that the femoral component is implanted about 10° flexed and 7° varus relative to the diaphyseal axis. It is therefore flexed about 10° and in neutral varus/valgus relative to the mechanical axis. The linkage does not control the mediolateral position of the femoral component. This has to be selected manually so that the drill hole is central on the condyle.

The femoral component is flexed 10° relative to the bone for a number of reasons. It increases the contact area between the femoral component and the bearing in high flexion (Fig. 6.16). It also facilitates accurate balancing of the knee. In order to assess ligament tension without the influence of the posterior capsule, the extension gap is measured at 20°. Ultimately the flexion gap should be measured 90° flexed relative to this at 110°. If adjustment of the extension gap is not to influence the flexion gap, then the femoral peg, along the direction of which the extension gap is adjusted, should be parallel to the tibial component in about 110° flexion. If the tibial component is flexed 7° relative to the tibial axis, this is best achieved by flexing the femoral component about 10°.

The reason why the femoral component is at 7° varus relative to the diaphyseal axis is that its peg is then approximately parallel to the mechanical axis. The intramedullary rod is very thin so therefore does not accurately control orientation, indeed errors of 3 – 5° are commonly seen. However, due to the spherical nature of the femoral component, these are of no consequence (Fig. 6.15). This would not be true were the surface of the femoral component cylindrical.

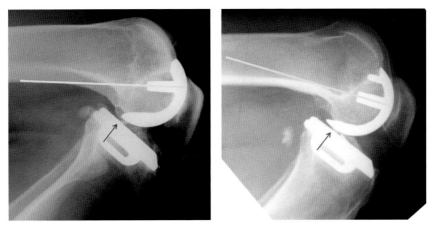

Figure 6.16 Radiographs showing increased contact area in flexion with a flexed femoral component.

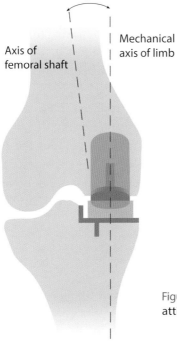

7°

Axis of femoral shaft

Mechanical axis of limb

Figure 6.17 Femoral component attitude: varus-valgus.

Femoral component design

The original (Phase 1) femoral component had a single oblique peg with faceted surfaces because the femoral condyle was prepared with a saw. The Phase 2, and subsequently the Phase 3, had a single peg parallel to the flat posterior surface, which allowed incremental milling (see Fig. 1.3). These components were designed to be implanted in neutral flexion/extension. When the cementless femoral component was designed, it included a second peg for more stable fixation and an anterior extension of about 17° (see Fig. 7.20(a) & (b)). A two-peg cemented femoral component of similar design to the cementless was introduced at the same time. The anterior extension meant that the femoral component could be implanted 10° to 20° flexed. It was also advantageous for cementless components as, in high flexion, the joint contact force was less likely to loosen the component. The anterior extension also ensures that, for both cemented and cementless components, high stresses in the bearing caused by contact with the posterior/proximal edge of the femoral component in high flexion are less likely. The components with the anterior extension do not fit within the milled surface until anterior bone has been removed to prevent impingement. This is advantageous as it ensures that anterior bone is removed. However it means that, for initial balancing, a one-peg trial component is needed.

The Microplasty method reliably implants the femoral components about 10° flexed. If surgeons wish to implant components more flexed, a 15° Microplasty adaptor is available. This is used by some surgeons in Asia whose patients require full flexion. Studies in these patients have not shown any clinical advantage of flexing the component 15° or more. However, we have seen a dislocated bearing which had a transverse groove caused by end loading retrieved from a patient with full flexion in whom the femoral component was not flexed 15°. Therefore there may be an advantage, in the long term, of flexing the component 15° in patients with full flexion.

As the cemented two-peg component was introduced in the USA at the same time as Microplasty and as it was felt there was no need to flex the component in the USA more than 10°, the two-peg component without the full anterior extension was used. This component, which has a 7° extension to support the second peg, fits within the milled surface. Therefore, a trial component based on the definitive component can be used for balancing (see Fig. 7.20).

References

1. Tokuhara Y, Kadoya Y, Nakagawa S, Kobayashi A, Takaoka K. The flexion gap in normal knees. An MRI study. *J Bone Joint Surg Br* 2004; **86**(8): 1133-6.
2. Monk AP, Choji K, O'Connor JJ, Goodfellow JW, Murray DW. The shape of the distal femur: a geometrical study using MRI. *Bone Joint J* 2014; **96-B**(12): 1623-30.
3. Gulati A, Chau R, Simpson DJ, Dodd CA, Gill HS, Murray DW. Influence of component alignment on outcome for unicompartmental knee replacement. *Knee* 2009; **16** (3): 196-9.
4. Chau R, Gulati A, Pandit H, Beard DJ, Price AJ, Dodd CA, Gill HS, Murray DW. Tibial component overhang following unicompartmental knee replacement – does it matter? *Knee* 2009; **16(5)**: 310-3.
5. Goodfellow J, O'Connor J. The anterior cruciate ligament in knee arthroplasty. A risk-factor with unconstrained meniscal prostheses. *Clin Orthop Relat Res* 1992; **(276)**: 245-52.

7

Surgical technique:
Cemented or cementless implantation with Microplasty instrumentation

Videos

Videos and surgical animations relevant to this chapter can be found at http://www.oxfordpartialknee.com.

Preoperative planning

The trays containing the tibial instruments, templates and trial components and those used with all sizes of femur are shown in Figure 7.1. A numbered list of illustrations of all the instruments, trial components and templates can be found at the end of this chapter. When a component or instrument is mentioned first in the following text, its number will be printed with square brackets.

The five sizes of femoral component have different spherical radii of curvature. For each femoral size, there is a matching set of men iscal bearings in seven thicknesses, from 3 mm to 9 mm. There is a separate tray of instruments for each femoral size. The trays, one of which is shown in Figure 7.2, contain colour coded instruments and trial components specifically for use with one size of femoral component. They must not be mixed up so it is safer just to open one size.

In addition to the instruments in the set, it is important to have the thigh support designed for the OUKA and appropriate saw blades. Three saw blades, reciprocating, oscillating and keel cut have been designed specifically for the OUKA and can be obtained in a three pack or individually (Fig 7.3). The reciprocating and oscillating saws have markings to guide the surgeon to the correct depth. The keel cut saw has two parallel blades with some of the teeth bent in. The saw will not only accurately cut the slot but also remove the residual bone between the cuts. Two sets of Microplasty tibial templates are available. Surgeons just wanting to use cemented components should use cemented templates and cemented keel cut saws. Surgeons who want to use cemented or cementless components should use cementless templates and the cementless keel cut saw blade. (Three-blade saws are available but are more difficult to use in hard bone than the two-blade saws.)

The surgical technique is basically the same for cemented or cementless fixation. Where there are differences, these are highlighted.

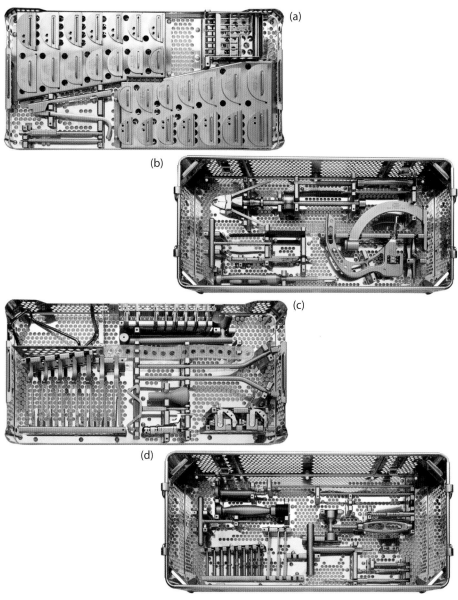

Figure 7.1 (a), (b), (c) Tibial instrument trays and (d) femoral tray used for all femoral sizes.

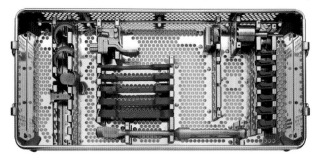

Figure 7.2 Tray for medium femoral components.

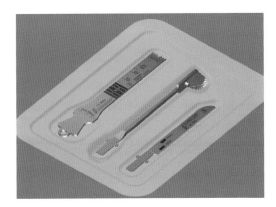

Figure 7.3 The three blade pack.

The size of the femoral component

The size of the femoral component can be estimated pre-operatively from the height and gender of the patient (Table 7.1). During the operation, based in part on the size of the femoral condyle and tibial component, the size may be adjusted. Pre-operative X-ray templating is less and less used.

Table 7.1 A guide to the size of femoral component based on information about height and gender and the size of the tibial component.

Women			Men		
Height	Femur	Matching tibia	Height	Femur	Matching tibia
<60" <153 cm	X-Small	AA, A or B	<63" <160 cm	Small	A, B or C
61–65" 153–165 cm	Small	A, B or C	63–67" 160–170 cm	Medium	C or D
66–69" 165–175 cm	Medium	C or D	67–73" 170–185 cm	Large	E, F
>69" >175 cm	Large	E	> 73" >185 cm	X-Large	F

A medium-size femoral component is appropriate for most patients. (It was, in fact, the only size used in the Phase 1 and 2 implants.) However, in small women, it is better to employ the small size and, in large men, the large size. The extra-large and extra-small sizes are rarely used in Western populations. In Asia the extra-small is used frequently. If there is doubt between small/medium, or large/medium, it is usually safer to use the medium. Similarly, if there is doubt between the extra-small and the small, or between the extra-large and the large, use the small or the large. The size is confirmed by the tibial size: Tibia A & B = usually small femur, Tibia C & D = usually medium femur, Tibia E & F = usually large femur. It is important to remember that all femoral and tibial sizes are fully interchangeable.

Positioning the limb

A thigh tourniquet is applied and the leg is placed on a thigh support with the hip flexed to about 40° and abducted, and the leg hanging freely. When the leg hangs freely, the knee should flex to about 110°. The knee must be free to be flexed to at least 135° (Fig. 7.4). The thigh support must not intrude into the popliteal fossa to ensure that risk of damage to the great vessels is minimised.

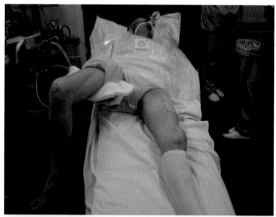

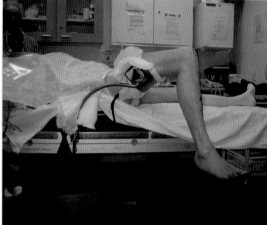

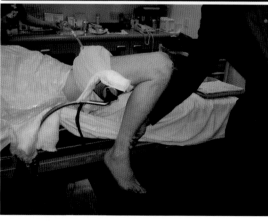

Figure 7.4 Positioning the limb on the thigh holder.

Incision

A paramedial skin incision is made from just above the medial pole of the patella to a point 3 cm distal to the joint line just medial to the tibial tubercle – two thirds above the joint line to one third below (Fig. 7.5). Surgeons who are starting the procedure should make a longer incision starting level with the upper pole of the patella. The medial margin of the patella is identified. The retinacular incision is made along the medial side of the patella and patella tendon. The anterior tibia is exposed. At its upper end, the retinacular incision is extended proximally for 2 to 3 cm into the vastus medialis.

Part of the retropatellar fat pad is excised and the anterior portion of the medial meniscus removed. Self-retaining retractors are inserted into the synovial cavity.

The ACL, lateral side and PFJ can now be inspected. If the ACL appears damaged, check its integrity by pulling on the ligament with a tendon hook. (Absence of a functioning ACL is a contraindication and the operation should be abandoned in favour of a total knee replacement.) A full thickness ulcer on the medial side of the lateral condyle and exposed bone in the PFJ can be ignored (see Chapter 5).

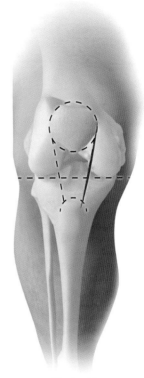

Figure 7.5 The incision.

Excision of osteophytes

Large osteophytes must be removed from the medial margin of the medial femoral condyle and from both margins and roof of the intercondylar notch (Fig. 7.6). Full clearance of the lateral side and apex of the notch must be achieved so as to ensure the ACL is not damaged and that the fixed flexion deformity corrects. Care should be taken while removing osteophytes from the anteromedial corner of the notch because the origin of the PCL can be damaged. The assistant extends and flexes the knee, moving the incision up and down, so that the various osteophytes come into view.

A narrow chisel (6 mm) is needed to remove the femoral osteophytes from beneath the medial collateral ligament (Fig. 7.7) and from the posterolateral

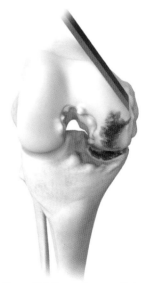

Figure 7.6 Removing medial margin osteophytes.

margin of the medial condyle (to make room to insert the saw blade into the inter-condylar notch at the next step).

Osteophytes should not be removed from the medial tibia as this may damage the MCL. These osteophytes tend to be removed with the resected tibia.

Osteophytes are removed from the anterior tibia because they interfere with seating of the tibial saw guide. In addition, there is usually an anvil shaped osteophyte anterior to the insertion of the ACL on the tibia. This should be removed.

Large medial patellar osteophytes should be removed to improve access but the odd facet should be retained. If the patella cannot be sub-luxed laterally, causing difficulty with access, the incision in the capsule and muscle should be extended proximally.

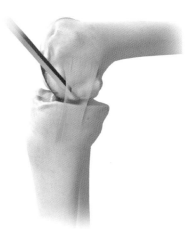

Figure 7.7 Removing femoral osteophytes beneath the medial collateral ligament.

Tibial saw cut

With the knee in 110° flexion, insert the femoral sizing spoon [23] (of appropriate size based on the pre-operative estimate) and 1 mm thick under the centre of the medial condyle. Its handle should lie approximately parallel with the long axis of the femur. With all retraction removed, assess the ligament tension by twisting the spoon. It should freely twist about 20° in both directions. Usually the 1 mm thick femoral sizing spoon achieves the proper ligament tension; if not, replace it with a thicker sizing spoon until the proper tension is achieved. The optimal size of the femoral component is confirmed by examining the relationship of the front of the spoon and the surface of the eburnated bone. Ideally it should be 3 to 5 mm above the surface approximately where the cartilage surface of the femur would have been before the arthritis. Once the appropriate spoon is inserted, apply a self retaining retractor which locks it in place.

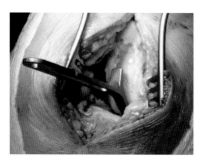 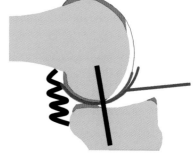

Figure 7.8 (a) The correct femoral sizing spoon in place with a gap of about 5 mm between the spoon and the eburnated bone. (b) Femoral spoon (the grey spoon is the correct size; the pink is too large).

Apply the tibial saw guide assembly [21, 25 & 53], with its shaft parallel with long axis of the tibia in both planes (Fig. 7.9). The ankle yoke [25] should be pointing towards the ipsilateral anterior superior iliac spine (ASIS). The tibial saw guide has 7° of posterior slope built in. The zero shim [20] should be in place.

The femoral sizing spoon, tibial saw guide and G-clamp [27], when used together, will accurately establish the level of bone resection (this can be seen in the video at www.oxfordpartialknee.com). Select either the 3 or the 4 G-clamp and apply to the femoral sizing spoon and to the medial side of the tibial saw guide to ensure access to pin holes in the guide. Although there is an option to adjust the height of the tibial cut using different shims [20], the zero shim must always be used with the G-clamp. In general, a 3 G-clamp is used for Extra Small and Small femurs and 4 for the rest although surgeons starting out with the OUKA should use the 4 G-clamp.

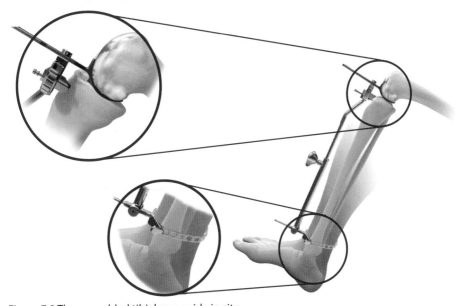

Figure 7.9 The assembled tibial saw guide in situ.

Confirm that the knee is flexed to 110°. Manipulate the upper end of the guide so that its face lies against the exposed bone. Push the guide laterally so its recess accommodates the patellar tendon (Fig. 7.10). Engage the cam on the G-clamp, by pulling the lever downwards, to lock the three components together. Fix the saw guide in place using a headed pin [4] through the central or lateral hole in the tibial saw guide. Unlock the G-clamp and remove along with the femoral sizing spoon.

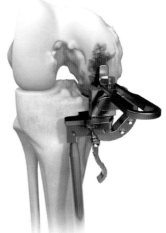

Figure 7.10 Tibial saw guide and femoral sizing spoon assembled in situ and held together by the G-clamp.

The vertical tibial cut

Identify the apex of the medial tibial spine with a diathermy (bovie) and make a mark just medial to the apex. Use the reciprocating saw designed for the OUKA with a stiff narrow blade, round end, and depth markings (Fig. 7.3) to make the vertical tibial saw cut. The saw cut should be just medial to the apex of the medial tibial spine. It will pass through the edge of the ACL insertion. Point the blade towards the ASIS, the position of which can be demonstrated by the assistant (Fig. 7.11(b)) or align the blade in the tibial flexion plane. The saw must reach the back of the tibial plateau and a little beyond. This is achieved by lining up the appropriate mark on the saw with the anterior tibial cortex (a series of marks appropriate to each size of tibial component exist on the saw blade). Advance the saw vertically down until it rests on the surface of the saw guide (Fig. 7.11(c)). The saw must remain parallel to the guide. Do not lift the saw handle as this will damage the posterior cortex and increase the risk of tibial plateau fracture.

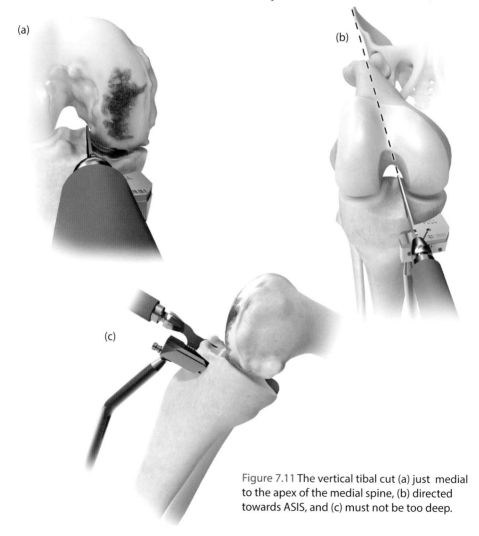

(a)

(b)

(c)

Figure 7.11 The vertical tibal cut (a) just medial to the apex of the medial spine, (b) directed towards ASIS, and (c) must not be too deep.

The horizontal tibial cut

Before making the horizontal cut remove the shim from the tibial resection guide and insert the slotted zero shim (Fig. 7.12). Also insert a medial collateral ligament (MCL) retractor [19] (sometimes called a Z or curly-whirly retractor). Ensure this retractor lies between the saw and the MCL, protecting the deep fibres of the ligament.

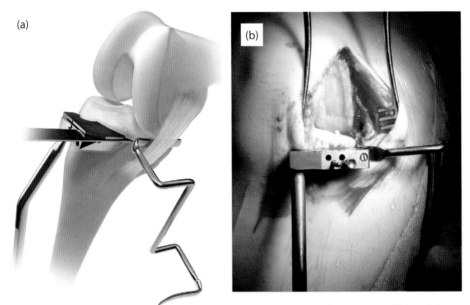

(a)

(b)

Figure 7.12 The horizontal cut with the Z-retractor used to protect the MCL (a and b), and the slotted shim (a).

Use the 12 mm wide oscillating saw blade, designed for the OUKA, with appropriate markings, to excise the plateau (Fig. 7.13). Ensure the saw blade is guided along the MCL retractor to cut the medial cortex completely without damaging the MCL. Slightly undermine the vertical cut. To cut the posterior cortex, advance the saw cut until the appropriate mark on the saw blade is aligned with the anterior cortex. When the cut is complete, the plateau usually moves. If it cannot be moved, the saw cuts have to be repeated. Remove the slotted shim, lever the plateau up with a broad osteotome to disrupt soft tissue attachments and remove with the knee in extension. If the plateau cannot be removed, soft tissue attachments posteromedially may need to be cut with a knife and occasionally posterior osteophytes need to be removed with an osteotome.

The excised plateau should show the classical lesion of anteromedial osteoarthritis: erosion of cartilage and bone in its mid and anterior parts and preserved cartilage posteriorly. Osteophytes around the edge of the plateau remain attached after its removal (see Fig. 4.4).

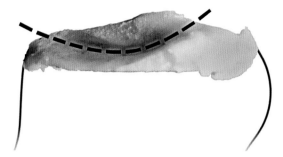

Figure 7.13 The excised plateau with the lesion outlined.

Lay templates [1] of the opposite side on the cut surface of the excised plateau to choose the tibial component with the appropriate width ignoring medial osteophytes. If the component of the appropriate width appears short, consider repeating the vertical cut 2 mm further laterally so that a wider and longer component may be used.

Horizontal cut first

Occasionally, using the standard technique, the vertical cut may go too deep posteriorly which weakens the tibia and increases the risk of tibial plateau fracture. An alternative is to do the horizontal cut first and then insert a shim in the cut to prevent the vertical cut from going too deep. The recommended steps are set out below.

Using a diathermy, identify the apex of the medial spine and mark the optimal site of the vertical cut just medial to the apex of the spine and in the direction of the ASIS. Insert the slotted zero tibial saw shim and MCL retractor. Perform the horizontal cut in the standard fashion except that it should be extended laterally so as to undermine the site of the vertical cut by about 5 mm. Remove the MCL retractor and slotted shim then insert a standard zero shim. A protective shim should then be inserted into the horizontal cut and held in place under the vertical cut whilst the vertical cut is being undertaken to prevent it from going too deep. Prototype protective shims are currently being tested and will be available for general use soon. In the interim, a horizontal cut saw blade, a steel rule, or an 'angel wing' may be used as a protective shim.

The femoral drill holes and alignment

With the knee in about 45° flexion, make a hole into the intramedullary canal of the femur with the 4 mm drill [54]. It should aim for the ASIS. This should be completed with the 5 mm awl [33] (Fig. 7.14(a)).

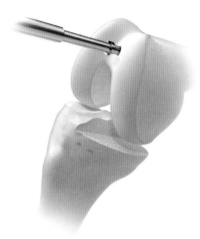

Figure 7.14(a)

The hole must be situated 1 cm anterior to the anterior edge of the intercondylar notch and in line with its medial wall (Fig. 7.14(b)).

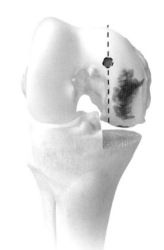

Figure 7.14(b)

Insert the intramedullary (IM) rod with the introducer until the introducer stops against the bone (Fig. 7.14(c)) [24, 29]. If the rod cannot easily be inserted do not hit it with a hammer as it may perforate the cortex. Instead enlarge the hole and perhaps move it further anterior.

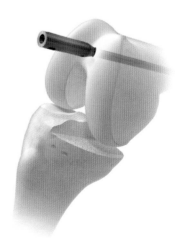

Figure 7.14(c)

Flex the knee to 110°. This must be done with care, because the medial border of the patella abuts the IM rod. Using a marker or diathermy, draw a line down the centre of the medial femoral condyle.

Confirm the size of the femoral component based on the size of the tibial component (Table 7.1). Insert the femoral drill guide [41] for the appropriate size, set to the size of the G-clamp used, either 3 or 4 (Fig. 7.15(a)). (See Chapter 6 for advice on the adjustment of the drill guide.) If the correctly adjusted femoral drill guide cannot be inserted or feels tight, remove about 1 mm of cartilage off the posterior femur using a sharp chisel. There should be no need to re-cut the tibial plateau.

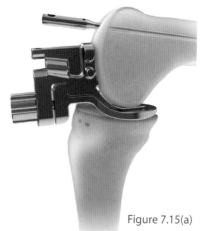

Figure 7.15(a)

Insert the IM link [26] into the IM rod and into the lateral hole of the femoral drill guide (Fig 7.15(b)). If necessary, tap it gently in with a hammer. The link ensures correct alignment of the guide. It will not necessarily position the guide in the correct medial/lateral position. This needs to be adjusted (Fig. 7.15(c)).

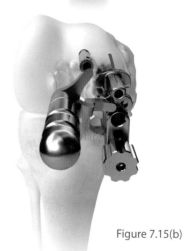

Figure 7.15(b)

The 6 mm hole must lie in the centre of the medial condyle, halfway between its medial and lateral borders. This is done by ensuring the medial and lateral bollards of the drill guide adjacent to the 6 mm hole on the guide are equidistant from the condyle edges. It can be confirmed by looking into the 6 mm hole and verifying that the line previously drawn down the centre of the condyle is in the centre of hole (Fig 7.15(c)). Ensure the cowl indicating the front of the component does not overhang medially. If it does, move the guide laterally.

Once the guide is centrally positioned, the 4 and 6 mm holes are drilled. The drill guide and link can then be removed.

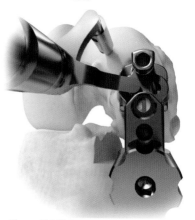

Figure 7.15(c)

Femoral saw cut

Insert the posterior resection guide
[46] into the drilled holes and tap
home (Fig. 7.16 (a)). Do not hit hard
because the guide can tilt.

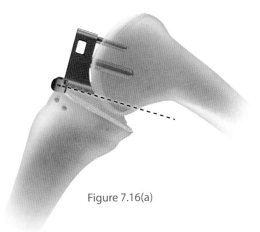

Figure 7.16(a)

Insert a retractor to protect the MCL.
Using the oscillating saw blade, excise
the posterior facet of the femoral
condyle. The saw blade should be
bent slightly by dropping the saw to
ensure it is guided by the underside
of the posterior resection guide (Fig.
7.16(b)). Take care to avoid damage
to the medial collateral and anterior
cruciate ligaments.

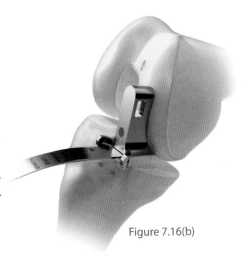

Figure 7.16(b)

Remove the guide with the slap hammer [9], ensuring that it is withdrawn in
line with the femoral drill guide holes so as to not damage them. (Use of the slap
hammer is counterintuitive. The handle should be pushed towards the knee so
as to lock the device onto the component while the hammer is used to pull the
component off.) Remove the bone fragment.

There is now good access to the back of the joint and any remnants of the medial
meniscus should be removed. In the region of the MCL, a small cuff of meniscus
should be left to protect the MCL from the tibial component. The posterior horn
should be completely removed.

First milling of the condyle

Insert the 0 spigot [36], which has the thickest collar, into the large drill hole and tap until the collar abuts the bone (Fig. 7.17). This ensures that the dual reference at the bottom of the hole and on the surface of the condyle are aligned.

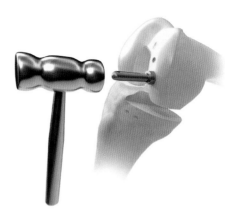

Figure 7.17

By extending the knee slightly and retracting the soft tissues, manoeuvre the spherical mill [43] onto the spigot (Fig. 7.18(a)) and into the wound so that the teeth touch the bone (Fig. 7.18(b)). Take care to avoid trapping soft tissues.

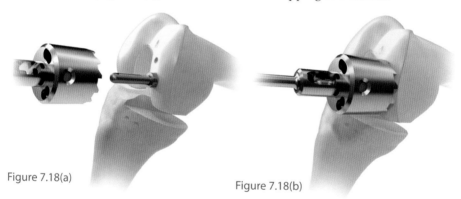

Figure 7.18(a)

Figure 7.18(b)

When milling, push firmly in the direction of the spigot axis, taking care not to tilt the mill as this will damage the hole. Mill until the cutter will no longer advance and the spigot can be seen, in the window, to have reached its end stop (see Fig. 6.9). If in doubt, continue to mill; the mill cannot continue beyond the amount permitted by the collar of the selected spigot.

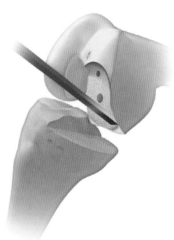

Remove the mill and the spigot and trim off the bone protruding from the posterior corners of the condyle that lie outside the periphery of the cutting teeth (Fig. 7.19). These corners should be removed tangentially to the spherically milled surface with a half inch (12 mm) chisel, taking care not to damage the flat posterior surface of the femoral condyle. In addition, any retained posteromedial osteophytes on the femur should be removed.

Fig. 7.19 Removing the posterior corners of the condyle after the first milling.

Measuring the flexion gap

Insert the tibial template [1] and apply the single peg femoral trial component [40] or, if available, the 2-peg without anterior extension (2-peg femoral US), to the milled condyle, tapping it home while holding the femoral impactor [31] angled at 45° to the femoral axis (Fig 7.20).

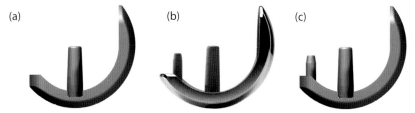

(a) (b) (c)

Figure 7.20 (a) Oxford single peg femoral component, (b) two-peg femoral component and (c) two-peg femoral component (US).

With the knee in about 110° of flexion and retractors removed, carefully measure the flexion gap with the gap gauges [47] (Fig. 7.21(a)). (In the unlikely event that the 3 mm gauge cannot be inserted, replace the tibial cutting guide and redo the tibial cut without the shim.) The gauge thickness is correct when natural tension in the ligaments is achieved. In these circumstances, the gap gauge when held between finger and thumb will easily slide in and out, but will not tilt. Confirmation of the correct thickness is obtained by demonstrating that a 1 mm thicker gauge is firmly gripped and a 1 mm thinner gauge is toggling loosely.

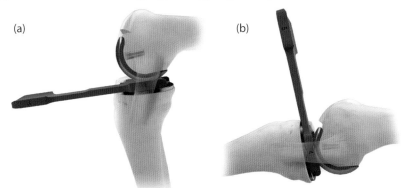

(a) (b)

Figure 7.21 (a) The flexion gap is measured at 110° knee flexion and (b) the extension gap in 20° knee flexion.

Measuring the extension gap

Having measured the flexion gap (say 4 mm), remove the gap gauge, fully extend the knee then flex to about 20° flexion. The surgeon should hold the leg and apply a gentle valgus load to take up any slack in the MCL. Use the gap gauges to measure the extension gap (say 1 mm) which is always less than, or equal to, the flexion gap. Confirm the size of the gap by using a gap gauge 1 mm thicker and 1 mm thinner. If a 1 mm gauge is too tight or cannot be inserted, assume the extension gap is zero. Calculate the amount of bone to remove by subtracting the extension gap from the flexion gap (4 − 1 = 3). It is therefore necessary to remove a further 3 mm of bone from the inferior femoral condyle (see pages 129 & 130). The spigots (numbered 1–7) allow bone to be removed in measured quantities (in mm) from the level of the first mill cut. The number 3 spigot removes 3 mm, so should be used. If the surgeon is not certain how much bone to remove it is best to be cautious and remove too little rather than too much.

Second milling

With the appropriate spigot in place (in this case a 3), use the spherical mill to remove the required additional thickness of bone from the condyle. Remove the corners of bone with a chisel tangential to the milled surface. If a collar of bone has appeared around the 6 mm hole, this should be removed with the bone collar remover [35]. Reinsert the trial femoral component and remeasure the gaps. The flexion gap should not have changed. The extension gap should now equal the flexion gap. Occasionally if the extension gap is still too narrow, a third milling is necessary.

Third milling

By subtracting the extension gap from the flexion gap the amount of bone to be removed is determined (say 1 mm). Add this to the size of the spigot used for the second milling (3) to determine the size (4) needed for the third milling. Insert the appropriate spigot, but do not hammer it in. As the small central collar of bone has been removed the spigot should not be touching the surface of the bone but is referenced off the bottom of the hole. Repeat milling and reassess gaps.

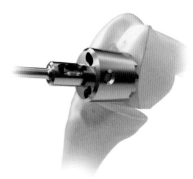

Figure 7.22

Preventing impingement

Apply the anti-impingement guide [45] to the condyle (Fig. 7.23(a)), and use the anterior mill assembly [28, 32, 42] to remove anterior bone and create clearance for the front of the bearing in full extension. Take great care to ensure the mill does not damage the tibia or patella. Before starting the mill, engage it on the peg and ensure the spring loaded mechanism moves freely. When milling, push firmly in the direction of the peg axis, taking care not to tilt the mill. Mill until the cutter will not advance further.

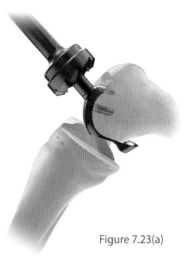

Figure 7.23(a)

Leave the anti-impingement guide in place and use the osteophyte chisel [49] to remove any posterior osteophytes (Fig. 7.23(b)). This should be done medially and laterally as well as centrally. Remove the guide and, using the osteophyte chisel, break off any attached osteophytes and sweep them down off the posterior capsule, and remove them. If possible palpate, with a little finger, the proximal part of the condyle to ensure all posterior osteophytes are removed.

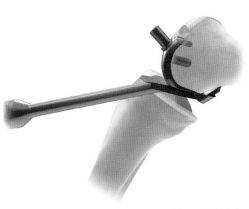

Figure 7.23(b)

Insert the tibial template, the twin peg femoral trial component [44 or 50] and a trial bearing [48] of appropriate thickness (as determined when measuring flexion and extension gaps). With these components in place, manipulate the knee through a full range of motion to ensure there is no impingement of bone against the bearing in full extension and full flexion (Figs. 7.24(a) and (b)). If the bearing impinges in flexion, the knee will open up like a book. If this happens, the osteophyte chisel should be used again to ensure all posterior osteophytes are removed.

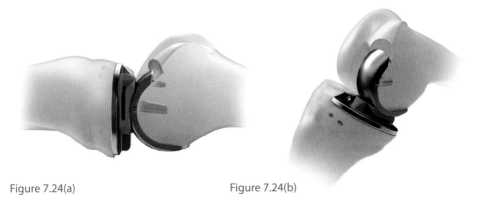

Figure 7.24(a)   Figure 7.24(b)

Ensure the bearing is not jammed against the vertical wall. If a narrow dissector put between the bearing and the wall is gripped by the bearing, consider redoing the vertical tibial cut 2 mm more laterally.

Remove the trial bearing and femoral trial component using the appropriate extractor [15] and slap hammer [9].

Note: Gap gauges are used to measure the gaps because they do not stretch the ligaments. The meniscal bearings have a 3 mm high posterior lip which, after multiple insertions, may stretch the ligaments.

Final preparation of the tibial plateau

To ensure the correct size, position the tibial template with its posterior margin flush with the posterior tibial cortex (Fig. 7.25(a)). This is facilitated by pushing the template too far back and passing the universal removal hook [14] over the posterior cortex of the tibia.

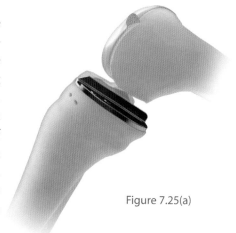

Pull the hook and thus the template forward until it is flush with the posterior cortex. The tibial template should be flush with the medial cortex (ignoring osteophytes) or overhanging slightly. If it overhangs by 2 mm or more use a smaller size tibial template. The front of the tibial template should also be within 3 mm of the front of the tibia. If it is not, redo the vertical cut so that a larger size template can be used. Note where the anterior margin of the template is.

Figure 7.25(a)

Force the tibial template laterally against the vertical cut and hammer the tibial template nail [6] into place, ideally in the posterior hole. Hold the nail throughout sawing to prevent movement of the template.

Introduce the keel cut saw into the front of the slot and saw until it has sunk to its shoulder (Fig. 7.25(b)). The saw blade is lifted up and down as it is advanced posteriorly. Confirm the cut is complete by holding the pin and feeling the saw hit the front and back of the keel slot. Once the saw cuts are complete, remove the tibial template, and wash the cut surfaces.

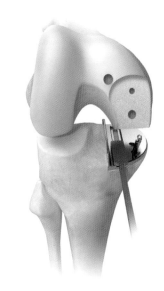

Figure 7.25(b)

Cemented/cementless differences

Select the appropriate keel cut saw. The standard Microplasty instruments are designed for the cementless saw and this should be used whether cemented or cementless fixation is used. In some countries, such as the USA, where cementless fixation is not yet available, Microplasty cemented templates are used with cemented keel cut saws.

If the cemented keel cut saw has been used, after removing the tibial template, excavate the groove to the correct depth by scooping out the bone with the blade of the cemented tibial groove cutter [18], taking care not to damage the anterior and posterior cortices (Fig. 7.26). The safest way to prepare the back of the groove is to feel the posterior cortex with the tibial groove cutter and then move it anteriorly by 5 mm before pushing down and bringing forward to empty the groove.

If the cementless keel cut saw has been used, the slot should have been accurately cut so the groove cutter should not be needed for cementless or cemented fixation. However some surgeons who use cemented fixation prefer to widen the slot with the cemented tibial groove cutter. The slot will then be the same width as the slot in long term studies.

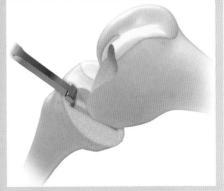

Figure 7.26

Insert the trial tibial component [7] and tap with the tibial impactor [12] until fully seated (Fig. 7.27).

Ensure that the component is flush with the bone and that the posterior margin of the component is flush with the back of the tibia. If the component does not seat fully remove it and clean the keel slot out with the appropriate tibial groove cutter. The cementless groove cutter is designed to be used through the Microplasty template whereas the cemented groove cutter should be used without the template.

Use only the small toffee hammer [34] to avoid the risk of plateau fracture.

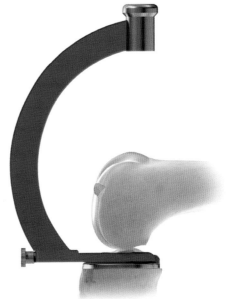

Figure 7.27

Final trial reduction

Insert the twin peg femoral trial component [44 or 50] and ensure it is fully seated by tapping home with the femoral impactor (Fig. 7.28).

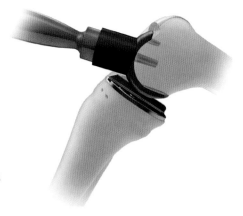

Figure 7.28

Insert a trial meniscal bearing of the chosen thickness (Fig. 7.29).

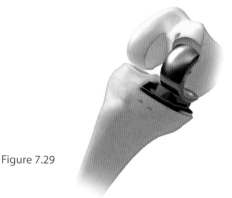

Figure 7.29

With the bearing in place, manipulate the knee through a full range of motion to demonstrate the stability of the joint, the security of the bearing and the absence of impingement. The thickness of the bearing should be such as to restore the ligaments to their natural tension, so that, when the bearing inserter/extractor is applied and gently lifted, the front of the bearing lifts 2 to 3 mm. In addition when a valgus force is applied to the knee, the artificial joint surfaces should distract a millimetre or two. This test should be done with the knee in 20° of flexion. In full extension, the bearing will be firmly gripped because of the tight posterior capsule.

Remove the trial bearing with the bearing extractor [15] (Fig. 7.30).

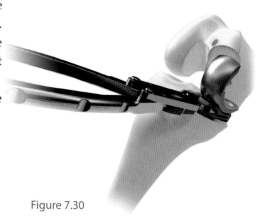

Figure 7.30

Cementing the components

Roughen the femoral and tibial surfaces including the posterior condyles, by making multiple small drill holes with the cement key drill [38] (Fig. 7.31). Clean the bone surface with a pulse-lavage and dry.

When surgeons start using the Oxford prosthesis, we strongly recommend that the components are fixed with two separate mixes of cement, because this makes it easier to retrieve any cement extruded posteriorly.

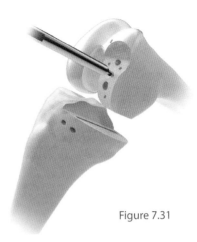

Figure 7.31

The tibial component

Place a small amount of cement on the tibial bone surface and flatten to produce a thin (about 1 mm thick) layer covering the whole surface. Insert the component and press down, first posteriorly and then anteriorly, to squeeze out excess cement at the front. As there is evidence to suggest that early application of cement to implant aids fixation, an alternative approach is to spread a thin layer of cement on the undersurfaces of the tibial component in addition to the layer on the tibia. If this is done, an osteotome should be used to force the cement into the surface of the tibia and sweep the remaining cement off the tibial surface.

Use the right-angled tibial impactor (Fig. 7.27) with the toffee hammer, applied from posterior to anterior, to complete the insertion. Ensure there is no soft tissue under the component. Remove excess cement with a Woodson cement curette [11] from the margins of the component. Insert the femoral trial component and pressurise cement by flexing the knee to 45° and then inserting the appropriate thickness feeler gauge. With the feeler gauge inserted, hold the leg in 45° of flexion while the cement sets. Do not fully extend or flex the leg as this may rock the component and compromise the fixation.

Once the cement has set, remove the feeler gauge and trial femoral component and look carefully for, and remove, cement that may have extruded. Finally slide the flat plastic probe [13] along the tibial articular surface, feeling for cement at the edges and posteriorly.

The femoral component

From the second mix, force cement into both femoral drill holes and fill the concave surface of the femoral component with cement. Apply the loaded component to the condyle and impact with the impactor held at 45° to the long axis of the femur. Remove excess cement from the margins with a Woodson cement curette. Pressurise the cement by inserting the appropriate feeler gauge with the knee at 45° of flexion and holding the leg in this position. Do not fully extend or flex the knee as this may rock the components and may loosen them. Once the cement has set, remove the feeler gauge. Clear the medial and lateral margins of the femoral component of any extruded cement. The posterior margin cannot be seen directly but can sometimes be seen reflected on the tibial surface and can be palpated with a curved dissector.

Experienced surgeons may wish to cement both tibial and femoral components with one mix. This is acceptable provided they are comfortable that they can do this and leave minimal cement to be removed from the back of the knee. A cement with a long working time should be used. An assistant should apply cement to the components. After the tibial cement has been briefly compressed with the femoral trial and feeler gauge, these should be removed and then excessive cement removed from around the tibia. The femur should then be cemented. Final pressurisation is achieved with a gap gauge inserted with the knee at 45° flexion.

Cementless

Component impaction

The cementless implants are impacted into the bone, tibial component first. It is essential that a small toffee hammer is used for impaction – a heavy hammer can cause a fracture. The tibial implant is assembled into the introducer/impactor [16] by locating its lugs into the recesses on the underside of the implant and tightening the thumb wheel (Fig 7.32).

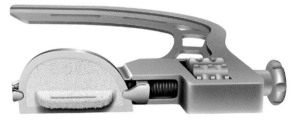

Figure 7.32

The component is then carefully impacted into the bone (Fig. 7.33).

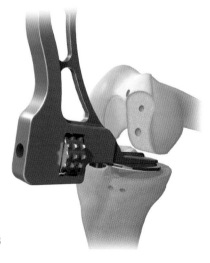

Figure 7.33

The keel is carefully driven into the keel slot from the front. The knee is fully flexed so the upper surface of the impactor is parallel to the posterior femoral saw cut thus increasing the available space. The component is impacted at an angle to the tibial surface so its posterior edge slides along the tibial surface thus pushing soft tissue out of the way. When the front of the component has reached the position where the front of the template was, the component is impacted down.

Before the implant is fully seated, the introducer/impactor is removed by unscrewing the thumb wheel. Using a small dissector, any soft tissue interposed between the implant and bone is swept out. Small adjustments can be made to the AP position of the component by using the side of the handle of the plastic cement removal chisel or a punch. Final impaction of the tibial component is achieved with the standard tibial impactor, placed over the centre of the keel.

Often the tibial component does not seat down fully and may be 0.5 mm proud. This should be accepted as it will subside with time. Attempting to hit it hard with a heavy hammer may cause a fracture.

Impaction of the femoral component is achieved with the standard impactor (Fig 7.28), used in line with the main peg hole. It is essential that a light hammer is used for impaction – a heavy hammer can be a cause of fracture. Both components are examined to ensure they are fully seated.

Bearing insertion

Reassess the gap by inserting a gap gauge and then a trial bearing. Using the bearing extractor, the front of the bearing should be gently lifted. A bearing of correct size should lift 2 to 3 mm. Occasionally a thinner bearing is needed than had previously been selected due to gap closure from the cement mantle. Complete the reconstruction by snapping the chosen bearing into place (Fig. 7.34).

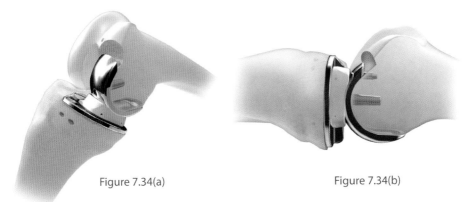

Figure 7.34(a)   Figure 7.34(b)

Close the wound in a routine manner. See Chapter 9 for post-operative management.

Instruments

(not shown to scale)

1   Tibial Tray Template

2   Quick-Release Drill Bit

3   Tibial Resection Headless Pin

4   Bone Pin

5   Pin Inserter/Extractor

6   Tibial Template Nail

7   Tibial Trial

8   Quick Release Drill Chuck

9   Slap Hammer

10   Tibial Groove Cutter (Cementless)

11   Woodson Cement Curette

12   Tibial Introducer/Impactor

13   Cement Removal Chisel

14   Universal Removal Hook

15   Trial Tibial Bearing Inserter/Extractor

16   Cementless Tibial Introducer/Impactor
17   Hex Driver

18   Tibial Groove Cutter (Cemented)

19   MCL Retractor

20   Tibial Shim

21   Microplasty Tibial Resector Body Tube

22   Silicone Ankle Strap

23   Femoral Sizing Spoon

24   IM Rod Pusher

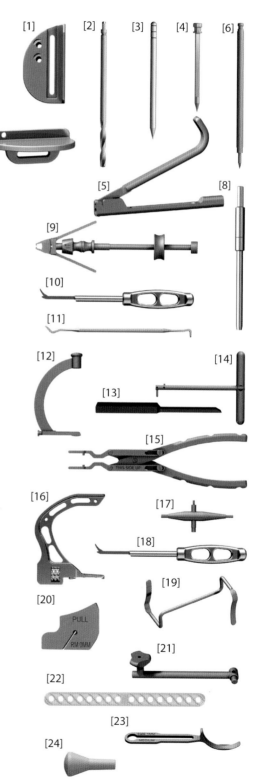

25   Ankle Yoke

26   IM Link

27   G-clamp

28   Anterior Bone Removal Shaft (Outer)

29   Cannulated IM Rod 300 mm

30   Cannulated IM Rod 200 mm

31   Femoral Impactor

32   Anterior Bone Removal Shaft (Inner)

33   Concise IM Awl

34   Toffee Hammer

35   Bone Collar Remover

36   Spigot

37   Metal Gap Gauge

38   Cement Key Drill

39   Quick Release Femoral Drill Bit

40   Single Peg Femoral Trial

41   Femoral Drill Guide

42   Anterior Bone Mill

43   Spherical Mill

44   Twin Peg Femoral Trial (US)

45   Anti-impingement Guide

46   Posterior Resection Guide

47   Gap Gauge, Medium

48   Trial Bearing, Medium

49   Osteophyte Chisel

50   Twin Peg Femoral Trial (not US)

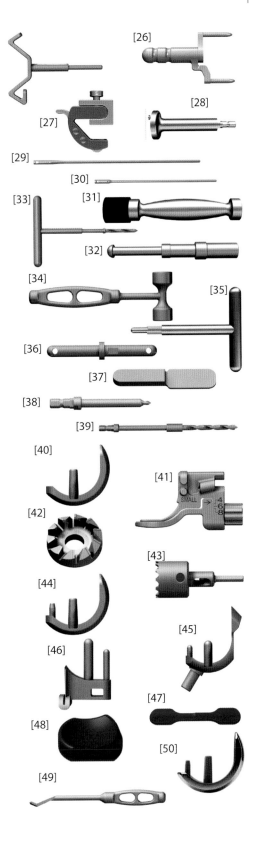

51 Femoral Drill Guide, Lateral Extension

52 Saw Blades (Reciprocating, oscillating and keel cut)

53 Tibial Saw Guide (upper part)

54 4 mm Drill

[51]

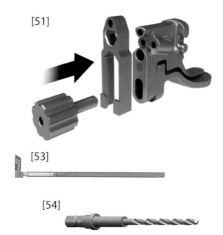

[52]

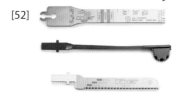

[53]

[54]

8

Medial Indications other than AMOA

Anteromedial OA (AMOA) accounts for more than 90% of the knees we consider suitable for OUKA. However, there are some other pathologies for which the operation may be appropriate.

Focal spontaneous osteonecrosis of the knee (SONK)

Avascular necrosis (AVN) of the medial femoral condyle or, more rarely, of the medial tibial plateau presents anatomical features very similar to those of AMOA (focal loss of bone and cartilage in the medial compartment with the ligaments intact) and therefore is theoretically suitable for OUKA (Fig. 8.1). The aetiology of AVN in the knee is poorly understood although factors such as steroid use, arthroscopy, systemic lupus erythematosus or trauma are sometimes implicated.

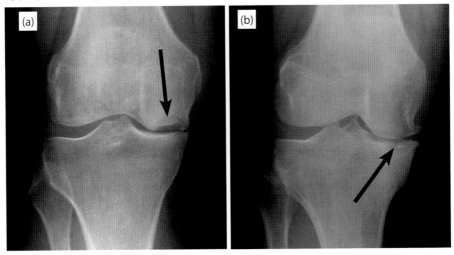

Figure 8.1 Avascular necrosis lesions in (a) femoral and (b) tibial condyles.

Early disease can usually be treated conservatively. However, once the disease is established, particularly if there is collapse, arthroplasty is usually required. Preoperative investigation should include MRI in addition to radiographs. Unlike AMOA, varus stressed radiographs of knees with AVN lesions usually do not show full-thickness cartilage loss, as the tibial cartilage is often preserved. The MRI substantially overestimates the extent of the damage because of the surrounding oedema associated with the condition in the acute phase. When assessing the extent of the disease the oedema should be ignored (Figs. 8.2(a) and (b)). MRI is useful for confirming the diagnosis and also ensuring there are no other lesions.

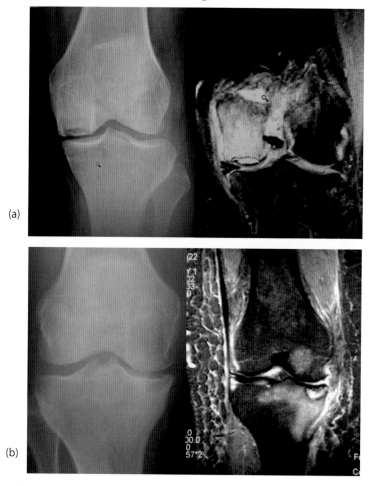

(a)

(b)

Figure 8.2 Plain AP radiograph and MRI scan showing (a) AVN of the medial femoral condyle and extensive oedema and (b) AVN of the medial tibial plateau and extensive oedema.

The surgical technique is similar to that of AMOA. Apart from the damage to the medial condyle, the rest of the knee is usually completely normal. If there is a very deep femoral defect, care has to be taken to ensure that too much bone is not milled from the femoral condyle. Therefore, the primary milling with the 0 spigot should be stopped when the mill is seen, in the window, to be about 2 mm from the end stop. Even if there is a deep defect, we have found, particularly with the two peg femoral component, that good fixation can be achieved. Traditionally we have used cemented fixation and have filled the defect with cement. We have recently started using cementless fixation but do not as yet have enough data to determine if this is reliable. There is also concern that there may be an increased risk of tibial plateau fracture if a cementless tibia is used.

Marmor [1] reported generally good results after UKA in 34 knees but with four failures at a mean follow-up of 5.5 years.

Langdown et al. [2] reported the results of 29 knees with medial compartment osteonecrosis (26 femoral and three tibial) treated by OUKA (Phases 2 and 3). The mean follow-up time was 8.2 years (range 1–13 years). There were no revisions, and the mean postoperative Oxford Knee Score (OKS) (37.8 ± 7.6, where 0 = poor; 48 = excellent) was not significantly different from the score for a similar group of osteoarthritic knees, matched for age, sex, and time since surgery, also treated by OUKA. We recently reviewed 33 cases with SONK treated with OUKA and matched them to 68 cases with OA followed up for 6.2 years (range 1 – 14). The OKS was 40 (SD 8) in SONK and 39 (SD 9) in OA and in SONK the 10-year survival was 97% (95% CI 81 - 100). In an independent series from Yoshida et al. [3] in Japan, there was a 10 year survival of 100% in 45 SONK cases with mean 6 year (range 1 – 14) follow up and OKS of 41. When the two series are combined, the survival of 99% at 10 years is relatively reliable as there are 78 cases.

We therefore conclude that although rare, SONK is a good indication for the OUKA.

ACL deficiency

If the ACL is ruptured and there is medial osteoarthritis, the erosions tend to extend to the back of the tibia so the disease is called posteromedial OA. In addition, there is usually cartilage loss on the posterior femur. The pathoanatomy is however different depending on whether the primary condition was anteromedial OA with secondary ACL rupture or primary ACL rupture with secondary OA.

With primary AMOA the disease begins anteriorly and centrally on the tibia with a varus deformity in extension. As the disease progresses posteriorly and the ACL fails, the varus deformity occurs also in flexion. The MCL shortens and the varus deformity becomes fixed. In addition the lateral subluxation of the tibia becomes fixed with increasing damage to the lateral side. Once these fixed deformities and lateral damage have occurred, the only solution is TKA.

In primary traumatic ACL rupture with secondary medial compartment arthritis, the cartilage defect and bony erosion tend to be central and posterior on the tibial plateau. This is likely to be due to recurrent episodes of giving way in which posterior femoral subluxation in the medial compartment can place a heavy load on the posterior horn of medial meniscus and posterior articular cartilage of the tibia, producing meniscal tears and arthritis. In some cases, the rest of the knee joint remains essentially intact with no shortening of the MCL. This is probably because, in extension, the intact distal femoral cartilage is in contact with the intact anterior tibial cartilage, so the varus deformity is corrected and the MCL is of normal length.

We, and others, treat such cases, in relatively young patients, by replacement of the ACL with a tendon graft and resurfacing of the medial compartment with OUKA. The operation is attractive to this group of patients who want to be active and hope to delay or avoid TKA. The ligament replacement and the resurfacing procedure can be done at the same time or in two stages. Pain is the usual presenting complaint. If this is the case, we address both pathologies offering a simultaneous UKA and ACL reconstruction. Occasionally, the patient presents with instability as the primary complaint and in these rare cases we offer ACL reconstruction first and only do UKA if pain subsequently becomes a problem.

Surgical technique for ACLR and OUKA

The set up is identical to the standard technique with the patient's thigh supported on the leg holder. A standard incision is employed extending the distal portion below the tibial tubercule to facilitate hamstring graft harvest.

The OUKA is undertaken first. The spoons/clamp do not predictably help define the tibial resection height and more anterior bone is usually removed because the defect is posteromedial in location. Care is taken to identify the medial tibial spine and the vertical cut is made just off the apex of the spine. Femoral preparation and balancing are undertaken in the usual manner. The joint line may be raised slightly, as the foot of the femoral drill guide references off bone posteriorly, not normal articular cartilage. As a result a larger spigot than normal may be required to balance the knee. The anti-impingement device is then used to remove posterior osteophytes and adequate anterior bone. Care is taken to use as large a tibial component as possible and to ensure it is supported by cortical bone all around its periphery and the keel cut is made using the 'keel cut' saw. Attention is then turned to the ACL reconstruction.

We favour a hamstring graft for the ACL reconstruction. The tendons are harvested from the lower portion of the wound and sized in standard fashion. An appropriate sized femoral tunnel is positioned anatomically through the wound with the knee hyperflexed in a figure of four position. Care is taken to position the tibial tunnel to exit in the posterior half of the ACL footprint lateral to the vertical tibial cut. The tunnel is generally more vertical than usual. The Oxford components are then fixed either using cement or cementless and an appropriate sized bearing is snapped home. The ACL reconstruction is fixed to the femur using the surgeon's fixation of choice. Finally the ACL is fixed to the tibia ensuring that the knee fully extends.

Results of combined ACLR & OUKA

We [4, 5] and others, have achieved good results in this young, active and highly demanding subgroup of patients. In our series of 52 cases with mean follow up of 5 years (range 1 – 10), the mean age was 51 (range 36 - 57). The mean OKS was 41, 98% were pleased and the 10 year survival was 91%. In 11 cases, the ACL reconstruction had been done before the OUKA. The results were independent of how well the original ACL reconstruction was performed so we tend to accept the original ACL reconstruction providing it is functioning. A kinematic study comparing OUKA with intact and reconstructed ACL demonstrated that the kinematics following ACL reconstruction were nearly normal. The relationship between patella tendon angle and knee flexion was normal although the position of the bearing was slightly more posterior on the tibia with a reconstructed ACL than in OUKAs with an intact ACL [5].

OUKA with absent ACL

Although we have always advised surgeons not to do OUKA with a non-functional ACL, we have occasionally done this. These may be elderly unfit patients with correctable deformities but without an ACL. We would have justified this because the risks of UKA were substantially less than those of TKA. Also there are patients who are very keen to have a UKR rather than a TKR even though they have ACL damage. We have reviewed the outcome of these cases, with mean age of 65 years. At average follow up of 5 years, there was one failure as a patient developed lateral compartment OA at 3.4 years, needing a TKA [6]. A kinematic study has shown that ACLD patients function less well (slower step up) than those with an intact ACL [7]. Furthermore, the kinematics are less predictable with atypical bearing movements in mid flexion.

Despite the abnormality in kinematics the results in this small cohort are acceptable. However, the indications for OUKA without ACL are not defined. The indications are very narrow as it is only appropriate for a very small percentage of patients with OA and ACLD. If the indications were too broad, then a high failure rate would be expected as in previous studies [8]. Furthermore the surgery is more difficult with a deficient ACL because of the damage to the posterior tibia. We therefore continue to recommend that an OUKA should not be implanted with an absent or non-functional ACL (non-functional is demonstrated by ACL rupture when pulled with a tendon hook during surgery).

Failed upper tibial osteotomy

We, and others, have used OUKA for the revision of knees with persistent symptoms after valgus osteotomy of the upper tibia, although there have been few reports on the outcome.

Thornhill and Scott [9], using the Brigham implant, referred to some successes but noted technical problems with ligamentous instability.

Vorlat et al. [10] reviewed 38 medial OUKAs, of which six were performed on knees with failed high tibial osteotomy (HTO). Two of these had to be revised because of progression of arthritis in the lateral compartment. The failure rate of 33% in the HTO group was compared with a 6.3% failure rate in the group with primary OA.

Rees et al. [11] collected data (from three sources) on 631 OUKAs, 18 of which had been performed for failed HTO and the remainder for primary anteromedial OA. The reason for revision of the original HTO was persistent medial pain in every case, and in all but one there had been undercorrection of the varus deformity. The mean cumulative follow-up times of the the failed HTO and primary AMOA groups were similar (5.6 years and 5.4 years, respectively) and there were no significant differences between their mean ages or sex ratios. The mean time to revision was 2.9 years for the HTO group (five knees) and 4.1 years for the primary OA group (19 knees). The cumulative survival rates at 10 years were 66 % and 96 %, respectively (log rank comparison $P < 0.0001$). The reason for all the OUKA failures in the HTO group was persistent pain and accelerated lateral wear. The explanation for this mode of failure may be biomechanical. OUKA corrects the varus deformity intra-articularly. If the varus has already been corrected (even partially) by an extra-articular osteotomy, valgus alignment may result, with overloading of the lateral compartment. The failure rate was independent of the type of osteotomy.

We believe that previous tibial osteotomy is a contraindication to OUKA. The revision rate of 34 % at a mean follow-up of 5.4 years is much worse than the results reported for TKA after HTO by Meding et al. [12]. They reported one implant failure in 33 knees followed for a mean of 8.7 years after TKA revision of failed tibial osteotomies.

Valenzuela et al. [13] compared clinical and radiological outcomes between UKA after HTO (n=22); TKA after HTO (n=18); and primary UKA (n=22). OKS, AKSS, hip/knee/ankle angles, mechanical axis and patella height were evaluated pre- and postoperatively. At a mean of 64 months (range 19 - 180) postoperatively, the mean OKS were 43.8, 43.3 and 42.5 respectively (p=0.73) with similar AKSS-O and AKSS-F. The authors' conclusion, which was different to ours, was that UKA can be safely performed after HTO. There may therefore be a role for OUKA after failed HTO. However, the indications for this are unclear so we still do not recommend it.

Post-traumatic osteoarthritis

Tibial plateau fracture might intuitively lend itself to UKA and some cases have been treated in this way. The number is low because the medial condyle is less often fractured than the lateral condyle. Limitation of the flexion range is not uncommon after intra-articular fracture and excludes some cases, as would coincidental liga-ment damage.

We have occasionally successfully implanted OUKA in patients with medial OA following malunion of femoral or tibial shaft fracture. This is only appropriate if the angular malunion is small. If the varus deformity at the fracture is large, it is probably best to correct the deformity first because this may help the symptoms rather like an HTO.

Overall the results of the OUKA in post-traumatic osteoarthritis have been vari-able, and we have too little data either to support or reject this pathology as an occasional indication

Bicompartmental replacement

We currently do not perform or recommend primary bicompartmental replacement using the OUKA. This may seem surprising considering the success of bicompartmental OUKA with an intact ACL achieved in the past (see Chapter 1) and as other surgeons are regularly perfoming bicompartmental replacement with fixed bearing UKA [14]. Bicompartmental replacement is commonly a medial and lateral UKA or a medial UKA and patellofemoral replacement (PFR).

In patients with AMOA, neither the state of the PFJ nor the presence of anterior knee pain influence the outcome. Therefore, a combined OUKA and PFR could not be expected to improve the outcome whatever the state of the PFJ or wherever the pain. Indeed, it could only make it worse by adding the relatively high failure rate of the PFR. The only exception might be in patients with severe lateral damage with grooving and subluxation. This is however so rare (<1%) that we would do a TKA in this situation.

In patients with medial compartment OA with an intact ACL, it is rare to find that the lateral compartment is not acceptable for a medial UKA (full thickness joint space on valgus stress and ignoring medial ulceration of the lateral condyle). If there is narrowing of the lateral compartment with full thickness medial loss, this is suggestive of an inflammatory condition so a TKA is probably best. The presence of a central lateral ulcer of full thickness on a valgus stress radiograph is a potential indication for bicompartmental surgery but this is rare. Therefore in general we see little role for a primary medial and lateral UKA. As discussed in Chapter 11, we would do lateral OUKA for arthritis progression after medial OUKA or a medial OUKA for arthritis progression after lateral OUKA.

Inflammatory arthritis

OUKA is contraindicated in the inflammatory forms of arthritis because they are diseases of the synovium and therefore cannot be limited to one compartment. Therefore, if an OUKA is implanted, progression of the disease to the other compartments is likely to occur. However, the loss of cartilage in early rheumatoid arthritis can be unicompartmental and has been mistaken for anteromedial OA and treated by OUKA [15]. The clinician needs to be aware of this pitfall because it results in early failure due to involvement of the other compartments of the knee.

With the widespread use of disease modifying drugs in inflammatory arthritis, the role of OUKA may change. It may be that it will be appropriate to use an OUKA in a patient with well controlled inflammatory arthritis. However, until there is evidence to support this, we do not recommend it.

References

1. Marmor L. Unicompartmental arthroplasty for osteonecrosis of the knee joint. *Clin Orthop Relat Res* 1993; (**294**): 247-53.

2. Langdown AJ, Pandit H, Price AJ, Dodd CA, Murray DW, Svard UC, Gibbons CL. Oxford medial unicompartmental arthroplasty for focal spontaneous osteonecrosis of the knee. *Acta Orthop* 2005; **76**(5): 688-92.

3. Yoshida K, Tada M, Yoshida H, Takei S, Fukuoka S, Nakamura H. Oxford phase 3 unicompartmental knee arthroplasty in Japan – clinical results in greater than one thousand cases over ten years. *J Arthroplasty* 2013; **28**(9 Suppl): 168-71.

4. Pandit H, Beard DJ, Jenkins C, Kimstra Y, Thomas NP, Dodd CA, Murray DW. Combined anterior cruciate reconstruction and Oxford unicompartmental knee arthroplasty. *J Bone Joint Surg Br* 2006; **88**(7): 887-92.

5. Weston-Simons JS, Pandit H, Jenkins C, Jackson WF, Price AJ, Gill HS, Dodd CA, Murray DW. Outcome of combined unicompartmental knee replacement and combined or sequential anterior cruciate ligament reconstruction: a study of 52 cases with mean follow-up of five years. *J Bone Joint Surg Br* 2012; **94**(9): 1216-20.

6. Boissonneault A, Pandit H, Pegg E, Jenkins C, Gill HS, Dodd CA, Gibbons CL, Murray DW. No difference in survivorship after unicompartmental knee arthroplasty with or without an intact anterior cruciate ligament. *Knee Surg Sports Traumatol Arthrosc* 2013 Nov; **21**(11):2480-6)

7. Pegg E, Mancuso F, Alinejad M, Mellon SJ, Hamilton T, Marks B, Dodd CAF, Murray DW, Pandit H. Behavior of anterior cruciate ligament (ACL) deficient knee after unicompartmental knee arthroplasty (UKA) (Poster #758). AAOS, Las Vegas, USA, March 2015.

8. Goodfellow JW, Kershaw CJ, Benson MK, O'Connor JJ. The Oxford Knee for unicompartmental osteoarthritis. The first 103 cases. *J Bone Joint Surg Br* 1988; **70**(5): 692-701.

9. Thornhill TS, Scott RD. Unicompartmental total knee arthroplasty. *Orthop Clin North Am* 1989; **20**(2): 245-56.

10. Vorlat P, Verdonk R, Schauvlieghe H. The Oxford unicompartmental knee prosthesis: a 5-year follow-up. *Knee Surg Sports Traumatol Arthrosc* 2000; **8**(3): 154-8.

11. Rees JL, Price AJ, Lynskey TG, Svard UC, Dodd CA, Murray DW. Medial unicompartmental arthroplasty after failed high tibial osteotomy. *J Bone Joint Surg Br* 2001; **83**(7): 1034-6.

12. Meding JB, Keating EM, Ritter MA, Faris PM. Total knee arthroplasty after high tibial osteotomy. A comparison study in patients who had bilateral total knee replacement. *J Bone Joint Surg Am* 2000; **82**(9): 1252-9.

13. Valenzuela GA, Jacobson NA, Buzas D, Koreckij TD, Valenzuela RG, Teitge RA. Unicompartmental knee replacement after high tibial osteotomy: Invalidating a contraindication. *Bone Joint J* 2013; **95-B**(10): 1348-53.

14. Parratte S, Pauly V, Aubaniac JM, Argenson JN. Survival of bicompartmental knee arthroplasty at 5 to 23 years. *Clin Orthop Relat Res.* 2010 Jan;**468**(1):64-72.

9

Postoperative Management and Radiography

Pain control

In the early postoperative period, good pain control is essential. Regimes of pain management appropriate for total knee arthroplasty may not be suited to the very rapid mobilisation that is possible after UKA through a minimally invasive approach. A multimodal approach is best with minimal opiate use. Different regimes are used successfully in different institutions.

Intraoperative local anaesthesia

We have found that a useful technique is a local anaesthetic block injected into the damaged tissues in the last stages of the operation. Our technique was developed from that of Kohan L and Kerr D [1].

Ropivacaine 300 mg, ketorolac 30 mg, and epinephrine 0.5 mg are made up to a total volume of 100 ml with normal saline. Adrenaline is added to a ratio of 1:200,000. The mixture is put into two 50-ml syringes. Before the components are implanted, the mixture is injected through a 19 gauge spinal needle into any tissue that was damaged during the operation. This is done methodically so that no area is missed, with particular attention being paid to the posterior capsule , the periosteum around the implant, and the margins of the incision in the quadriceps muscle. The skin is infiltrated up to 3 cm from the margins of the wound and 10 ml is reserved until the end of the procedure to inject around the drain site, if a drain is used.

This treatment usually results in very little pain when the patient wakes from the anaesthetic, allowing immediate resumption of knee flexion and walking. Occasionally, however, the local anaesthetic is slow to work and patients awake with severe pain. Pain immediately after the operation can be more reliably avoided by regional nerve blocks given at the beginning of the procedure. They have the additional advantage of minimising the dose of general anaesthetic required, which helps with more rapid recovery. However, femoral and sciatic nerve blocks with bupivacaine, and epidural anaesthesia, may have motor effects that delay mobilisation. Therefore, we now use prilocaine nerve blocks or a short-acting spinal anaesthetic. The effects of these have usually worn off 2–3 hours after the operation when the patients start to walk.

Severe pain may occur on the second day when all these drugs have ceased to act (so called 'rebound pain'). This can be controlled by instilling local anaesthetic into the joint through a fine (epidural) catheter inserted into the knee before wound closure. The catheter should be fitted with a bacterial filter to minimise the risk of infection. The morning after surgery, 20 ml of 0.5% bupivacaine is instilled into the joint. (If a suction drain was used it should be clamped.) The catheter (and drain) are then removed. In a randomised controlled trial, we found that this technique can provide good pain relief for a further 24 hours [2].

In recent years, long acting local anaesthetic (liposomal bupivacaine) has been used for pain relief after UKA. It is reported to last for up to 72 hours, allowing UKA to be performed as a day case in the majority of cases (J Barrington - personal communication). We do not have experience with the use of liposomal bupivicaine as it is not licensed for use in the UK.

In addition to the local anaesthetic, we use high doses of oral non-steroidal anti-inflammatory drugs with a gastroprotective agent such as ranitidine or omeprazole.

Blood loss

The amount of blood lost is small and transfusion is rarely required. We routinely use a thigh tourniquet for the operation. Occasionally, in a patient with a compromised circulation, we have carried out the procedure without a tourniquet but it is much more difficult.

We insert a vacuum drain into the joint at the end of the operation. It is placed in the lateral gutter of the knee so that it does not interfere with early knee flexion. Occasionally, in the absence of a drain, there are acute haemarthroses in the post-operative period which can delay rehabilitation. The drain is removed the morning after surgery (or 4–5 hours postoperatively if the patient is to go home on the day of operation).

We have recently started to use Tranexamic acid. The evidence suggests that whether this is used topically or intravenously just before the tourniquet is released, it is effective at decreasing blood loss [3]. With this approach a drain is not necessary [4].

It is our belief that unless patients are very high risk, and have for example had a previous DVT/PE, that anticoagulent drugs such as Warfarin or Low Molecular Weight Heparin are not necessary. This is because the risk of thromboembolism is low with rapid mobilisation the UKA patient. Furthermore they tend to cause knee and leg swelling and bruising which slows recovery. Unfortunately we currently are required to use this kind of medication.

Rehabilitation

Range of motion

Patients recuperate from UKA more rapidly and more predictably than after TKA and do not require formal exercise regimes or outpatient physiotherapy appointments to recover knee movement. Vigorous exercises are counterproductive by making the knee more painful and swollen.

On the day of the operation, while the local anaesthetic block is providing good pain relief and the drain is in place, most patients can easily perform an active straight leg raise and flex the knee to 110°. Thereafter, the joint tends to become more swollen, pain relief is less complete, and flexion is more difficult. Exercises to encourage flexion at this stage may make the knee worse, and patients should be allowed to limit knee movement within the range that is comfortable. Education of physiotherapists may be necessary especially if the unit is new to UKA. They may well treat the patient as though they have a TKA which is understandable but counterproductive as the patient often loses confidence if pushed too hard. By the end of the first week, pain and swelling subside. Motion is gradually regained in succeeding weeks, usually recovering to what it was preoperatively after a month and often improving further thereafter.

Ambulation

Most patients can start to walk about 2–3 hours after the operation. Early walking seems to improve the pain relief. If there is quadriceps weakness, splinting the knee may help.

Early discharge

With rapid recovery, it is possible to discharge patients from hospital early. Repicci and Eberle [5] were able to treat 80% of their patients with less than 24 hours in hospital.

We undertook a randomised study, within the setting of the UK National Health Service 10 years ago, to compare the effect of discharge on the day after operation with our practice at that stage which was discharge on day 4 or 5 [6,7]. In appropriately selected patients, discharge on the day after operation did not prejudice the speed of recovery or increase the incidence of complications. However, it did result in a significant cost saving [8]. In order that patients are suitable for early discharge, they must be relatively fit and live locally, there must be a support system so that patients can telephone if they have problems and be readmitted if necessary.

Increasingly, patients having the OUKA are being discharged on the day of surgery. Up to 80% of patients undergoing UKA in some centres are discharged on the same day. These patients undergo a prior rigorous health check up, have a detailed outpatient consultation including counselling about advantages of day case surgery and are provided adequate support (including visits and 24 hour telephone service) after surgery. Education of patients and staff is essential. In addition reliable pain control and postoperative support is required. Early outcomes have been shown to be better than or as good as those with conventional discharge without any increase in readmission rates or mortality or morbidity [9].

Duration of recovery

The early rapid recovery of function after UKA tends to slow down in later weeks. Often, at 6 weeks, patients are disappointed that they still have symptoms (although these are usually less severe than those experienced at the same stage after TKA). Therefore, we warn patients before discharge that their rapid rate of recovery may not continue and that they may still have some pain medially, numbness laterally, swelling of the knee, stiffness and restriction of extension and flexion for three months. Night pain around the six week mark is a not uncommon complaint. The patients recover quickly, and therefore stop taking pain relief medication and become increasingly active. As a result they may have increasing symptoms. They should be warned not to stop night time medication too soon. If a patient does have increasing symptoms, they should decrease their level of activity.

Overall, most of the recovery occurs within the first three months. After that the symptoms continue to improve slowly for about a year.

Postoperative radiology

Good postoperative radiographs are necessary as a baseline for comparison with later films and to allow 'quality control' of the surgical technique.

For these purposes, the standard methods of aligning the X-ray beam are neither sufficiently accurate, nor repeatable enough. To assess the positions of the two metal components, the X-ray beam must be centred on one component and aligned with it in two planes. The resulting projection of the other component can then be used to deduce their relative positions. We therefore suggest that fluoroscopically aligned radiographs are taken (screened X-rays). If this is not possible, reasonably good radiographs can be obtained using a digital system. Low dose images are used to adjust the position. When good alignment is achieved, a standard image is obtained.

In the anteroposterior projection, the patient lies supine on the X-ray table and the leg and the X-ray beam are manipulated under fluoroscopic control until the tibial component appears exactly end-on in silhouette. The radiograph is then taken (Fig. 9.1).

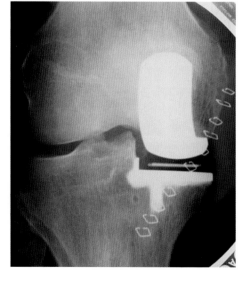

Figure 9.1 Fluoroscopically centred anteroposterior radiograph.

In this projection, the alignment of the beam with the flat orthogonal surfaces (horizontal tray and vertical lateral wall and keel) allows great accuracy and reproducibility.

In the lateral projection, the patient lies supine on the couch with the knee flexed 20°–30°. The fluoroscope is rotated through 90° so that the X-ray beam is parallel to the floor and centred on the femoral component (Fig. 9.2). (The tibial implant is not so useful in this projection because it offers no vertical surface and its horizontal surface is obscured by its lateral wall.) Therefore, the lateral projection is not as precise or as reproducible as the anteroposterior projection.

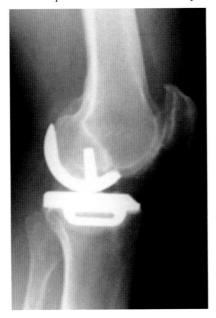

Figure 9.2 Fluoroscopically centred lateral radiograph.

Radiographs taken in this way can be repeated at any time interval in the knowledge that (at least in the anteroposterior films) the projections of the tibial component are always the same. Therefore, small changes in the relationships of the components to one another and to the bones can be detected. Furthermore, because the X-ray beam is parallel to the tibial plateau, the state of its bone/implant interface is always reliably imaged. Without properly aligned postoperative films for comparison, later radiographs are difficult, or impossible, to interpret. Subsequent radiographs should be undertaken using the same technique to allow accurate comparison.

The postoperative radiographs can be used to measure the accuracy with which the prosthesis has been implanted. As the femoral component is spherical and the bearing spherically concave, the orientation of the components are not critical. Our studies suggest that 10° of mal-orientation of the femoral component and 5° mal-orientation of the tibial component do not compromise the outcome [10]. However, the positioning of the components is important (as is the way the soft tissues are balanced but this cannot be assessed radiographically).

Tibial component

On the anteroposterior projection, the vertical cut should be just medial to the apex of the medial spine. The component should appear approximately perpendicular (±5°) to the tibial axis (Fig. 9.3). The medial margin should always reach to the medial tibial cortex and may overhang a little (no more than 2 mm as greater overhang may cause soft tissue irritation). The bone/implant interface should show a complete cement layer with a few millimetres penetration into the bone. (Cement penetration is deeper laterally and around the keel than medially, where the subchondral bone is less porous.) If the vertical saw cuts have been made too deep (increasing the risk of fracture), they may be outlined by opaque cement or show up as vertical lucent lines. (The horizontal saw cut may undermine the tibial eminence laterally but this has no serious consequences.)

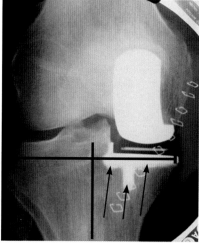

Figure 9.3 See text for details

With cementless implants, often a narrow radiolucency may be present on the immediate post-operative radiograph. It is typically partial and suggests incomplete seating of the tibial component. This is of no consequence as, with the passage of time, the component will settle and the radiolucency will disappear.

(a)

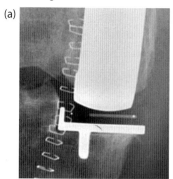

(b)

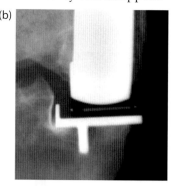

Figure 9.4 Post-operative radiograph (a) of a cementless tibial component showing a radiolucent zone at the interface which had disappeared by the time the one-year radiograph (b) was obtained.

On the lateral projection, the tibial component should slope downwards and backwards at about 7° (±5°) to the tibial axis (Fig. 9.5). The posterior edge of the component should reach to the posterior cortex but should not overhang. Overhang implies that the posterior cortex was damaged when the groove for the keel was excavated. Extra care must be taken whilst preparing the keel slot in female patients with small bones.

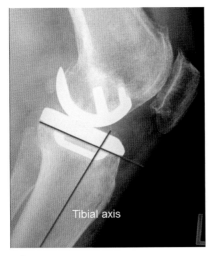

Figure 9.5 Tibial component at 7° slope to tibial axis

Femoral component

On the anteroposterior projection, the femoral component usually has the appearance of a 'bucket seat' (Fig. 9.6), with the component internally rotated relative to the tibia. The explanation for this results from the obligatory 'screw home' mechanism of the knee in extension. The components are implanted in a neutral position relative to each other in flexion. The radiograph is taken in extension. With extension there is internal rotation of the femur (see Figs. 3.2 - 3.4) and thus of the femoral component relative to the tibial component. The femoral component should be parallel to the mechanical axis, but ±10° of varus/valgus positioning is acceptable (see Fig. 6.15).

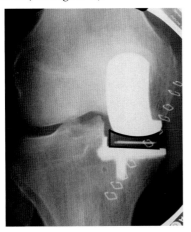

Figure 9.6 See text for details

On the lateral projection, the fixation peg should be flexed to the long axis of the femur (Fig. 9.7). With the introduction of a two peg femur and the microplasty technique, we aim for the femoral component to be flexed by 10° (±10°) to the femoral axis.

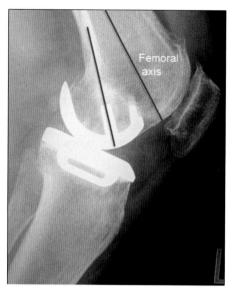

Figure 9.7 Femoral component flexed relative to the femoral axis.

The bone/implant interfaces of the femoral component are not as readily seen as those of the tibial implant. The inner surface of the inferior facet of the femoral component is concave, so that interface is hidden by the metal. The only interface that is readily imaged is at the flat posterior facet. If the radiographic technique has resulted in a true lateral silhouette, that interface is visible. It should present a thin parallel-sided layer of cement, with shallow penetration of the dense femoral bone. The central peg of the implant should appear solidly cemented in the drill hole.

Meniscal bearing

On the anteroposterior projection, the mediolateral position of the bearing on the tibial plateau is deduced from the position of the radio-opaque markers. In the current bearings, there is a line across the front and two small balls at the back corners (Fig. 9.6). The bearing should lie with its lateral edge 2–3 mm away from the vertical wall of the tibial implant. Its position is explained by remembering that the bearing was positioned 1 mm from the wall with the knee flexed. The radiograph is taken with the knee extended, and extension causes the bearing to glide not only forward on the plateau but also medially, away from the wall (Chapter 6, Fig. 6.17).

Impingement

The proper function of the OUKA depends upon the unimpeded freedom of the bearing to translate on the surfaces of the fixed components. The limits to its movement must be set by tension in the cruciate and collateral ligaments and in the posterior capsule, not by impingement against bone, retained osteophytes or fragments of cement.

The lateral projection may reveal retained posterior osteophytes on the femur or extruded cement at the back of the tibial component, either of which may impinge on the posterior edge of the bearing in flexion (Fig. 9.8).

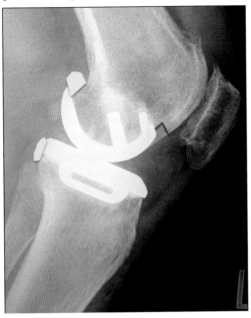

Figure 9.8 The sites of possible impingement of the bearing are indicated.

Impingement anteriorly, due to inadequate removal of femoral bone from in front of the component, is the most frequent finding in retrieved bearings, but radiographs do not show this site well.

Impingement between an 'anvil' osteophyte just anterior to the ACL insertion on the tibia and osteophytes in the roof of the notch may occur and limit extension. Confirm that the anvil osteophyte is removed.

Radiolucent lines

The geometry of the tibial implant and the method of fluoroscopically controlled radiography that we have employed to image it, have provided abundant evidence of the radiographic appearances of the bone/cement/implant interface under that component. The radiolucent 'line' seen on a radiograph is the image of a thin layer of relatively lucent material that can be seen only if the X-ray beam is parallel to it[11]. The degree of accuracy required cannot be regularly achieved without the use of screened alignment (Fig. 9.9).

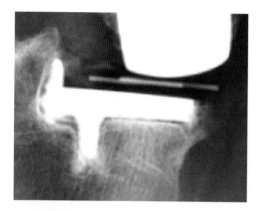

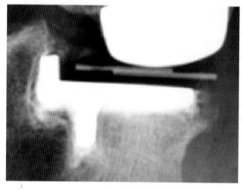

Figure 9.9 Two fluoroscopic images of the same knee taken one after the other. In the lower film the X-ray beam was tilted 2°, and the complete radiolucent line beneath the medial part of the plateau has disappeared.

Cemented components

The almost ubiquitous appearance of radiolucency beneath the tibial components of the biocompartmental cemented Oxford Knee (Phase 1) when using the fluoroscopic technique was reported in 1984 [12]. A radiolucent line was observed under at least one of the tibial components in 77 of 80 knees (96%) in which radiodense cement had been used. Most of the radiolucencies were incomplete. The most common site was medial to the keel in the medial implants and lateral to the keel in the lateral implants. Radiolucency was also common around and under the keel. The radiolucent line was usually no more than 1 mm thick and none exceeded 3 mm.

The radiodense line

A striking feature of the radiographs was the presence of a thin radiodense line in the bone immediately adjacent to the radiolucencies. It was present in all but three of the 77 knees with radiolucent lines. It was also present, and more readily seen, in all the 11 knees in which the components had been fixed with radiolucent cement (precluding the demonstration of the radiolucent line, the presence of which was inferred). In all these knees, a thin bone shell completely surrounded both tibial components, and the bone trabeculae could be seen inserting into it, as they do into the normal subchondral bone plate.

Time of appearance

The radiolucent and the radiodense lines appear at the same time, usually between 6 and 12 months after the arthroplasty. Once developed, they do not progress.

Natural history

Although the study referred to above was of bicompartmental Phase 1 Oxford prostheses (and some prototype devices implanted before late 1978) [12], our subsequent experience has confirmed nearly all the conclusions drawn from it. The incidence of radiolucencies in cemented unicompartmental replacement with the Phase 2 and 3 implants is somewhat lower (75%) than that mentioned above which referred to knees not compartments. No correlation has ever been found between clinical symptoms and the presence of radiolucency, and Röntgen stereometric analysis (RSA) studies have shown no association with the rate of subsidence of the tibial component [13].

In a study of 26 knees examined radiographically 1 year and 10+ years after OUKA (Phases 1 and 2), 21 had partial or complete radiolucent lines around the tibial implant Fig. 9.10) [14]. All but one were ≤1 mm thick. Only two had progressed between the early and late reviews, and only one of these was 2 mm thick.

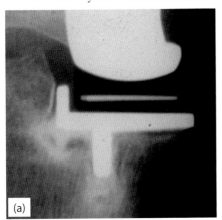 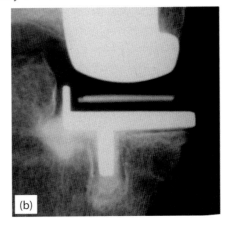

(a) (b)

Figure 9.10 Physiological radiolucent and radiodense lines at (a) 1 year and (b) 10 years after implantation.

Berger et al. [15] reported an incidence of 49% partial or complete radiolucency around the tibial component of the Miller–Galante unicompartmental implant at 3–7 years review. None of them progressed after the third year and there was no instance of loosening of a component. The radiographs were not screened for alignment, which may explain the lower incidence. An RCT (56 knees in 48 patients) looking at fixed (Miller-Galante) versus mobile UKA (OUKA) showed a significantly lower incidence of radiolucent lines at the bone/implant interface with the mobile as compared to fixed UKA (8% vs. 37% respectively, $p<0.05$) at two-year follow up [16].

Significance

We conclude that radiolucent lines around the tibial component of the cemented OUKA are the rule not the exception, and that the radiographic technique mainly determines how frequently they are observed. They are probably as common around the femoral component, but are more difficult to demonstrate there. They do not appear to be the cause of symptoms nor evidence of loosening of the component. Therefore, we refer to the radiographic appearances described above as 'physiological radiolucency'. They can usually be distinguished from the pathological lucency that surrounds an infected or a loose component by thickness and the presence of the radiodense line. The physiological lucent line is almost always <2 mm thick and defined by a thin radiodense bone plate; the pathological lesion is thicker, and the margins of the radiolucent zone are characteristically ill defined.

Cementless OUKA

Pandit et al. [17] reported on a RCT comparing 62 patients who received either cemented (n = 32) or cementless (n = 30) versions of the OUKA. The tibial interfaces were studied with fluoroscopically-aligned radiographs. At one year there was no difference in clinical outcome between the two groups. Narrow radiolucent lines were seen at the bone-implant interfaces in 75% of cemented tibial components. These were partial in 43%, and complete in 32%. In the cementless implants, partial radiolucencies were seen in 7% and complete radiolucencies in none. These differences are statistically significant (p < 0.0001) and imply satisfactory bone ingrowth into the cementless implants. These results continued to show the same trends at five years with no complete radiolucencies in the cementless group (28% in the cemented implants), confirming stable and superior fixation with the cementless OUKA as compared to the cemented OUKA.

Radiolucencies are commonly seen beside the vertical wall but we consider them to be of no significance as this is non-weightbearing.

We have seen very few cases of complete radiolucencies around cementless components so we know little about their significance. The cases we have seen have been associated with tibial subsidence and pain, at about three to six months post surgery. With time, the symptoms settled and the radiolucency disappeared, suggesting that the implant had become securely fixed (Fig. 9.4). We would not have expected this to occur with a cemented component. We have not seen complete radiolucencies around cementless components in the long term.

References

1. Kerr DR, Kohan L. Local infiltration analgesia: a technique for the control of acute postoperative pain following knee and hip surgery: a case study of 325 patients. *Acta Orthop* 2008; **79**(2): 174-83.

2. Weston-Simons JS, Pandit H, Haliker V, Dodd CA, Popat MT, Murray DW. Intra-articular local anaesthetic on the day after surgery improves pain and patient satisfaction after Unicompartmental Knee Replacement: a randomised controlled trial. *Knee* 2012; **19**(4): 352-5.

3. Patel JN, Spanyer JM, Smith LS, Huang J, Yakkanti MR, Malkani AL. Comparison of intravenous versus topical tranexamic acid in total knee arthroplasty: a prospective randomized study. *J Arthroplasty* 2014; **29**(8): 1528-31.

4. Zhang Q, Zhang Q, Guo W, Liu Z, Cheng L, Zhu G. No need for use of drainage after minimally invasive unicompartmental knee arthroplasty: a prospective randomized, controlled trial. *Arch Orthop Trauma Surg* 2015; **135**(5): 709-13.

5. Repicci JA, Eberle RW. Minimally invasive surgical technique for unicondylar knee arthroplasty. *J South Orthop Assoc* 1999; **8**(1): 20-7; discussion 7.

6. Beard DJ, Murray DW, Rees JL, Price AJ, Dodd CA. Accelerated recovery for unicompartmental knee replacement–a feasibility study. *Knee* 2002; **9**(3): 221-4.

7. Reilly KA, Beard DJ, Barker KL, Dodd CA, Price AJ, Murray DW. Efficacy of an accelerated recovery protocol for Oxford unicompartmental knee arthroplasty – a randomised controlled trial. *Knee* 2005; **12**(5): 351-7.

8. Shakespeare D, Jeffcote B. Unicondylar arthroplasty of the knee – cheap at half the price? *Knee* 2003; **10**(4): 357-61.

9. Gondusky JS, Choi L, Khalaf N, Patel J, Barnett S, Gorab R. Day of surgery discharge after unicompartmental knee arthroplasty: an effective perioperative pathway. *J Arthroplasty* 2014; **29**(3): 516-9.

10. Gulati A, Chau R, Simpson DJ, Dodd CA, Gill HS, Murray DW. Influence of component alignment on outcome for unicompartmental knee replacement. *Knee* 2009; **16**(3): 196-9.

11 O'Connor J, Goodfellow J, Perry N. Fixation of the tibial components of the Oxford Knee. *Orthop Clin Nth America*. 1982;13:65-87.

12. Tibrewal SB, Grant KA, Goodfellow JW. The radiolucent line beneath the tibial components of the Oxford meniscal knee. *J Bone Joint Surg Br* 1984; **66**(4): 523-8.

13. Kendrick BJ, Kaptein BL, Valstar ER, Gill HS, Jackson WF, Dodd CA, Price AJ, Murray DW. Cemented versus cementless Oxford unicompartmental knee arthroplasty using radiostereometric analysis: A randomised controlled trial. *Bone Joint J* 2015; **97-B**(2): 185-91.

14. Weale AE, Murray DW, Crawford R, Psychoyios V, Bonomo A, Howell G, O'Connor J, Goodfellow JW. Does arthritis progress in the retained compartments after 'Oxford' medial unicompartmental arthroplasty? A clinical and radiological study with a minimum ten-year follow-up. *J Bone Joint Surg Br* 1999; **81**(5): 783-9.

15. Berger RA, Nedeff DD, Barden RM, Sheinkop MM, Jacobs JJ, Rosenberg AG, Galante JO. Unicompartmental knee arthroplasty. Clinical experience at 6- to 10-year followup. *Clin Orthop Relat Res* 1999; (**367**): 50-60.

16. Li MG, Yao F, Joss B, Ioppolo J, Nivbrant B, Wood D. Mobile vs. fixed bearing unicondylar knee arthroplasty: A randomized study on short term clinical outcomes and knee kinematics. *Knee* 2006; **13**(5): 365-70.

17. Pandit H, Jenkins C, Beard DJ, Gallagher J, Price AJ, Dodd CA, Goodfellow JW, Murray DW. Cementless Oxford unicompartmental knee replacement shows reduced radiolucency at one year. *J Bone Joint Surg Br* 2009; **91**(2): 185-9.

10

Clinical Results

The results of UKA can be gathered from three main sources: the reports of the national registers, observational studies (both comparative and case series), and randomised controlled trials. In this chapter, we attempt an overview of the clinical results of UKA in general and OUKA in particular. It is important to note that the 'result' is of the whole arthroplasty which includes the indications, the technique as well as the implant.

National registers

In Joint Registries, longitudinal data is collected from large numbers of participating institutions before being assembled centrally. In most cases, a report is issued annually and raw data are released on request for research studies. The principal aim of joint registries is to facilitate the identification of poorly-performing implants at the earliest possible stage, allowing modification or abandonment of such implants before large numbers are implanted. Registers collect data when a joint replacement implant is inserted, ideally from the surgeons. Although there is some variation between registers, a revision operation is usually considered to have occurred the second time an implant is inserted in a particular joint. Using this information, cumulative revision rates (CRR) can be calculated. They are our best source of information on the epidemiology and demography of arthroplasty.

The first national joint registry was established in Sweden in 1975. Since then, national joint registers have been established in Finland (1980), Norway (1987), Denmark (1995), Australia, and New Zealand (both 1998), amongst others. The National Joint Registry for England and Wales (NJR) was established in 2003 and is currently the largest database of joint replacements in the world.

The principal advantage of national joint registers is the large number of cases they report. In some cases, participation is near-universal (and in some cases is obligatory) which minimises the problems of reporting and publication bias. The fact that national joint registers study the population as a whole allows great diversity within cases studied in terms of implant type, surgical technique and experience, patient selection and postoperative regimen. The large overall number of cases allows the study of these subgroups with acceptable power. National registers have additional benefits in allowing surgeons to compare their results with their peers', and allowing easy identification of implants in need of recall.

However, national registers remain imperfect tools to measure outcome. The large number of cases reported, and the reliance on operating units to report their cases, limits the quantity of data that can be gathered on each patient. In all national registers, the primary measure of outcome is the rate of revision surgery; whilst this has the benefit of being objective and easy to measure, it has several deficiencies. When a revision occurs, the implant is considered to have failed. If it has not been revised, it is considered to have survived and be a success even if it is painful and has poor function. Implant survival is a solid end-point and has been described as the point at which both the surgeon and the patient agree that revision is preferable to continuing with the prosthesis *in situ*. As a result of the way data is collected by the registers, revision is considered to occur if a new implant is inserted. The commonest revision is therefore removal of a joint replacement and replacement with a new one. The addition of an extra component, such as secondary resurfacing (after TKA), the addition of a lateral or patellofemoral replacement (to a medial UKA with osteoarthritis progression) or exchange of a bearing (for a dislocation or a washout) are therefore also considered to be a revision whereas replacement of the original bearing after a dislocation is not. Using the same definition, an amputation, a knee fusion or death resulting from surgery would not be considered a "revision" and so that the knee arthroplasty would be considered a success.

It is therefore important to consider a whole series of different end points other than just revision to assess success or failure of a joint replacement. These could include all adverse events such as reoperations, complications, mortality and morbidity and patients with poor outcome scores and/or dissatisfaction.

Comparison of UKA and TKA

All national registers have found that the revision rate of UKA is about three times that of TKA. As a result, it is generally concluded that UKA have more poor results than TKA and therefore that UKA should not be used. This conclusion is probably not justified. There are many reasons why the revision rate of UKA is higher than that of TKA. Perhaps the most important is that the threshold for revision of UKA is much lower than that of TKA and therefore the higher revision rate does not necessarily suggest that UKA have worse outcomes than TKA.

Figure 10.1 shows a graph based on presented data from the Trent Regional Arthroplasty Register comparing the long term outcome of seven different total knee arthroplasties [1]. As would be expected, most of the knee replacements have a survival of 90 to 95% at 15 years. However, there is a single implant with a survival rate of 100% at 15 years. This implant appears to be so much better than the other knee replacements that all surgeons should use it. However, this implant, the Sheehan knee (Fig. 10.2), is a hinged knee replacement with long stems which is no longer available because of its poor performance. Due to the size of the implant and the damage it caused when it failed, revisions were very difficult. Therefore, surgeons would try to avoid revising it even if it was loose and was causing the patient significant symptoms.

This suggests that for different types of implant there are different thresholds for revision and that these thresholds have a profound effect on the revision rate of the implant. This effect can be so large that comparison of revision rates between implants may lead to misleading conclusions.

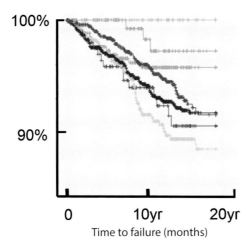

Figure 10.1 Graph showing survival data of seven TKAs from the Trent Regional Arthroplasty Register [1].

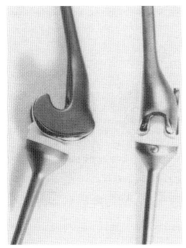

Figure 10.2 Sheehan Total Knee Replacement (G F McCoy, N W McLeod and J R Nixon, Experience with the Sheehan knee replacement. *Ulster Med J* **1983**; 52(1): 35-39).

There is evidence to suggest that the threshold for revision influences the comparison between UKA and TKA. The New Zealand Joint Registry (NZJR), as well as collecting data about revision, also collects Oxford Knee Scores (OKS) six months after the operation. The OKS is subcategorised into poor, fair, good and excellent [2,3] (Fig. 10.3). Data from the NZJR demonstrates that UKA not only have more excellent results but also fewer poor results than TKA. Therefore, the high revision rate of UKA is not because UKA have more poor results.

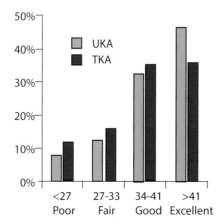

Figure 10.3 Proportion of UKR and TKR achieving four classes of OKS outcome.

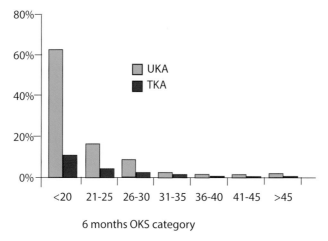

6 months OKS category

Figure 10.4 Two year revision rates for UKA and TKA having different PROMS results at six months post-surgery [3].

The NZJR also compares the six month OKS with the subsequent revision rate [4]. We have used data derived from the NZJR to draw the graph shown in Figure 10.4 [3]. The graph demonstrates that, for each outcome score, the revision rate of UKA is about five times higher than that of TKA. This suggests that factors independent of outcome score increase the revision rate by five times. The most important factor is likely to be a different threshold for revision.

The most striking difference in revision rate occurs in patients who are likely to have a worse score postoperatively than preoperatively (OKS less than 20). These patients have a 10% chance of being revised if they have had a TKA and a 60% chance of being revised if they have had a UKA. This is not surprising because the revision of a UKA is usually a simple conversion to a primary TKA and the outcome of this is generally expected to be good. In contrast, a revision of a TKA is often complex, requiring the use of stems, wedges and stabilised implants and the outcome of this type of revision is known to be unpredictable. We therefore conclude that the higher revision rate of UKA is not because they have more poor results but because they have a lower threshold for revision.

Most surgeons would agree that it is an advantage of UKA over TKA that UKA is relatively straightforward to revise if there is a problem. The consequence of it being easy to revise is that the threshold for revision is lower and therefore the revision rate is higher. The higher revision rate of UKA should thus not be considered to be a problem because it is a manifestation of an advantage.

Matched comparisons of UKA and TKA

When national registers compare different implants, they tend to use raw, unmatched data. Based on raw data, the revision rate of UKA is about three times higher than that of TKA. Raw data relating the death rate after UKA and TKA is also contained in the registers and shows that the death rate five years after a total knee is about twice as high as after a partial knee [4]. This difference in death rate is clearly not a simple manifestation of the different types of operation and demonstrates how invalid a comparison using raw data is. Furthermore, if a comparison based on raw data is invalid for death, then it will also be invalid for revision. The reason for the dramatic difference in the death rate is that UKA tend to be implanted in younger and more active patients than total knees. An identical explanation must at least in part explain the difference in the revision rate because young and active patients tend to have a high revision rate.

Liddle et al. [5] compared adverse events in matched UKA and TKA. Data was obtained not just from the NJR for England and Wales, but also the Hospital Episodes Statistics (HES) database and the Office for National Statistics (ONS). Patients were matched, using a propensity score analysis, on 20 variables including preoperative score, patient demographics, co-morbidities and deprivation indices. 25,334 UKA were matched against 75,996 TKA. Almost all the UKA with data were matched to TKAs. All patients who were treated with UKA could alternatively have been treated with a TKA so the conclusions are generalisable.

Based on the matched cohort, it was found that there were many advantages of UKA compared to TKA. For example, the length of stay was 1.38 (95% CI 1.33-1.43) days shorter with a UKA. The re-admission rate within the first year 0.65 (95% CI 0.58 – 0.72), intra-operative complications 0.73 (95% CI 0.58 - 0.91), and transfusions 0.25 (95% CI 0.17 - 0.37) were all less. Complications also occurred significantly less frequently, for example the incidence of thromboembolism with the UKA was 0.49 (95% CI 0.39 – 0.62) that of TKA, infection was 0.5 (95% CI 0.38 – 0.66), stroke was 0.37 (95% CI 0.16 – 0.86) and myocardial infarct was 0.53 (95% CI 0.30 – 0.90).

The mortality following UKA was also significantly lower (Fig. 10.5). For example, during the first 30 days, the hazard ratio was 0.23 (95% CI 0.11 – 0. 50 p<0.001) and during the first 90 days it was 0.46 (95% CI 0.31 – 0.69 p<0.001). The difference in mortality was not just seen in the short term. The survival curves progressively separated for about four years and thereafter remained parallel until the study stopped at eight years suggesting that the effect of surgery on mortality lasted for four years (Fig. 10.5). At eight years, the mortality following UKA was 0.87 that of TKA (95% CI 0.80 – 0.94 p<0.001). Overall there was an appreciable difference in death rate. If 62 patients (95% CI 43 – 116) were treated with a UKA rather than a TKA, over the eight year period one life would be saved. Furthermore, if within the National Health Service, the proportion of knee replacements that were UKA increased from about 7% to 20%, then about 160 deaths per year would be saved.

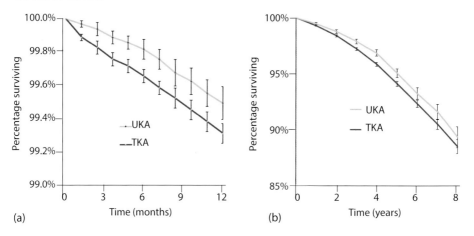

(a)　　　　　　　　　　　　　　　　　　(b)

Figure 10.5 Post-operative mortality: for matched UKA and TKA (a) for the first year and (b) for eight years.

In the matched comparison, it was found that the revision rate and reoperation rate were still higher after UKA than TKA. At eight years, the revision rate was 2.12 (95% CI 1.99 - 2.26) times higher and the overall reoperation rate was 1.38 (95% CI 1.31 - 1.44) times higher with UKA. However, to put the adverse outcomes in perspective, it was concluded that "if 100 patients receiving TKA received UKA instead, the result would be around one less death and three more reoperations in the first four years after surgery" [5].

It has been suggested that this analysis is biased [6]. The data is, however, freely available and, if the analysis were to be repeated, similar results would be obtained. Futhermore, there is another similar study done under the auspices of the NJR assessing 45-day mortality that found results virtually identical to ours [7].

Liddle *et al.* in a separate matched study, compared the patient reported outcome scores (PROMS) of UKA and TKA [8]. 3,519 UKA were matched with 10,557 TKA. The main outcome measure was the Oxford Knee Score (OKS). Excellent matching was achieved with the preoperative knee scores (UKA being 21.8 (SD 7.6) and TKA being 21.7 (SD 7.7)). At six months following UKA, the OKS was significantly better (p<0.0001) with the UKA being 38 and the TKA 36. Although this difference in Oxford Score is relatively small, many more patients achieved an Excellent OKS (> 41) with UKA rather than TKA (Odds ratio 1.59 95% CI 1.47 – 1.73, p<0.001).

EQ-5D™ (EuroQuol, Rotterdam, The Netherlands) was also collected and a significantly better overall score was achieved with UKA rather than TKA (p<0.001). Furthermore, the four subscales relating to mobility, pain, function and self care were significantly better but, in the subscale of anxiety, there was no significant difference. The level of patient satisfaction was also assessed and more patients achieved Excellent satisfaction with UKA compared to TKA (Odds ratio 1.3 times CI 1.3 (SD 1.2 – 1.4, p<0.0001)) .

As far as we are aware, there are no other matched comparisons of UKA and TKA based on PROMS from national registers. Unmatched comparisons based on data from the New Zealand Joint Registry showed a significantly better OKS with UKA compared to TKA (UKA 39, TKA 37 p<0.0001) [9]. Similarly, an unmatched comparison by Baker *et al.* [10] from the NJR showed significantly better OKS compared to TKA (35.5 (95% CI 34.5 – 36.4) to 34.0 (95% CI 33.0 – 34.2)) although, in this study, no significant difference was found in the improvement in OKS between UKA and TKA when adjusted for other factors.

Addressing the high revision rate

The revision rate of the UKA is much higher in national registers than in most published series. Although some authors [11] have implied that this is due to biased or even fraudulent reporting of the cohort studies by the designer surgeons, the main reason is likely to be due to surgical experience. In the national registers, most surgeons are found to be doing very small numbers whereas, in published series, surgeons tend to do large numbers. The data from the NJR would suggest that about half the surgeons doing knee replacement do some unicompartmental replacement. For those doing unicompartmental replacement, the most common number implanted per year is one and the second most common number is two (Fig. 10.6) [12]. The average number is five.

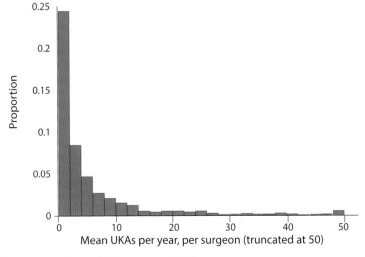

Figure 10.6 Surgeon numbers of UKA per year in NJR.

When the number of UKA performed per surgeon per year were compared to the revision rate, it was found, not surprisingly, that the surgeons doing small numbers have a very high revision rate (Fig. 10.7). The surgeons doing one or two UKA per year have a 4% failure rate per year which would equate to about a 60% survival at 10 years. The revision rate dramatically decreases with increasing numbers. Surgeons doing about 10 UKA per year have a revision rate of 2% per year whereas surgeons doing about 30 per year or more have a revision rate of 1% per year (Fig. 10.7). The data would suggest that surgeons should do at least 10 per year and ideally at least 30 per year. When surgeons perform at least 30 per year, the re-operation rate is the same with UKA and TKA out to eight years.

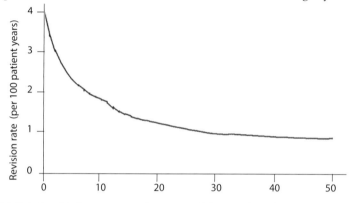

Figure 10.7 Relationship between revision rate and the number of UKA done per surgeon per year in NJR [12].

Over the years we, and others, have encouraged surgeons to increase their numbers of UKA but these efforts have had little effect. This is not surprising because surgeons cannot easily increase the size of their practice. However, there is an alternative way of increasing the number of UKA: increasing the proportion of their knee replacements that are unicompartmental. In order to do this, they would have to broaden their indications for UKA.

Figure 10.8 shows the relationship between the revision rate and the percentage of a surgeon's knee replacements that are UKA, which we have called usage. The shape of the graph is not what would be expected. In 1989, Kozinn and Scott defined the ideal indications for UKA and implied that surgeons who extended the indications would have a higher revision rate [13]. Subsequently Stern et al. [14], and Ritter et al. [15], found that, based on Kozinn and Scott criteria, about 5% of patients would be considered ideal for unicompartmental replacement. It would therefore be expected that the lowest revision rate would be achieved when surgeons did 5% per year and that the revision rate would increase with higher usage. This is far from what actually happens: the revision rate for surgeons with a 5% usage is very high, about 3% per year, which equates to a 70% survival at 10 years. As the usage increases, the revision rate dramatically decreases until 20% usage. Thereafter, for the OUKA, with increasing usage there is a slow but steady decrease in the revision rate with the optimal usage being around 50%.

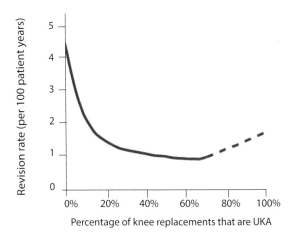

Figure 10.8 Annual Revision Rate for OUKA plotted against the proportion of a surgeon's practice that is unicompartmental (based on Liddle *et al.* [16]).

With usage higher than about 65%, the revision rate increases although the data at these high usage rates is unreliable because of the small numbers of surgeons doing these rates and because these surgeons tend to have atypical referral practices.

There are two main reasons why the revision rate decreases with increased usage up to 50%. Firstly with increased usage, surgeons do increased numbers and their results improve. Secondly, their indications change. Surgeons doing small numbers tend only to use UKA when there is early disease and the rest of the knee is pristine. In these circumstances, particularly with partial thickness cartilage loss, the revision rate is very high [17, 18]. To achieve good results, surgeons not only need to do reasonable numbers but also to use the appropriate indications. The evidence would suggest that, if surgeons have a low usage, they should either stop doing UKA or change their indications so they are doing at least 20%. We would consider usage of 20% or more to be acceptable. For optimal results, surgeons should increase their usage to about 50%. If the recommended indications for the OUKA are adhered to, then about 50% of a surgeon's knee replacements would be UKA.

Liddle *et al.* [5] in their propensity matched cohorts of UKA and TKA, assessed the effect of usage. Overall, in the unmatched cohort, the revision rate of UKA was 3.2 times higher than TKA but, when the patients were matched, the hazard ratio for revision became 2.12 (95% CI 1.99 – 2.26) that of TKA. However, in the subset of patients in whom the surgeons were considered to have optimal usage rates (40 – 60%), the revision rate of UKA was only 1.4 times higher than TKA. Revision is in some ways a biased outcome measure and reoperation rate is probably a fairer measure with which to compare UKA and TKA. Out to eight years for unicompartmental replacements done by surgeons with 40 – 60% usage, there was no significant difference in reoperation rate between matched UKA and TKA (Fig 10.9) [12].

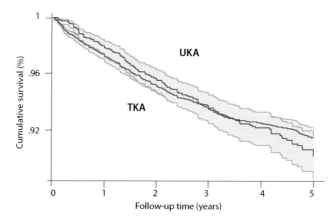

Figure 10.9 Revision/reoperation rates for matched cohorts of UKA and TKA for UKA surgeons with optimal usage between 40% and 60%.

Results of Oxford UKA in registries

We have always been interested in how the OUKA has been performing in the national registers and how its revision rate compares with that of other UKA. We have, however, found this data difficult to interpret, as it is very contradictory. For example when the Swedish Knee Arthroplasty Register (SKAR) first reported the results of the OUKA in 1995 [19], it was performing very badly with a revision rate about twice that of the Marmor. As SKAR thought they had identified a bad implant, they wrote to all the Swedish surgeons using the OUKA advising them to stop using it. Ten years later (Table 10.1), in 2005, the OUKA was the best performing UKA in SKAR. This clearly demonstrates that registers cannot reliably achieve their primary aim of identifying poorly performing implants.

Table 10.1 shows the results of UKA performed in Australia and New Zealand as well as in Sweden in 2005. The OUKA was not only the best in Sweden but also in New Zealand. It was, however, significantly worse than the three comparators used in Australia (comparators selected because they were the best performing implants done in large numbers). More strikingly, the Repicci was the best in Australia and worst in Sweden. Clearly registers cannot reliably compare different implants. The reason for these apparently contradictory results is that the results of a joint replacement depend not only on the implant but also the indications and surgical technique.

Registers collect very little data about indications and technique so cannot adjust for these. Surgical experience is in some ways a surrogate for indications and technique. We were able to obtain data from the Australian Orthopaedic Association National Joint Replacement Registry (AOANJRR) to try and help explain why the comparator implants were doing significantly better than the OUKA. We found that the OUKA was being done in hospitals doing smaller numbers than the hospitals doing the comparators. When adjustments were made for this, the significant difference in results disappeared.

For completeness, although it is difficult to interpret, we present the outcomes reported in the most recent registry reports. SKAR does not report the revision rate of the OUKA, but it is not significantly different from their comparator [20]. They acknowledge that the results of the OUKA have improved with teaching. In the NJR the survival rate was 88% at 10 years. In ANJR the survival rate was 85% at 10 years [21]. They acknowledge that the high revision rate was due to surgeons implanting small numbers. In the Danish Knee Arthroplasty Register (DKAR) the five-year survival is 90% [22]. The register acknowledges that survival is not a good endpoint with which to compare UKA and TKA. In the NZJR, the revision rate of the cemented OUKA is 1.37/100 component years [23]. The cementless OUKA (see page 206, Clinical results of cementless Oxford UKA) has the lowest revision rate of any UKA at 0.72/100 component years.

Table 10.1 UKA tabulated in order of their revision rate, with the lowest at the top, in the Swedish (SKAR), Australian (AOANJRR) and New Zealand (NZJR) joint registries in 2005. The comparator or comparators are shown in italics. * indicates that the revision rate is significantly different from the comparators.

SKAR (10yr)	AOANJRR (4yr)	NZJR (3yr)
Oxford	*Repicci*	Oxford
Link–Uni	GRU	Genesis
Genesis	*Unix*	Repicci
Miller-Galante*	*Miller-Galante*	Miller-Galante
Allegretto	PFC	Preservation
Brigham *	Link-Uni	
Marmor*	Oxford *	
Duracon *	Genesis	
PFC *	Allegretto *	
Repicci*	Preservation Fixed *	
	Natural Knee *	
	Preservation Mobile*	

Non-registry studies

UKA v TKA

We have been able to identify 13 published clinical studies comparing the outcomes of total and unicompartmental knee replacement. Two studies are randomised controlled trials (RCTs), six are cohort studies, three are case-control studies and two are self-controlled studies of patients receiving TKA in one knee and OUKA in the other. In the following paragraphs, key results from these studies are summarised.

Ackroyd et al. [24] performed the first RCT comparing UKA to TKA. Between 1989 and 1992, 102 knees suitable for UKA were randomised to receive either a St Georg Sled UKA or a Kinematic modular TKA. The early results demonstrated that the UKA group had fewer complications and more rapid rehabilitation than the TKA group. At five years, there was an equal number of failures in the two groups but the UKA group had more excellent results and a greater range of movement. At 15 years, 43 patients (45 knees) had died with their prosthetic knees intact [24, 25]. The

Bristol knee scores of the UKA group throughout the review period were better and, at 15 years, 15 (71.1%) of the surviving UKAs and 10 (53.1%) of the surviving TKAs had achieved an excellent score. The 15-year survival rate based on revision or failure for any reason was 90% for UKA and 79% for TKA. During the 15 years of the review, four UKAs and six TKAs failed.

Sun et al. [26] randomised 56 patients to either an OUKA, or an AGC TKA (both Biomet, Warsaw, USA) and reported the results with a mean follow-up of 52 months. The UKA group had a shorter operative time, less blood loss, a lower transfusion requirement and fewer DVTs than TKA. KSS-Obj and mean range of movement was higher in the UKA group, but neither are described as being statistically significant. Seven patients in the UKA group required revision for tibial loosening (six patients) or subsidence. The authors attribute this to the learning-curve effect, as all were performed within the first two years of use of the OUKA. There were no revisions in the TKA group.

A case-control study, by Lombardi et al. [27], compared early (mean 31 months) outcomes for TKA and UKA, with particular emphasis on speed of recovery. 103 consecutive UKA patients (115 knees) were matched to the same number of TKA patients (and knees) on the basis of age, gender, BMI and bilaterality. The number of revisions was similar as were the number of complications. Stiffness requiring manipulation under anaesthetic (MUA) was significantly more common in TKA (7/115 v 0/115, $p=0.007$). Patients with UKA had a higher mean haemoglobin at discharge (12.1 g/dL v 11.3 g/dL, $p<0.001$), shorter hospital stays (1.4 days v 2.2 days, $p<0.001$) and a better mean range of movement (77° of flexion v 67°, $p<0.001$). There was no statistically significant difference in KSS-Fcn or KSS-Obj.

Amin et al. [28] matched 54 consecutive UKAs with 54 TKAs on age, gender, BMI, range of movement and pre-operative function. At a mean follow-up of 59 months, there was a superior range of movement, but inferior survival, in UKA compared to TKA. There were no differences in the outcome scores.

Sweeney et al. [29] performed a retrospective cohort comparison of 317 OUKAs to 425 Advance TKAs (Wright Medical Technologies, Arlington, TN) from a single institution. The authors used hierarchical linear modelling to estimate the treatment effect of UKA and TKA at different time-points, allowing for clustering by surgeon and adjusting for age and gender. At six months, there was no significant difference between TKA and UKA.

Walton et al. [30] retrospectively compared 183 UKAs with a non-matched group of 142 TKAs, reporting a mean OKS of 37.8 in the UKA group and 35.5 in the TKA group, a significant difference ($p=0.04$). Weale et al. [31] retrospectively compared cohorts of patients undergoing OUKA (31 patients) and AGC TKA (130 patients), reporting inferior survival in the UKA group but with functional outcomes similar to TKA.

Three studies have been published comparing outcomes for UKA and TKA in the same patient. Costa et al. [32] performed simultaneous bilateral knee replacement in 34 consecutive patients, performing UKA in one knee and TKA in the other. Five knees from the UKA group (all received the EIUS system (Stryker, Marwar, NJ)), were revised, four for peri-prosthetic fractures and one with unexplained pain. There was no difference between the groups on the basis of KSS-Fcn or KSS-Obj scores. Dalury *et al.* [33] performed a retrospective review of all patients in a single centre who had received a TKA on one side and a UKA on the other. Range of motion was greater in the UKA group (123° v 120°), but there was no difference in functional scores between the groups. Of the 23 patients, 12 expressed a preference for their UKA knee and none expressed a preference for their TKA knee. A study by Laurencin *et al.* [34] compared TKAs to UKAs in patients who had received both, reporting a superior range of motion in the UKA (123° v 110°). In this study, 44% of patients expressed a preference for their UKA, 12% for their TKA and 44% could perceive no difference between the function of their knees.

Rougraff *et al.* [35] retrospectively compared 120 UKAs to 81 TKAs, finding superior survival in UKA (the end point being any reoperation) and significantly superior combined KSS scores in the UKA group.

In the USA, an independent telephone survey done at Washington University compared the level of satisfaction with various activities (Fig. 10.10(a)) and extent of residual symptoms (Fig. 10.10(b)) in a series of 353 mobile UKAs, 104 fixed bearing UKAs and 661 TKAs implanted in four centres [36]. Overall, the results of mobile UKA were better than fixed UKA or TKA. The fixed bearing UKA did better than TKA on some questions and worse on others.

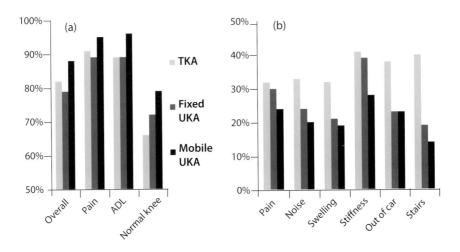

Figure 10.10 (a) Satisfaction of USA patients surveyed by telephone (ADL - activities of daily living; Normal knee - the knee with a replacement felt like a 'normal knee'); (b) Residual symptoms experienced.

TOPKAT (Total Or Partial Knee Arthroplasty Trial)

In order to overcome various issues (including small sample size, short follow up, bias in patient selection) associated with the studies described above, TOPKAT was set up [37]. The aim of TOPKAT is to assess the clinical and cost effectiveness of TKAs compared to UKAs in patients with medial compartment osteoarthritis. The design of the study is a single layer multicentre superiority type randomised controlled trial of unilateral knee replacement patients. It aimed to recruit 500 patients from approximately 28 secondary care orthopaedic units from across the UK including district general and teaching hospitals. The study is pragmatic in terms of implant selection for the knee replacement operation. Participants will be followed up for 5 years. The primary outcome is the Oxford Knee Score, which will be collected via questionnaires at 2 months, 1 year and then annually to 5 years. Secondary outcomes will include cost-effectiveness, patient satisfaction and complications data. Patient recruitment has been completed. Preliminary analysis of the one year data does show small but significant advantages of UKA with some outcome measures. No firm conclusions can be drawn from this study until five year data is available [89].

Health economic studies

Various studies have compared cost-effectiveness of UKA and TKA. In 2006, Soohoo et al. [38] analysed cost-effectiveness using a decision model. The study supported UKA as a cost-effective alternative for the treatment of unicompartmental arthritis when the durability and function of a UKA are assumed to be similar to those of a primary TKA. Using non-matched data from the NJR, Willis-Owen et al. [39], at a three year follow up, reported cost savings of £1761 (about $2650) per knee treated with UKA compared to TKA, data which is supported by other observational studies [40,41]. Longer term assessment has been provided by Slover et al. [42] who, focusing on the elderly low demand population and using the Norwegian Arthroplasty Register, demonstrated that UKA had a lower mean cost and higher mean number of quality adjusted life years gained compared to TKA. Conversely, Koskinen et al. [43], using the Finnish Arthroplasty Register, report that in the short term UKA was associated with lower costs, but in the long term, due to the higher revision rate, TKR was the more cost effective.

In 2007, Confalonieri et al. [44] in a study involving 64 patients, compared the midterm outcome and cost-effectiveness of UKA with minimally invasive computer assisted TKA in patients matched for age, gender, time to follow up, pre-operative arthritis and range of movement. The authors concluded that UKA cost at least 3100 Euros (approximately US $4100) less than computer assisted TKA due to shorter surgical time and shorter in-patient stay. In 2015, Ghomrawi et al. [45] assessed the effect of age on cost-effectiveness of UKA vs TKA using a Markov decision analytic model. They considered lifetime costs, quality-adjusted life-years (QALYs), and incremental cost-effectiveness ratios (ICERs) from a societal perspective for patients undergoing surgery at 45, 55, 65, 75 or 85 years of age. Transition probabilities were estimated from the literature; survival, from the Swedish Knee Arthroplasty Register; and costs, from the literature and the Healthcare Cost and Utilization Project (HCUP) database. The authors concluded that, for patients sixty-five years of age and older, UKA was more cost-effective with lower lifetime costs and higher QALYs. In the 45 year group, UKA became cost-effective when its 20-year revision rate dropped from 28% to 26% and in the 55 year old group when it changed from 28% to 27%. The OUKA implanted by experienced surgeons would therefore be cost effective in all age groups as the 20-year survival would be expected to be better than 75% even in the young (see Chapter 5).

Cohort studies of Oxford unicompartmental knee arthroplasty

In this section, we first summarise the 20-year and longer results of the Oxford Knee. These results relate primarily to the Phase 1 and Phase 2 Oxford Knee because the Phase 3 was introduced only in 1998. We then summarise the 10 and 15-year results of the Phase 3 Oxford Knee. There are numerous short term studies of the Oxford Knee. We will not discuss these in depth but we will present the results of a meta-analysis of all published Phase 3 studies [46].

Dr Ulf Svard is a surgeon who works in Skövde in Sweden. In 1983, he visited Oxford and learned how to use the Oxford Knee. He has been using it since then and following his patients. Initially a group of four surgeons did the operations but more recently he has done them alone so the majority of the patients had their surgery done by him. Currently he has implanted Oxford Knees in more than 1100 patients (mean age 69). At the time of his various reviews, none were lost to follow up. His 20-year data was first presented in 2006 [47]. At that stage, there were 638 OUKA and the 20-year survival was 92% (95% CI 77 – 100). At 10 years when 187 patients were reviewed, 90% had good or excellent HSS scores. This data was updated and subsequently published in 2011 [48] with a 20-year survival of 91%. There had been 29 revisions, 10 for lateral arthrosis, nine for component loosening, five for infection, two bearing dislocations and three for unexplained pain.

The next review was based on the first 1000 implants (125 Phase 1, 271 Phase 2, and 604 Phase 3), and at 20 years the survival rate was 87% (95% CI 79 - 95). The survival was also 87% at 22 years. Dr Svard also reviewed his 125 Phase 1 implants [49]. These had been implanted between 1983 and 1988. At the time of review, 80% were dead and the remainder were reviewed with an average follow up of about 25 years. At time of death, or last review, 90% had not been revised and had a good or excellent Hospital for Special Surgery (HSS) Score. This demonstrates that, when used correctly with the correct indications, the Oxford Knee could be considered to be a definitive knee replacement. We are not aware of any other implant, either unicompartmental or total, that has achieved as good, or better, results.

At 20 years, about 2% of cases had failed from progression of the disease in the lateral compartment [48]. It is generally believed that arthritis will inevitably progress in the lateral compartment after medial unicompartmental replacement. The very low incidence of progression demonstrates that this is not the case and that progression should be considered to be a rare event. The incidence of progression was higher in the Phase 2, than the Phase 1, OUKA. Analysis of the post-operative radiographs demonstrated that, following Phase 2, the knees were in slightly more valgus than Phase 1. The Phase 2 tibial resection guide had an extension that passed around the medial side of the tibia (Fig. 10.11). To insert this, a small medial release was required. In contrast, the Phase 1 did not have this extension so no medial release was required. It was thought that this medial release might have contributed to the higher incidence of lateral compartment arthritis.

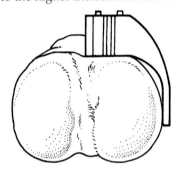

Figure 10.11 Plan view of OUKA (Phase 2) tibial saw guide.

Barrington and Emerson [50] also presented 20 year results of the Oxford Knee and in this study, which was originally started as part of an Investigational Device Exemption (IDE) study in the USA for the Phase 2, there were 54 knees in 48 patients. At 20 years, the survival was 85%. Nine knees in seven patients had been revised, six for disease progression. As part of the surgical technique, a medial release was undertaken to allow for insertion of a retractor. This may have contributed to the incidence of progression of lateral compartment arthritis.

The 15-year results of the first consecutive 1000 cemented medial Oxford Phase 3 UKA implanted by two designer surgeons have been reviewed with a mean follow up of 10 years [51]. At 10 years, the mean Oxford Knee Score (OKS) was 40 (SD 9) with 79% of the knees having excellent or good outcome. There were 52 implant related re-operations at a mean of 5.5 years (range 0.2 – 14.7 years). Progression of arthritis in the lateral compartment (2.4%) followed by bearing dislocation (0.7%) and unexplained pain (0.7%) were the most common indications for revision. When implant-related re-operations are considered failures, the 15-year survival is 91% (95% CI 83 – 98). When the end point is revision for failure of the tibial or femoral components, the 15-year survival is 99% (95% CI 96 - 100). When revision requiring TKA components are considered failures, the 15-year survival is 99.7% (95% CI 98 – 100). There were no cases of a revision performed for wear, progression of PFJOA or bearing fracture. When all implant-related re-operations are considered to be failures with 3 or 4 mm bearings (n = 712), the 15-year survival was 94.3%

(95% CI 87.1 - 100), with 5 mm or greater (n = 86) 15-year survival was 75.0% (95% CI 28.5 - 100). Although the reasons for these differences are not fully understood, it seems sensible to aim for a 3 or 4 bearing. If this is achieved, the 15-year survival is as good as the best TKA.

Tables of results

Table 10.2 shows the published 10, 15 and 20-year results of the Phase 1 and Phase 2 OUKA. The 10 year survival rate ranges from 82% to 98%. The series with the second lowest survival rate, by Vorlat et al. [52], had broad indications and included patients who had undergone previous HTO or had inflammatory arthritis. Similarly, in the series by Kumar et al. [53] four of the seven revisions were attributed to loosening, two were for disease progresion and one was for tibial fracture. Seven of a cohort of 100 cases were subsequently found to have inflammatory arthritis. There were no revisions for wear. In the designer series, which should be indicative of the best results that can be achieved, the survival was 98% [54].

Table 10.3 includes all the published and presented series with 10-year survival rates of the Phase 3 medial OUKA. The authors were contacted to determine what percentage of their knee replacements were OUKA. The nine papers include over 6000 patients with an estimated average survival rate at 10 years of about 95% (range 91 - 97%). Although most series were performed by one or two surgeons, in two a large number of surgeons were involved. In one series from Oxford (Bottomley et al. [55]), which did not include designer surgeons, there were 56 surgeons. In the series from Basingstoke (Briant-Evans et al. [56]), there were 35. Despite the high numbers of surgeons, many of whom were trainees, the 10-year results were good, suggesting the indications for the operation are very important. In these institutions, it is likely that there was a standard set of indications, whereas the surgical skill among the trainees is probably somewhat variable. Further evidence that the indications are important relates to the usage of the device. In the nine series, somewhere between 20% and 60% of the surgeons' knee replacements were OUKA. This fits well with the registry data because it shows that, to obtain good results with the OUKA, usage between 20% and 50% should be aimed for. To achieve this, the recommended indications should be used.

In addition to these series including 10-year results, there are other shorter series reporting the results of the OUKA. Hamilton et al. are conducting a meta-analysis of published phase 3 OUKA results. The authors identified 47 studies and contacted the authors to determine what percentage of their knee replacement practice was UKA [46]. There were marked differences between those who use the UKA in a small proportion of their knee replacement practice compared with those who use it in a high proportion. For <10% usage, UKA revision rate per 100 observed component years was 2.13 (SD 1.36). For >10% and <30%, it was 1.47 (SD 0.92). For $\geq$ 30%, it was 0.67 (SD 0.52). A Kruscal-Wallis test revealed statistically significant differences between the three groups (p = 0.021).

Table 10.2 Survival Rates for Oxford Medial Arthroplasties Phase 1 & 2 at 10, 15 & 20 years. Only the most recent report of a series is included.

Implant	Principle Surgeon* or Author	Date	Ref	No. of Knees	Age	Time (yrs)	Survival	No. of Revisions	Reasons for Revision	Score	Pre-op	Latest post-op
Phase 2	Emerson*	2010	50	54	64	20	84%	9	Disease progression (6), loosening (1), hemarthrosis (1), bearing impingement (1)	KSS		'KSS-Obj 75 KSS-Fn 90'
Phase 1-2	Murray	1998	54	143	71	10	98%	5	Disease progression (2), infection (1), loosening (1), pain (1)	HSS & KSS		89% good or excellent72
Phase 2	Rajasekhar	2004	57	135	71	10	94%	5	Loosening (3), pain (1), dislocation (1)	KSS		'KSS-Obj 92 KSS-Fn 76'
Phase 1-2	Kumar	1999	53	100	71	10	85%	7	Loosening (4), disease progression (2), fracture (1)	KSS	'KSS-Obj 62 KSS-Fn 45'	'KSS-Obj 91 KSS-Fn 71'
Phase 2	Vorlat	2006	52	149	66	10	82%	24	Disease progression (9), loosening (7), bearing dislocation (4), bearing fracture (2), instability (1), unknown (1)			
Phase 1-2	Koskinen	2007	59	1113	64	10	80%	51	Not reported			
Phase 1-3	Svard*	2011	48 & 88 (scores)	682	70	20	91%	29	Disease progression (10), loosening (9), infection (5), pain (3), bearing dislocation (2)	HSS	56.5	86

Table 10.3 Reported 10-year survival of Oxford Phase 3.

Principle Surgeon * or author	Date	Ref	No. of surgeons	No. of Knees (at start)	10 year survival	% of Knee Replacements that are UKA
Pandit	2011	(60)	2	1000	96%	>50%
Yoshida*	2013	(61)	1	1344	97%	>50%
Wagner-Kristensen*	2012	(62)	1	765	95%	20-25%
Bottomley	2012	(55)	56	1084	94%	50%
Kim*	2012	(63)	1	400	94%	>50%
Butler-Manuel*	2012	(64)	1	124	90%	25-30%
Keys*	2013	(65)	1	107	97%	30%
Briant-Evans	2013	(56)	35	827	91%	14%
Faour-Martin	2013	(66)	1	511	95%	

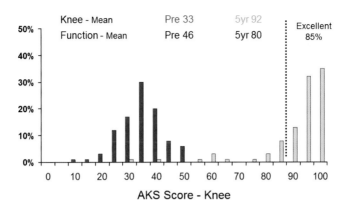

Figure 10.12 Change in Knee Society Score (Objective) for 101 knees, pre-op in red, mean five-year follow-up in green.

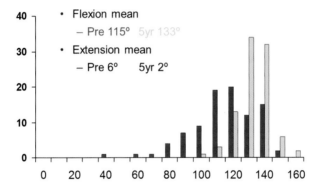

Figure 10.13 Maximum flexion in 101 knees (pre-op in red, mean follow-up of five years in green).

Functional outcome

The clinical outcome of the Phase 3 OUKA was reported in 2006 [51]. The mean objective Knee Society Score improved from 33 to 92, the mean function score improved from 46 to 80, with 85% considered Excellent (Fig. 10.12). The mean flexion deformity decreased from 6° to 2° and the mean flexion limit increased from 115° to 133° (Fig. 10.13). The Knee Society Score is not a good tool for assessing the outcome of UKA. For example it does not give credit for flexion beyond 125°. A study by Choy et al. [67] from Korea of 188 knees in 166 patients, with a mean follow up of 6.5 years, found that the mean flexion limit increased from 135° preoperatively to 150° (140° to 165°) postoperatively; 81% of the patients could squat and 91% could sit cross-legged, both activities that require full flexion in Korea. The very high preoperative range of motion reflects the social practices of that country.

Another problem with the Knee Society Score is that points are deducted for malalignment. Although this is appropriate for TKA where the aim is usually to restore neutral alignment, it is not appropriate for the OUKA where the aim is to restore pre-disease alignment. Gulati et al. [68] found that 18% of patients had mild varus postoperatively (about 5° from neutral) and 8% had marked varus (about 10° from neutral). As the OKS was no worse in those with varus than those with neutral alignment, the deductions are unjustified. Removing the deduction increased the postoperative KSS-objective) from 77 (SD 15) to 89 (SD 14) in the mild varus group and from 70 (SD 13) to 94 (SD 8) in the marked varus group. We favour the OKS for assessing outcome and find that, on average, the preoperative score is about 25 (SD 9) and the postoperative score at 10 years is about 40 (SD 9)

Price *et al.* [69] compared the rate of recovery (measured by the time taken to achieve straight-leg raising, 70° of flexion, and independent stair climbing) in 40 OUKAs performed through a short incision medial to the patellar tendon, without dislocation of the patella, using Phase 3 instrumentation, with 20 OUKAs implanted through an open approach with dislocation of the patella. Both groups were compared with 40 AGC (Biomet, Swindon, UK) TKAs performed for osteoarthritis during the same time period. The average rate of recovery after the short-incision UKA was twice as fast as after open UKA and three times as fast as after TKA.

Studies of other UKA and comparison of OUKA and others

Table 10.4 summarises the studies of UKA other than the Oxford Knee that give 10-year survival or longer. Argenson reports a 20-year survival in a series of 160 Miller-Galante of 74% (95% CI 67 – 81) [70]. This series is independent. In the designer series of 68 reported by Foran, the survival was 90% [71]. A single large series of St Georg Sled from Bristol has been reported at various time intervals. The 10-year survival was 88% and, of those reaching 10 years, 86% survived to 20 years. This suggests the overall survival at 20 years was 75% [25].

Six studies report the results of the Marmor with 10-year survival ranging from 70% – 93%. The majority of revisions (42/70, 60%), were for loosening or subsidence with a particular problem reported for smaller sizes. Of the remaining reasons for revision, the commonest was disease progression. Five 10-year studies exist on the Miller-Galante with survival ranging from 74% - 95%. The commonest reason for revisions (25/47, 53%) was disease progression either in the lateral or patellofemoral joint. Wear (17%) and loosening (13%) are other major reasons for revision.

Parratte *et al.* [72] compared the long-term survival and function of 79 fixed and 77 Phase 2 mobile bearing UKAs implanted between 1989 and 1992 (mean age was 63 years). The mean Knee Society Scores and range of movement were not significantly different in the two groups. At final follow up, considering revision for any reason, 12 of 77 (15%) UKAs were revised (for aseptic loosening, dislocation, and arthritis progression) in the mobile-bearing group and 10 of 79 (12%) in the fixed-bearing group (for wear and arthritis progression). The authors concluded that although there were no differences in the outcome or survivorship between fixed and mobile bearing UKAs, the failure mechanisms were different (wear for fixed bearing and progression of arthritis for the mobile bearing).

Table 10.4

Prosthesis	Year	Author	Knee (lateral)	Age	Time (years)	Survival (%)	No. of revisions	Reason for revision	Outcome measure	Pre-op scores	Latest scores
Genesis	2012	Heyse[73]	251 (78)	54	15	86	15	Wear/loosening (6), disease progression (4), pain (3), instability (2)	KSS	'KSS-Obj 50 KSS-Fn 44'	'KSS-Obj 94 KSS-Fn 95'
LCS	2004	Keblish[74]	177 (21)	68	10	82	32	Bearing wear (26) Loosening (6)	HSS	60	89.6
Marmor	2005	O'Rourke[75]	136 (14)	71	20	84	19	Disease progression (9), loosening (8), pain (2)	KSS		'KSS-Obj 72 KSS-Fn 53'
									HSS		58
Marmor	1999	Squire[76]	140 (15)	68	15	87	14	Disease progression (7) tibial subsidence (6), pain (1)	KSS	'KSS-Obj 31 KSS-Fn 85'	'KSS-Obj 42 KSS-Fn 71'
									HSS	57	82
Marmor	1998	Tabor[77]	73	61	15	79	11	Subsidence (6), disease progression (2), inflammatory disease (2), not stated (1)	KSS		'KSS-Obj 91 KSS-Fn 77'
Marmor	1996	Cartier[78]	207	65	10	93	7	Infections (3), femorotibial subluxation (3), disease progression (1)	KSS		'Obj 75% Excellent Fn 57% Excellent'
Marmor/C1/C2	1993	Heck[79]	294 (39)	68	10	91	16	Loosening (11), disease progression (4), infection (1)	KSS II HSS		'93 84'
Marmor	1988	Marmor[80]	87 (7)	63	10	70	21	Loosening (11), disease progression (8), other (2)	HSS		50% Excellent
Miller-Galante	2013	Argenson[70]	160	66	20	74	19	Disease progression (12), loosening (2), wear (5), infection (1)	KSS		'KSS-Obj 91 KSS-Fn 88'
Miller-Galante	2013	Rachha[81]	74 (5)	64	10	95	5	Disease progression (2), pain (2), infection (1), bearing change (2)			'KSS-Obj 76 KSS-Fn 80'
Miller-Galante	2012	Foran[71]	62 (3)	68	20	90	5	Disease progression (2), pain (1), component dislocation (1), not stated (1)	HSS		78
Miller-Galante	2011	John[82]	94 (9)	67	10	94	7	Disease progression (5), loosening (2)	Bristol Knee Score		44
Miller-Galante	2004	Naudie[83]	113	68	10	90	11	Disease progression (4), wear (3), pain (1), loosening (2), traumatic ligament rupture (1)	KSS	'KSS-Obj 48 KSS-Fn 53'	'KSS-Obj 93 KSS-Fn 80'
St Georg	1997	Ansari[84]	461	70	10	87	20	Disease progression (9), loosening (4), pain (3), prosthesis fracture (2), infection (1)	Bristol Knee Score		92% good or excellent
Unix	2013	Hall[85]	85 (20)	65	10	92	7	Tibial loosening (4), Disease progression (2), Infection (1)	OKS		38

Clinical results of cementless Oxford UKA

The current design of cementless components was first used in 2004. It was important to assess accurately the results of these components before they were widely used because cementless total knee replacements have not performed as well as cemented total knees. The planned assessment included a randomised controlled trial based on RSA to compare the migration with cemented and cementless implants. In addition, another RCT was undertaken to compare the fixation based on screened radiographs of the cemented and cementless implants together with clinical scores. A large multicentre cohort study was undertaken because these two randomised studies were relatively small and therefore could not identify complications or contraindications. Finally, the outcomes will be assessed in the Joint Registries.

We used a model-based RSA system to compare the migration of cemented and cementless Oxford UKA [86]. 43 knees were randomised. In RSA studies, the best predictor of long term loosening is increased migration in the second year. During the first year, both the cemented and cementless femoral components migrated 0.2 mm anteriorly and proximally. There was no significant difference between cemented and cementless. In the second year, there was no significant migration of either the cementless or cemented femoral components. During the first year, the cementless tibial components subsided significantly more than the cemented (0.3 mm v 0.1 mm p<0.01). However, during the second year, there was no significant difference in subsidence and both subsided 0.05 mm. The conclusion of the RSA study was that the cementless fixation was as good as the cemented.

In the clinical randomised study, 63 knees were randomised. Pre-operatively, there were no significant differences between the groups. The cementless procedure was 9 minutes quicker on average than the cemented. At 5 years, there was no significant difference between the OKS (cemented 39 (SD 10.4) and cementless 39.4 (SD 9.9)) and the KSS (Objective) (cemented 80.1 (SD 19.3) and cementless 78.8 (SD 14.0)). However, the KSS (Functional) was significantly better (p<0.01) for the cementless, (cemented 78.8 (SD 18.4) and cementless 92.0 (SD 12.7)). At 5 years, there was no significant difference in Tegner score although, at 2 years, the cementless was significantly better (p=0.04). There were no revisions.

The patients were assessed with fluoroscopically aligned radiographs. On the femoral side, there was no evidence of radiolucency or migration and no loosening. On the tibial side, there was also no evidence of loosening with no pathological radiolucencies or subsidence. However, there were physiological radiolucencies which were all less than or equal to 1 mm thick with a sclerotic margin [86]. With cemented components, 25% had complete radiolucent lines, 36% had partial radiolucent lines and 35% had no radiolucent lines. The cementless components had significantly fewer radiolucent lines (p<0.001), with no complete radiolucencies, 7% partial and 93% no radiolucencies (Fig. 10.16).

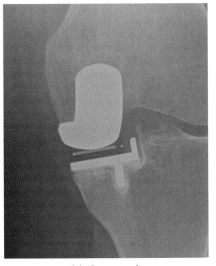
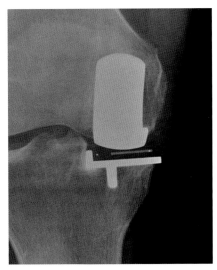

(a) Cemented   (b) Cementless

Figure 10.16 Radiographs demonstrating radiolucent lines under (a) a cemented tibial tray and their absence (b) with a cementless implant.

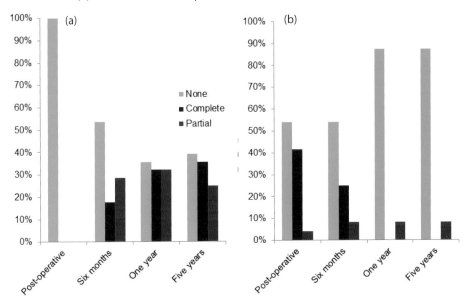

Figure 10.17 Progression of radiolucencies in (a) cemented and (b) cementless OUKA in the RCT.

In the cemented group, there were no radiolucencies on the postoperative radiographs but they appeared during the first year. In contrast, in the cementless group, there were some radiolucencies immediately postoperatively, suggesting the components were not fully seated, but these disappeared within the first year. This study therefore suggests that the fixation of the cementless was better than cemented. It also suggests that the appearance of the interfaces did not change after a year so a one year follow up should give a good indication of the quality of fixation. The functional outcome of the cementless was as good, if not better than, the cemented.

A multicentre prospective study of cementless OUKA was undertaken in Oxford, Belfast (Northern Ireland) and Christchurch (New Zealand) [83]. 1000 knees (881 patients) were reviewed with a minimum follow-up of one year and a maximum of eight years. All patients had the standard indications used for cemented OUKA and the standard operative technique and rehabilitation regime. There were 19 (1.9%) reoperations. These consisted of dislocations (0.6%), OA progression (0.5%), peri-operative tibial fractures (0.3%), infections (0.3%), a late fracture from trauma (0.1%) and lateral AVN (0.1%). The seven year survival, when all reoperations were considered to be failures, was 97% which was similar to the cemented. The average pre-operative OKS was 21 (SD 7.9) and at one year was 40 (SD 7.8). 6.3% had partial radiolucencies and the remainder had no radiolucencies. There were no complete radiolucencies. No subgroup did badly suggesting that there were no additional contraindications for cementless compared with cemented. The conclusion therefore is that complication rate, survival and outcome for the cementless was similar to that of cemented. As there were no complete radiolucencies at a year, this is suggestive of improved fixation compared to the cemented.

Data from both the NJR and the New Zealand Joint Registry would suggest that the results of the cementless implant are better than the cemented. In the NJR, the five year survival of all Oxford arthroplasties was 93% (CI 92.7 – 93.5%, n = 33,272) and the five year survival of the cementless was 97% (CI 95.2 – 98%, n = 2,011). In New Zealand, the five year survival of the cemented implant was 93% (n = 3,267) and the cementless was 98% (n = 795). In both registers, the five year revision rate of the cementless arthroplasty was less than half that of the cemented and the difference was highly statistically significant. Although this does suggest the results of the cementless are better than the cemented, the better results may at least in part be explained by the fact that more experienced surgeons tend to use the cementless and also tend to have better results. A matched analysis of cemented and cementless components based on the NJR found that the OKS was significantly better with cementless (37.9 with cemented, 40.2 with cementless) [12].

Conclusions

Over the past 40 years we have collected data on the Oxford Knee. This chapter should have provided the reader with an overview of the current and past results of UKA and a comparison with TKA.

The data from joint registers confirms that whilst patients undergoing TKA, in general, had lower revision rates, they had higher rates of morbidity and mortality, longer hospital stays, and inferior PROMs compared to UKA. Surgeons with a higher UKA caseload had significantly lower revision rates and superior patient-reported outcomes. Increasing usage (offering UKR to a greater proportion of knee replacement patients) appears to be a viable method of increasing caseload and therefore of improving results. Surgeons with optimal usage (20% to 50% of knee replacements) achieved revision/reoperation rates similar to matched patients undergoing TKA up to eight years postoperatively.

Cohort studies of the cemented OUKA have demonstrated that high levels of function and excellent long term survival can be achieved. In an independent study the 20+ year survival was similar to the best TKA. The proposed general contraindications for UKA (youth, obesity, activity, PFJ damage, chondrocalcino-sis) did not compromise the outcome. This suggests that if patients have AMOA, these proposed contraindications can be ignored. AMOA is present in about 50% of patients needing knee replacement. The importance of surgeons using the OUKA in a high proportion of patients is demonstrated by nine studies of the Phase 3, including 6000 patients, with 10 year survival of about 95% in which surgeons used the OUKA in 20% to 50% of their knee replacements.

Although the best 10 and 20-year results for mobile and fixed are similar, it is clear that, to achieve good long term results with the mobile, surgeons need a large usage, ideally somewhere between 20 and 50%. There is little evidence as to the optimal usage with the fixed but the evidence that exists would suggest that the usage should be much lower with much narrower indications. This is primarily due to problems with wear and progression of disease in the patellofemoral joint. The main conclusion of Argenson's 20-year study was that the fixed bearing should not be used with significant patellofemoral joint problems [70]. This is opposite to the evidence for the Oxford which suggests that, apart from very rare cases with severe damage to the lateral side patellofemoral joint with bone loss, it can be ignored.

Although the results of the cemented OUKA are good, there can be problems particularly in the hands of inexperienced surgeons. Cementing errors are common and even if there are no errors, radiolucent lines are often present. These may be misinterpreted and lead to unnecessary revisions. To address these problems the cementless OUKA was introduced. This appears to be at least as good as the cemented. There is some evidence to suggest that it has better fixation, better func-tion and better survival than the cemented.

References

1. Esler C, Roberts V, Harper W. 15 year outcome of 4665 primary knee arthroplasties: Results from a UK joint register. American Academy of Orthopaedic Surgeons Annual Meeting, San Francisco, USA, 2008.

2. Kalairajah Y, Azurza K, Hulme C, Molloy S, Drabu KJ. Health outcome measures in the evaluation of total hip arthroplasties--a comparison between the Harris hip score and the Oxford hip score. *J Arthroplasty* 2005; **20**(8): 1037-41.

3. Goodfellow JW, O'Connor JJ, Murray DW. A critique of revision rate as an outcome measure: re-interpretation of knee joint registry data. *J Bone Joint Surg Br* 2010; **92**(12): 1628-31.

4. 7th Annual Report, National Joint Registry for England and Wales. 2010.

5. Liddle AD, Judge A, Pandit H, Murray DW. Adverse outcomes after total and unicompartmental knee replacement in 101,330 matched patients: a study of data from the National Joint Registry for England and Wales. *Lancet* 2014; **384**(9952): 1437-45.

6. The swings and roundabouts of unicompartmental arthroplasty. In Knee Roundup. *Bone Joint J 360* 2015; **4**: 17.

7. Hunt LP, Ben-Shlomo Y, Clark EM, Dieppe P, Judge A, MacGregor AJ, Tobias JH, Vernon K, Blom AW, on behalf of the National Joint Registry for England and Wales. 45-day mortality after 467 779 knee replacements for osteoarthritis from the National Joint Registry for England and Wales: an observational study. *Lancet* 2014; Oct 18; **384**(9952):1429-36

8. Liddle AD, Pandit H, Judge A, Murray DW. Patient reported outcomes following total and unicompartmental knee replacement: a study of 14,076 matched patients from the NJREW. *Bone Joint J* 2015 Jun; **97-B**(6):793-801

9. Rothwell AG, Hooper GJ, Hobbs A, Frampton CM. An analysis of the Oxford hip and knee scores and their relationship to early joint revision in the New Zealand Joint Registry. *J Bone Joint Surg Br* 2010; **92**(3): 413-8.

10. Baker PN, Petheram T, Jameson SS, Avery PJ, Reed MR, Gregg PJ, Deehan DJ. Comparison of patient-reported outcome measures following total and unicondylar knee replacement. *J Bone Joint Surg Br* 2012; **94**(7): 919-27.

11. Labek G, Sekyra K, Pawelka W, Janda W, Stockl B. Outcome and reproducibility of data concerning the Oxford unicompartmental knee arthroplasty: a structured literature review including arthroplasty registry data. *Acta Orthop* 2011; **82**(2): 131-5.

12. Liddle AD. Failure of unicompartmental knee replacement [DPhil]. Oxford: University of Oxford; 2014.

13. Kozinn SC, Scott R. Unicondylar knee arthroplasty. *J Bone Joint Surg Am* 1989; **71**(1): 145-50.

14. Stern SH, Becker MW, Insall JN. Unicondylar knee arthroplasty. An evaluation of selection criteria. *Clin Orthop Relat Res* 1993; (**286**): 143-8.

15. Ritter MA, Faris PM, Thong AE, Davis KE, Meding JB, Berend ME. Intra-operative findings in varus osteoarthritis of the knee. An analysis of pre-operative alignment in potential candidates for unicompartmental arthroplasty. *J Bone Joint Surg Br* 2004; **86**(1): 43-7.

16. Liddle AD, Pandit H, Judge A, Murray DW. Narrow indications predict poor outcomes in unicompartmental knee replacement. International Society of Arthroplasty Registers (ISAR) Annual Meeting. Stratford-upon-Avon, UK; 2013.

17. Niinimaki TT, Murray DW, Partanen J, Pajala A, Leppilahti JI. Unicompartmental knee arthroplasties implanted for osteoarthritis with partial loss of joint space have high re-operation rates. *Knee* 2011; **18**(6): 432-5.

18. Pandit H, Gulati A, Jenkins C, Barker K, Price AJ, Dodd CA, Murray DW. Unicompartmental knee replacement for patients with partial thickness cartilage loss in the affected compartment. *Knee* 2011; **18**(3): 168-71.

19. Lewold S, Goodman S, Knutson K, Robertsson O, Lidgren L. Oxford meniscal bearing knee versus the Marmor knee in unicompartmental arthroplasty for arthrosis. A Swedish multicenter survival study. *J Arthroplasty* 1995; **10**(6): 722-31.

20. Annual Report, Swedish Knee Arthroplasty Register. Helsingborg, Sweden, 2013.

21. Australian Orthopaedic Association National Joint Replacement Registry, 2013.

22. Danish Knee Arthroplasty Register - Annual Report 2010. Aarhus, Denmark, 2010.

23. New Zealand Joint Registry 15 year Report. Christchurch, New Zealand, 2014.

24. Ackroyd CE, Whitehouse SL, Newman JH, Joslin CC. A comparative study of the medial St Georg sled and kinematic total knee arthroplasties. Ten-year survivorship. *J Bone Joint Surg Br* 2002; **84**(5): 667-72.

25. Steele RG, Hutabarat S, Evans RL, Ackroyd CE, Newman JH. Survivorship of the St Georg Sled medial unicompartmental knee replacement beyond ten years. *J Bone Joint Surg Br* 2006; **88**(9): 1164-8.

26. Sun PF, Jia YH. Mobile bearing UKA compared to fixed bearing TKA: a randomized prospective study. *Knee* 2012; **19**(2): 103-6.

27. Lombardi AV, Jr., Berend KR, Walter CA, Aziz-Jacobo J, Cheney NA. Is recovery faster for mobile-bearing unicompartmental than total knee arthroplasty? *Clin Orthop Relat Res* 2009; **467**(6): 1450-7.

28. Amin AK, Patton JT, Cook RE, Gaston M, Brenkel IJ. Unicompartmental or total knee arthroplasty?: Results from a matched study. *Clin Orthop Relat Res* 2006; **451**: 101-6.

29. Sweeney K, Grubisic M, Marra CA, Kendall R, Li LC, Lynd LD. Comparison of HRQL between unicompartmental knee arthroplasty and total knee arthroplasty for the treatment of osteoarthritis. *J Arthroplasty* 2013; **28**(9 Suppl): 187-90.

30. Walton NP, Jahromi I, Lewis PL, Dobson PJ, Angel KR, Campbell DG. Patient-perceived outcomes and return to sport and work: TKA versus mini-incision unicompartmental knee arthroplasty. *J Knee Surg* 2006; **19**(2): 112-6.

31. Weale AE, Halabi OA, Jones PW, White SH. Perceptions of outcomes after unicompartmental and total knee replacements. *Clin Orthop Relat Res* 2001; (**382**): 143-53.

32. Costa CR, Johnson AJ, Mont MA, Bonutti PM. Unicompartmental and total knee arthroplasty in the same patient. *J Knee Surg* 2011; **24**(4): 273-8.

33. Dalury DF, Fisher DA, Adams MJ, Gonzales RA. Unicompartmental knee arthroplasty compares favorably to total knee arthroplasty in the same patient. *Orthopedics* 2009; **32**(4).

34. Laurencin CT, Zelicof SB, Scott RD, Ewald FC. Unicompartmental versus total knee arthroplasty in the same patient. A comparative study. *Clin Orthop Relat Res* 1991; (**273**): 151-6.

35. Rougraff BT, Heck DA, Gibson AE. A comparison of tricompartmental and unicompartmental arthroplasty for the treatment of gonarthrosis. *Clin Orthop Relat Res* 1991; (**273**): 157-64.

36. Berend ME, Nunley R, Berend KR, Lombardi AV, Della Valle CJ, Barrack RL. Patient satisfaction and residual pain following TKR, fixed bearing and mobile bearing PKR. Closed Meeting of the Knee Society, Charlotte, NC, USA, September 2014.

37. Beard D, Price A, Cook J, Fitzpatrick R, Carr A, Campbell M, Doll H, Campbell H, Arden N, Cooper C, Davies L, Murray D. Total or Partial Knee Arthroplasty Trial - TOPKAT: study protocol for a randomised controlled trial. *Trials* 2013; **14**: 292.

38. Soohoo NF, Sharifi H, Kominski G, Lieberman JR. Cost-effectiveness analysis of unicompartmental knee arthroplasty as an alternative to total knee arthroplasty for unicompartmental osteoarthritis. *J Bone Joint Surg Am* 2006; **88**(9): 1975-82.

39. Willis-Owen CA, Brust K, Alsop H, Miraldo M, Cobb JP. Unicondylar knee arthroplasty in the UK National Health Service: an analysis of candidacy, outcome and cost efficacy. *Knee* 2009; **16**(6): 473-8.

40. Shakespeare D, Jeffcote B. Unicondylar arthroplasty of the knee--cheap at half the price? *Knee* 2003; **10**(4): 357-61.

41.Xie F, Lo NN, Tarride JE, O'Reilly D, Goeree R, Lee HP. Total or partial knee replacement? Cost-utility analysis in patients with knee osteoarthritis based on a 2-year observational study. *Eur J Health Econ* 2010; **11**(1): 27-34.

42.Slover J, Espehaug B, Havelin LI, Engesaeter LB, Furnes O, Tomek I, Tosteson A. Cost-effectiveness of unicompartmental and total knee arthroplasty in elderly low-demand patients. A Markov decision analysis. *J Bone Joint Surg Am* 2006; **88**(11): 2348-55.

43.Koskinen E, Eskelinen A, Paavolainen P, Pulkkinen P, Remes V. Comparison of survival and cost-effectiveness between unicondylar arthroplasty and total knee arthroplasty in patients with primary osteoarthritis: a follow-up study of 50,493 knee replacements from the Finnish Arthroplasty Register. *Acta Orthop* 2008; **79**(4): 499-507.

44.Confalonieri N, Manzotti A, Pullen C. Navigated shorter incision or smaller implant in knee arthritis? *Clin Orthop Relat Res* 2007; **463**: 63-7.

45.Ghomrawi HM, Eggman AA, Pearle AD. Effect of age on cost-effectiveness of unicompartmental knee arthroplasty compared with total knee arthroplasty in the US *J Bone Joint Surg Am* 2015; **97**(5): 396-402.

46. Hamilton T, Pandit H, Murray D. Oxford Unicompartmental Knee Replacement: a meta-analysis. 2016; in preparation.

47.Price AJ, Svard U. 20-year survival and 10-year clinical results of the Oxford medial UKA. 73rd Annual Meeting of the AAOS. Chicago, Il; 2006.

48.Price AJ, Svard U. A second decade lifetable survival analysis of the Oxford unicompartmental knee arthroplasty. *Clin Orthop Relat Res* 2011; **469**(1): 174-9.

49.Svard U. Phase 1: Perhaps the gold standard for new technology and surgical technique. Global Oxford Masters Symposium. Keble College, Oxford: Biomet; 2012.

50.Barrington JW, Emerson RH. The Oxford Knee: First report of 20-year follow-up in the US. AAOS. New Orleans; 2010. p. Paper no 422.

51.Pandit H, Hamilton TW, Jenkins C, Mellon SJ, Dodd CA, Murray DW. The clinical outcome of minimally invasive Phase 3 Oxford unicompartmental knee arthroplasty: a 15-year follow-up of 1000 UKAs. *Bone Joint J* 2015; **97-B**(11): 1493-500.

52.Vorlat P, Verdonk R, Schauvlieghe H. The Oxford unicompartmental knee prosthesis: a 5-year follow-up. *Knee Surg Sports Traumatol Arthrosc* 2000; **8**(3): 154-8.

53.Kumar A, Fiddian NJ. Medial unicompartmental arthroplasty of the knee. *Knee* 1999; **6**: 21-3.

54.Murray DW, Goodfellow JW, O'Connor JJ. The Oxford medial unicompartmental arthroplasty: a ten-year survival study. *J Bone Joint Surg Br* 1998; **80**(6): 983-9.

55. Bottomley NJ, Jones L, Rout R, Jackson WF, Beard D, Price A. The survival and functional outcome of unicompartmental knee arthroplasty undertaken by high or low volume users (poster #202). American Academy of Orthopedic Surgeons Annual Meeting, Las Vegas, USA, 2015.

56.Briant-Evans T, Gould A, Pearce A, Risebury M, Thomas N, Wilson A. The Oxford Phase 3 medial unicompartmental knee replacement. 10 year results from an independent centre: Survival, function and risk factors for revision. British Association for Surgery of the Knee (BASK) Annual Meeting. Derby, UK; 2013.

57.Rajasekhar C, Das S, Smith A. Unicompartmental knee arthroplasty. 2- to 12-year results in a community hospital. *J Bone Joint Surg Br* 2004; **86**(7): 983-5.

58. Price AJ, Dodd CA, Svard UG, Murray DW. Oxford medial unicompartmental knee arthroplasty in patients younger and older than 60 years of age. *J Bone Joint Surg Br* 2005; **87**(11): 1488-92.

59. Koskinen E, Paavolainen P, Eskelinen A, Pulkkinen P, Remes V. Unicondylar knee replacement for primary osteoarthritis: a prospective follow-up study of 1,819 patients from the Finnish Arthroplasty Register. *Acta Orthop* 2007; **78**(1): 128-35.

60. Pandit H, Jenkins C, Gill HS, Barker K, Dodd CA, Murray DW. Minimally invasive Oxford phase 3 unicompartmental knee replacement: results of 1000 cases. *J Bone Joint Surg Br* 2011; **93**(2): 198-204.

61. Yoshida K, Tada M, Yoshida H, Takei S, Fukuoka S, Nakamura H. Oxford phase 3 unicompartmental knee arthroplasty in Japan – clinical results in greater than one thousand cases over ten years. *J Arthroplasty* 2013; **28**(9 Suppl): 168-71.

62. Wagner-Kristensen P. Follow up on 800 patients having a medial Oxford prosthesis at Vejle Hospital, Denmark. . Oxford Global Masters Symposium. Oxford; 2012.

63. Lim HC, Bae JH, Song SH, Kim SJ. Oxford phase 3 unicompartmental knee replacement in Korean patients. *J Bone Joint Surg Br* 2012; **94**(8): 1071-6.

64. Davidson JA, Jha S, Edmondson M, Sandiford N, Miles K, East D, Apthorp H, Goddard R, Butler-Manuel PA. The use of the Oxford Partial Knee Replacement in the elderly population; a knee for life? Oxford Global Masters Symposium. Oxford; 2012.

65. Nagy M, Keys GW. Long-term outcome of unicompartmental knee replacement in a district general hospital (paper 234). AAOS. Chicago; 2013.

66. Faour-Martin O, Valverde-Garcia JA, Martin-Ferrero MA, Vega-Castrillo A, de la Red Gallego MA, Suarez de Puga CC, Amigo-Linares L. Oxford phase 3 unicondylar knee arthroplasty through a minimally invasive approach: long-term results. *Int Orthop* 2013; **37**(5): 833-8.

67. Choy WS, Kim KJ, Lee SK, Yang DS, Lee NK. Mid-term results of Oxford medial unicompartmental knee arthroplasty. *Clin Orthop Surg* 2011; **3**(3): 178-83.

68. Gulati A, Pandit H, Jenkins C, Chau R, Dodd CA, Murray DW. The effect of leg alignment on the outcome of unicompartmental knee replacement. *J Bone Joint Surg Br* 2009; **91**(4): 469-74.

69. Price AJ, Webb J, Topf H, Dodd CA, Goodfellow JW, Murray DW, Oxford Hip and Knee Group. Rapid recovery after Oxford unicompartmental arthroplasty through a short incision. *J Arthroplasty* 2001; **16**(8): 970-6.

70. Argenson JN, Blanc G, Aubaniac JM, Parratte S. Modern unicompartmental knee arthroplasty with cement: a concise follow-up, at a mean of twenty years, of a previous report. *J Bone Joint Surg Am* 2013; **95**(10): 905-9.

71. Foran JR, Brown NM, Della Valle CJ, Berger RA, Galante JO. Long-term survivorship and failure modes of unicompartmental knee arthroplasty. *Clin Orthop Relat Res* 2013; **471**(1): 102-8.

72. Parratte S, Pauly V, Aubaniac JM, Argenson JN. No long-term difference between fixed and mobile medial unicompartmental arthroplasty. *Clin Orthop Relat Res* 2012; **470**(1): 61-8.

73. Heyse TJ, Khefacha A, Peersman G, Cartier P. Survivorship of UKA in the middle-aged. *Knee* 2012; **19**(5): 585-91.

74. Keblish PA, Briard JL. Mobile-bearing unicompartmental knee arthroplasty: a 2-center study with an 11-year (mean) follow-up. *J Arthroplasty* 2004; **19**(7 Suppl 2): 87-94.

75. O'Rourke MR, Gardner JJ, Callaghan JJ, Liu SS, Goetz DD, Vittetoe DA, Sullivan PM, Johnston RC. The John Insall Award: unicompartmental knee replacement: a minimum twenty-one-year followup, end-result study. *Clin Orthop Relat Res* 2005; **440**: 27-37.

76. Squire MW, Callaghan JJ, Goetz DD, Sullivan PM, Johnston RC. Unicompartmental knee replacement. A minimum 15 year followup study. *Clin Orthop Relat Res* 1999; (367): 61-72.

77. Tabor OB, Jr., Tabor OB. Unicompartmental arthroplasty: a long-term follow-up study. *J Arthroplasty* 1998; **13**(4): 373-9.

78. Cartier P, Sanouiller JL, Grelsamer RP. Unicompartmental knee arthroplasty surgery. 10-year minimum follow-up period. *J Arthroplasty* 1996; **11**(7): 782-8.

79. Heck DA, Marmor L, Gibson A, Rougraff BT. Unicompartmental knee arthroplasty. A multicenter investigation with long-term follow-up evaluation. *Clin Orthop Relat Res* 1993; (286): 154-9.

80. Marmor L. Unicompartmental knee arthroplasty. Ten- to 13-year follow-up study. *Clin Orthop Relat Res* 1988; (226): 14-20.

81. Rachha R, Veravalli K, Sood M. Medium term results of the Miller-Galante knee arthroplasty with 10 year survivorship. *Acta Orthop Belg* 2013; **79**(2): 197-204.

82. John J, Mauffrey C, May P. Unicompartmental knee replacements with Miller-Galante prosthesis: two to 16-year follow-up of a single surgeon series. *Int Orthop* 2011; **35**(4): 507-13.

83. Naudie D, Guerin J, Parker DA, Bourne RB, Rorabeck CH. Medial unicompartmental knee arthroplasty with the Miller-Galante prosthesis. *J Bone Joint Surg Am* 2004; **86-A**(9): 1931-5.

84. Ansari S, Newman JH, Ackroyd CE. St. Georg sledge for medial compartment knee replacement. 461 arthroplasties followed for 4 (1-17) years. *Acta Orthop Scand* 1997; **68**(5): 430-4.

85. Hall MJ, Connell DA, Morris HG. Medium to long-term results of the UNIX uncemented unicompartmental knee replacement. *Knee* 2013; **20**(5): 328-31.

86. Kendrick BJ, Kaptein BL, Valstar ER, Gill HS, Jackson WF, Dodd CA, Price AJ, Murray DW. Cemented versus cementless Oxford unicompartmental knee arthroplasty using radiostereometric analysis: A randomised controlled trial. *Bone Joint J* 2015; **97-B**(2): 185-91.

87. Liddle AD, Pandit H, O'Brien S, Doran E, Penny ID, Hooper GJ, Burn PJ, Dodd CA, Beverland DE, Maxwell AR, Murray DW. Cementless fixation in Oxford unicompartmental knee replacement: a multicentre study of 1000 knees. *Bone Joint J* 2013; **95-B**(2): 181-7.

88. Price AJ, Waite JC, Svard U. Long-term clinical results of the medial Oxford unicompartmental knee arthroplasty. *Clin Orthop Relat Res* 2005; (435):171-80.

89. Beard D, Price A, Cook J, Maclennan G, Campbell M, Davies L, Murray D, TOPKAT Study Group. Total Or Partial Knn Replacement: One year results from a large multi-centre randomised controlled trial (TOPKAT). ESSKA, Geneva, Switzerland, June 2016.

11

Management of Complications

In this chapter we describe the common modes of failure of the OUKA and suggest ways of dealing with them. We also discuss why they occur and how they can be prevented.

Complications occur more commonly in the hands of learners than in those of the experienced surgeons whose reports are published in the literature. As a result, the incidence of complications is lower in published cohort series compared to national registers

In Table 11.1 we show the incidence of the various different complications in two different series, the NJR and our own series out to 15 years.

Table 11.1 Reasons for reoperation in the designer series and NJR based on Patient Time Incident Rate (PTIR).

Indication for re-operation / revision	Designer Series Phase 3, at mean 10 years	NJR Data at 10 years
Progression of arthritis in the lateral compartment	2.4 %	2.6 %
Bearing dislocation	0.7 %	0.1 %
Unexplained pain	0.7 %	1.9 %
Infection	0.6 %	0.5 %
Aseptic loosening	0.2 %	3.6 %
Fracture		0.2 %
PFJ problem		
Other	0.6 %	3.5 %

In the long term, the commonest cause of failure is progression of arthritis in the lateral compartment although the incidence is low. In the NJR, there is a much higher incidence of revision for pain or loosening than in the designer series. This is likely to be, at least in part, because of misinterpretation of tibial radiolucency. Inexperienced surgeons often consider the common stable radiolucency to be a source of pain or indicative of loosening when the evidence suggests it is not. The dislocation rate of 0.1% in the NJR is surprisingly low, perhaps because surgeons do not consider treatment of a dislocation to be a revision. There are no failures because of patellofemoral joint problems or wear in either series.

Infection

The incidence of infection after UKA is about half that after TKA [1]. The methods of investigation of suspected infection are the same in OUKA as in TKA except that radionuclide uptake studies are not helpful. After OUKA, activity in the bone beneath the implants persists for several years, so the presence of a 'hot' area on the scan is not necessarily evidence of infection (or loosening). The C-reactive protein or erythrocyte sedimentation rate are the most useful diagnostic tests but may not be positive in the first 2–3 weeks. We do not have any experience of using the new synovial fluid markers to diagnose suspected prosthetic joint infection after UKA.

Treatment

Acute infection

In the early postoperative period, acute infection is diagnosed and treated in the same way as after TKA. Early open debridement and change of meniscal bearing and intravenous antibiotics can arrest the infection and save the arthroplasty. The use of arthroscopic lavage is not recommended as it is not as reliable as open debridement and exchange of bearing.

Late infection

Failure of treatment of an acute infection, or infection of later onset, is diagnosed from the clinical and radiological signs and bacteriological studies, as in TKA. The earliest radiological signs may be in the retained compartment. Figure 11.1(a) shows thinning of the articular cartilage and juxta-articular erosions of the lateral joint margin of an infected knee after medial OUKA; evidence of chondrolysis by the infecting organism and chronic synovitis. (Note that acute rheumatoid synovitis can produce a similar appearance.) The eventual appearance of thick (>2 mm), ill-defined progressive radiolucencies beneath the components (Fig. 11.1(b)), quite different from the thin radiolucent lines with radiodense margins that outline most normally functioning OUKA, is diagnostic.

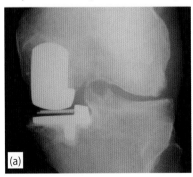 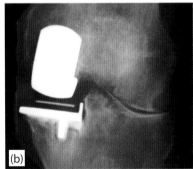

Figure 11.1 (a) The earliest radiographic sign of infection may be the appearance of subchondral erosions in the retained compartment of the knee. (b) The radiolucencies under the tibial plateau are more than 2 mm thick and are not defined by a radiodense line. They are different from the common 'physiological' radiolucent lines and suggest infection and/or loosening.

Treatment is by removal of the implant and excision of the inflammatory membrane, followed by one- or two-stage revision to TKA. We prefer the two-stage procedure, with removal of the implant and excision of the articular surfaces of the retained compartment at the first stage. An antibiotic-loaded spacer is left in the joint to maintain the gap and deliver high doses of antibiotic until the infection is eradicated and the second stage can be safely undertaken. Three types of spacers can be used (Fig. 11.2). We favour a bicompartmental spacer as this allows removal of all infected articular cartilage at the first stage. The spacer can be static or articulating depending on surgeon preference. The second-stage TKA may require a stemmed tibial implant (with additional medial augments) if there is substantial tibial bone loss.

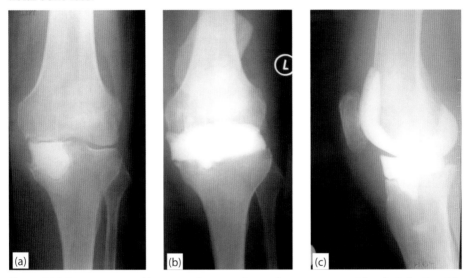

Figure 11.2 Spacers are used between the procedures of a two-stage revision for infection: (a) unicompartmental (not recommended as bacteria can persist in retained cartilage); (b) simple bicompartmental; (c) articulating.

Medial tibial plateau fracture

The 2014 NJR report gives a figure of 0.30 revisions for periprosthetic fracture per 1000 years (95% CI 0.24 – 0.37) in UKA (Fig. 11.3(a)) [2]. Registers however underestimate the incidence of fracture as many are internally fixed rather than revised. In our series of 1000 Phase 3 cemented OUKAs, we did not encounter a single fracture [3]. Similarly with the current design of cementless OUKA, we have not encountered any tibial plateau fracture. Fractures occur with all types of UKA, for example four plateau fractures occurred in 62 UKAs reported by Berger et al. [4] and there are other occasional reports in the literature [2, 6-9]. We have reported on a series of eight cases of tibial plateau fractures after Oxford UKA (which occurred over a period of seven years) collected from various institutions in the UK [8]. The study confirmed that these fractures are rare and tend to occur in inexperienced hands with both cemented as well as cementless implants.

Despite the very few fractures in the published reports of OUKA cohorts, several have been reported to us by other users and we believe that the complication is more common than the literature suggests, particularly among surgeons beginning to do unicompartmental arthroplasty, in populations with constitutionally small tibiae (e.g. Asian populations) and following cementless fixation.

Cause

It seems likely that plateau fractures either occur intraoperatively or are a result of severe weakening of the bone caused intraoperatively. They are either diagnosed intraoperatively or present later, commonly at 2–12 weeks postoperatively (Fig. 11.3(a)). If the fracture is initially undisplaced, it may not be visible on the immediate postoperative radiographs, only appearing later when weight-bearing has caused displacement, and postoperative pain and deformity have drawn attention to the problem.

Weakening of the condyle

Weakening of the condyle by removal of its articular surface and subchondral bone plate is probably the main reason for fracture. Since this is unavoidable, great care should be taken to avoid any additional weakening of the bone. We believe that the most potent cause of fracture is damage to the posterior tibial cortex and the cancellous bone by vertical saw cuts that go deeper than they need or if the keel slot breaks through the posterior cortex (Fig. 11.3(c)). Even the two small holes made in the anterior cortex by the nails that fix the tibial saw guide have been shown to decrease the strength of the tibial condyle [2, 6]. Although we have used this method of fixation in all phases of the OUKA without complication, we now use only one nail.

The more bone that is removed from the condyle, the weaker is the remainder; therefore the surgical objective should be to remove as little as possible. It is an advantage of meniscal-bearing arthroplasty that polyethylene only 3 or 4 mm thick can be used safely. This advantage should be exploited by removing as little tibial plateau as possible.

The smaller the tibia, the less bone can be safely removed from it. This may explain why more fractures have been reported to us from Asian countries where many adults are of small stature. It is particularly important in small patients that the horizontal tibial saw cut should aim to accommodate a thin bearing which can be as little as 3 mm thick (see Chapter 6). Cadaver studies have shown that the load to fracture is significantly lower following cementless fixation than cemented so surgeons must be more careful with cementless fixation [10]. This is a particular problem when surgeons with a large experience of the more forgiving cemented fixation swap to cementless.

Finite element analysis (FEA) work shows that the strain in the proximal tibia and thus the risk of fractures is significantly elevated by (a) a deep tibial resection; (b) too medial or too deep a vertical cut (Fig. 11.4) [11]. This in turn diminishes the area available for load transfer and, if the vertical cut violates the posterior cortex and/or the keel cut is made too deep, then a fracture may occur. The surgeon must not lift, and therefore tilt, the saw when performing the vertical cut. The vertical cut should be made just medial to the apex of the medial tibial spine. A simple way to ensure the vertical cut does not go too deep is to do the horizontal cut first and then insert a shim into the cut to act as an end stop for the vertical cut. (Extending the horizontal cut laterally tends to decrease the risk of fracture (Fig. 11.4).) The surgeon should also use the keel-cut saw blade and hold onto the pin fixing the template when performing the keel cut, to prevent the cut going too far posterior.

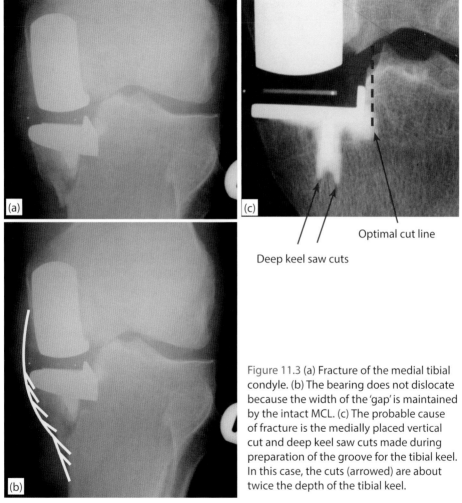

Optimal cut line

Deep keel saw cuts

Figure 11.3 (a) Fracture of the medial tibial condyle. (b) The bearing does not dislocate because the width of the 'gap' is maintained by the intact MCL. (c) The probable cause of fracture is the medially placed vertical cut and deep keel saw cuts made during preparation of the groove for the tibial keel. In this case, the cuts (arrowed) are about twice the depth of the tibial keel.

Application of excessive force may also cause fracture. The heavy hammer commonly used in TKA is not appropriate for UKA. A small hammer, in the hands of a surgeon alert to the risk, will seldom cause a tibial plateau fracture. This is a particular risk with cementless fixation as often the tibial plateau, after insertion, is left about 0.5 mm proud. This should be accepted as it will subside with time and integrate. Impacting it hard may cause a fracture.

(a) Excessive horizontal cut   (b) Excessive vertical cut

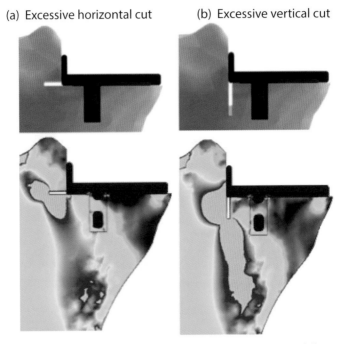

Figure 11.4 Finite element models showing the high risk of fracture (gray) following excessively deep vertical cuts [11].

Pathological anatomy

Figure 11.3(b) shows how the strong attachments of the MCL to the cortex of the medial tibial plateau maintain the components of the arthroplasty in their proper relationship. In particular, the gap between the femoral and tibial implants remains unaltered, and dislocation of the bearing does not occur. Displacement of the fragment distally allows the tibiofemoral axis to drift into varus.

Treatment

Management depends on the stage at which the fracture is diagnosed and the degree of varus deformity.

Intraoperative diagnosis

Several reports suggest that if the fracture is diagnosed during the operation it should be reduced and internally fixed. Thereafter, the UKA can be completed in the expectation of a good result [12]. If the medial fragment is comminuted, it is best fixed with a medial buttress plate. The alternative option is to use cancellous screws inserted through the medial fragment under image intensifier control.

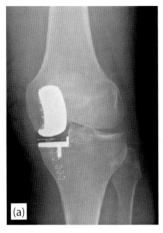
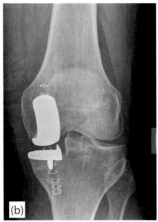
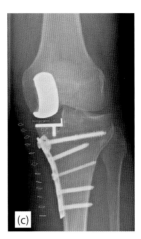

Figure 11.5 Tibial plateau fracture fixed with a buttress plate. : (a) post operation; (b) fracture; (c) post fracture.

Postoperative diagnosis

The following algorithm is suggested but may need to be modified according to the circumstances.

Within three months of surgery:

A.   If the fracture is minimally displaced, or undisplaced, employ external splinting to maintain alignment while awaiting union.

B.   If there is significant displacement, employ open reduction and internal fixation with an AO buttress plate or interfragmentary screws (Fig. 11.5).

Later than three months after surgery:

A.   If the fracture is united and the varus deformity is acceptable, no action is required.

B.   If the fracture is united but causing pain, suspect tibial component loosening. If this is confirmed, revise to a TKA.

C.   If the fracture is not united, revise to a TKA with a stemmed tibial component.

What constitutes 'acceptable' varus deformity? In this context, up to 5° of varus is probably acceptable. In UKA, varus malalignment does not have the same sinister implication as it has in TKA; indeed, many practitioners aim always to leave the operated limb in a few degrees of varus.

Dislocation of a mobile bearing

This complication was introduced into surgery with the invention of mobile-bearing knee arthroplasty [13]. In the NJR, the incidence is reported as 1.2 revisions for dislocation/subluxation per 1000 component years (95% CI 1.05 - 1.37) for mobile bearing UKA. This dislocation rate may be low because surgeons may not consider dislocation to be a failure. In a meta-analysis of published or presented studies on Phase 3 OUKA, it is 0.73% (34 studies, total number of knees 10,125 and 74 dislocations at a mean follow up of 54 months [range 24-138 months]). In our 1000 Phase 3 cohort, the dislocation rate was 0.5%. Most dislocations occur early [3].

Causes

Primary dislocations are usually caused by a combination of distraction of the joint and displacement of the bearing due to impingement. They are the most common type of dislocation. They occur early and are usually due to surgical error.

The following mistakes all increase the risk of dislocation (the mechanism of entrapment is explained in detail in Chapter 6).

1. Failure to remove osteophytes from the back of the femoral condyle causing impingement in flexion, stretching of the ligaments and anterior displacement of the bearing, particularly in patients who achieve high degrees of flexion.

2. Inequality of the 110° and 20° flexion gaps or MCL damage.

3. Retained cement protruding above the tibial plateau surface.

4. Femoral component (and therefore the bearing) sited too far from the lateral wall of the tibial component so that the bearing is free to rotate through 90°. This is unlikely to be a problem with anatomic bearings, which are now routinely used (see Fig. 6.14).

5. A bearing that is much too thin relative to gap width may, theoretically, dislocate, and beginners, fearful of dislocation, tend to insert the thickest bearing possible, but this is a mistake. 'Overstuffing' the knee should be avoided as it increases the risk of dislocation, pain and delayed recovery.

Secondary dislocation is the result of loss of entrapment from loosening (and subsidence) of the metal components. Spontaneous elongation of ligaments over time does not seem to occur unless there is impingement, when forced flexion or extension may stretch ligaments. Secondary dislocation is rare.

Traumatic dislocation has occasionally been encountered when a normally functioning OUKA has been forced into an extreme posture and the MCL has been momentarily stretched or damaged.

Diagnosis

Dislocation occurs when the knee is unloaded or at the moment when load is re-applied, for example rising from a chair or getting out of bed. It is usually a dramatic event and the patient seeks urgent advice, but dislocation can occur relatively silently. Walking may be resumed with the bearing displaced; the weight is borne (painlessly) through the opposed metal components.

Radiographs demonstrate the site of the displaced bearing, and may suggest its cause (e.g. osteophytes, retained cement, or displacement of a metal component).

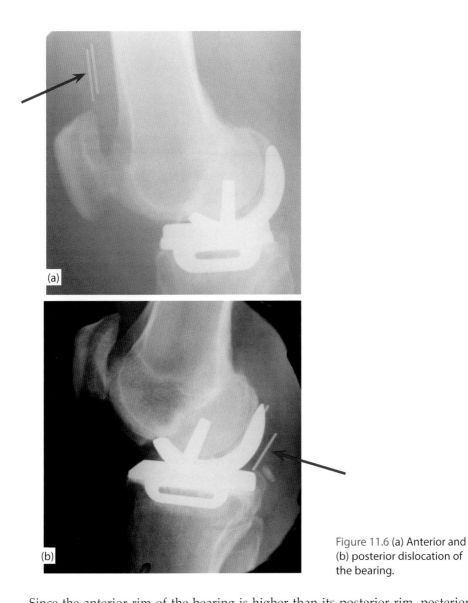

Figure 11.6 (a) Anterior and (b) posterior dislocation of the bearing.

Since the anterior rim of the bearing is higher than its posterior rim, posterior dislocation requires more distraction of the joint than anterior dislocation (5 mm compared with 3 mm). Therefore, the displaced bearing is most commonly found in the anterior joint space, and occasionally in the suprapatellar pouch (Fig. 11.6(a)). Displacement into the posterior joint space (Fig. 11.6(b)) suggests that the bearing has rotated through 90° (point (2) above), from which position it is as easy for it to dislocate backwards as forwards as the entrapment has decreased to 2 mm. Introduction of the anatomical bearing has significantly reduced the incidence of posterior dislocation, as the long lateral side prevents bearing rotation. Occasionally, the bearing is found to be tilted into the intercondylar space where it may stabilise in a subluxed position (see Chapter 12).

Treatment

Manipulation can result in relocation. On a few occasions reduction has occurred, more or less spontaneously, under anaesthesia. However, **arthrotomy** is almost always required to remove the bearing and to determine the cause of its displacement. The bearing can usually be retrieved through a small anterior incision, even if it is in the back of the joint, but an additional posterior arthrotomy has sometimes been needed. We are aware of two cases in which the bearing, which could not be retrieved from the back of the knee, was left in the knee and did not cause problems [14]. The femoral component was dislodged on one occasion while retrieving the bearing and was successfully re-cemented.

Primary dislocation

When both the metal components are found to be securely fixed to the bones, other causes of dislocation need to be sought.

Any bone or cement that might impinge on the bearing is removed. Retained posterior femoral osteophytes can be removed with the posterior osteophyte chisel. An anatomical bearing, usually one size thicker, is inserted (see Chapter 6, Figure 6.14). It is important not to over tighten the ligaments.

If there is recurrent dislocation, MCL damage or a serious mismatch between the 110° and 20° flexion gaps, TKA should be performed. Since the introduction of a fixed-bearing tibial plateau to articulate with the OUKA femoral component, some surgeons have converted to this in cases where instability of the mobile bearing is the only defect in the arthroplasty. However, it should be noted that Australian Orthopaedic Association National Joint Replacement Registry data demonstrate that revisions of failed UKA to another UKA have generally been less successful than revisions from UKA to TKA [15]. Recurrent dislocation is rare and should be treated by conversion to TKA.

Secondary dislocation

This is dealt with in the section below on loosening of a fixed component.

Traumatic dislocation

The few patients in which this has occurred have been successfully managed by either closed reduction of the displaced bearing or open insertion of a new bearing.

Loosening of a fixed component

Over the years we have gained a good insight into why loosening of cemented components occurs and how it can be prevented. It would seem factors causing loosening of cementless components are different and, as cementless loosening is rare, we have little insight into this. Loosening is one of the commonest causes of failure in the national registers. In the NJR, the loosening rate is 4.01 (CI 3.73 – 4.32) per 1000 patient years [2]. It is much less common in the published series. For example, our series of 1000 cemented OUKA with up to 15 years follow-up, we have encountered one case each of femoral and tibial loosening [16]. A possible reason for the high rate seen in registers relates to misdiagnosis of physiological radiolucencies (see Chapter 9). The incidence of loosening of cementless components is less than cemented in the registries.

Diagnosis

In OUKA, the only reliable radiographic evidence for loosening of a metal component is its displacement. For example, a loose tibial component may tilt (Fig. 11.7) or a femoral component rotate (Fig. 11.8). As has been discussed elsewhere, stable radiolucencies are very common at the bone–cement interfaces and are not evidence of loosening. Displacement is diagnosed by comparing two radiographs taken with a time interval between them; however, small changes in position can only be detected if the X-ray beam was aligned, on both occasions, in the same relation to one of the components. The required accuracy can only be achieved if both radiographs were taken with the beam aligned by fluoroscopy or by carefully adjusting it while taking multiple low dose images with a digital system (Fig. 11.7).

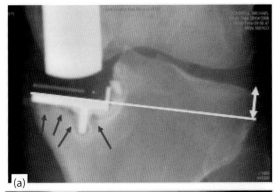

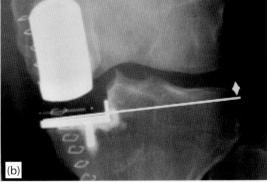

Figure 11.7 (a) Aligned radiograph showing a thick poorly defined pathological radiolucency around the tibial component. Comparison with a similarly aligned post operative radiograph (b) shows that the tibial component has tipped and is therefore loose.

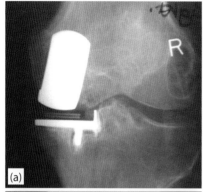

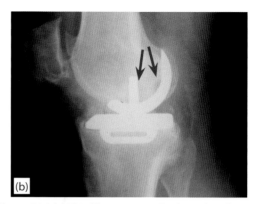

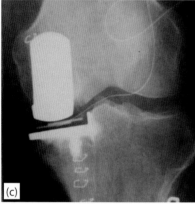

Figure 11.8 (a) This (fluoroscopically aligned) radiograph was misinterpreted as evidence of loosening of the tibial component. However, the radiolucencies beneath that component are thin and defined by a radiodense line, suggesting they are stable and benign. (b) Careful examination of the lateral radiograph shows a possible pathological radiolucency around the peg and posterior part of the femoral component. When the AP radiograph is compared with the (similarly fluoroscopically aligned) postoperative radiograph (c) it can be seen that there is displacement of the femoral component but the tibial component has not moved. At the revision operation, the tibial component was found to be firmly fixed and the femoral component was loose.

Misinterpretation of the 'physiological' lucencies, so commonly seen on aligned radiographs, has resulted in unnecessary revision by surgeons unfamiliar with their benign nature. Femoral component loosening is difficult to diagnose because the pathological radiolucencies can be difficult to see (Fig. 11.8). If it is suspected, it is recommended that lateral X-rays are taken in flexion and extension [17] (Fig. 11.9). These may show evidence of movement of the femoral component which is diagnostic of loosening.

Bone scans can be very misleading so it is recommended that they are not used. Typically, whether there is loosening or not, there is increased uptake under the tibial component, presumably due to remodelling, which persists for many years. On the femoral side, there is usually no increased uptake. The bone scan will be reported as indicative of tibial loosening. We are aware of a surgeon who revised an OUKA on the basis of a typical scan appearance and a report suggesting a loose tibial component and a secure femoral component, and found at operation, a secure tibia and loose femur.

Occasionally, dislocation of the bearing draws attention to a loose component.

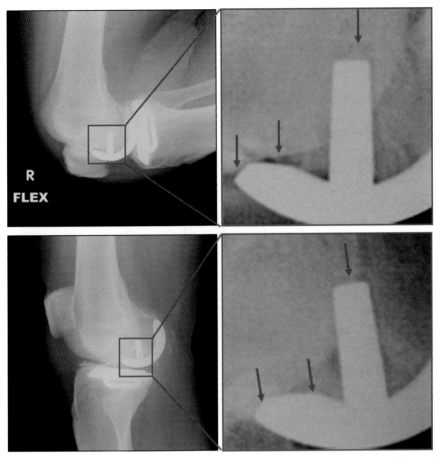

Figure 11.9 Flexion and extension radiographs with magnified views showing the femoral component moving which is diagnostic of loosening.

Causes

Early failures are probably the result of poor initial fixation. Immediate postoperative radiographs and retrieved specimens have often revealed unsatisfactory cementing of the tibial component. In addition, the tibial component is often too small and does not reach the posterior cortex. We have had several reports of sudden displacement of the femoral component in the immediate postoperative period, but usually it occurs a few years later and is associated with clunking, attributable (in retrospect) to poor initial fixation of its posterior facet and lack of cement in the 6 mm hole. It is hoped that use of the two-peg femoral component will decrease the incidence of femoral loosening. Some evidence from the retrieval studies suggests that late tibial loosening may be due to the accumulated effects of impact loading from impingement of the front of the bearing on the femoral condyle in full extension [18].

Treatment

In **early loosening**, if the bone has not been seriously eroded, cementing a new component is a possible option and has been successful on several occasions.

However, in **late loosening**, the bone will already be more extensively damaged and revision to TKA is better undertaken immediately.

Loosening of cementless components

We have little experience of loosening of cementless components as it seems to occur much less frequently than with cemented components. We are not aware of any cases of late femoral loosening but have heard of cases in which the femoral component was observed to be loose at the end of the operation and a cemented component was therefore implanted. These presumably occurred because the 6 mm hole was accidently enlarged during the operation. Care must be taken to avoid toggling instruments that go into the 6 mm hole.

We have not seen late tibial loosening but are aware of a number of cases in which the tibia has subsided early [19]. Typically, during the first month, the post-operative course and radiograph is normal. However, during the next few months, the patient complains of new or persistent pain and the radiograph demonstrates the tibial component has developed a complete radiolucency, has subsided into valgus and tipped posteriorly. If this is treated conservatively, the pain tends to settle spontaneously, the implant stops subsiding and the radiolucency eventually disappears as the component becomes securely fixed (Fig. 11.10).

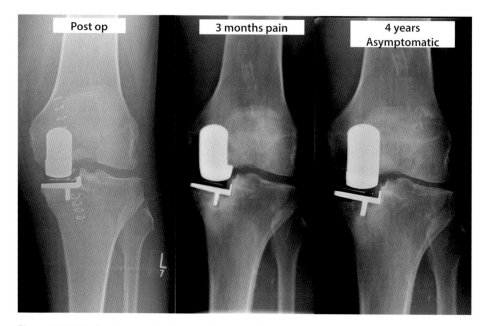

Figure 11.10 Early valgus subsidence and pain. Subsequently the pain settles and the tibial component becomes securely fixed.

Factors that may contribute to tibial subsidence are an undersized component that does not reach the posterior cortex, a deep resection, multiple and deep vertical cuts or damage to the back of the keel slot. Perhaps the most important factor is that the bearing may be jammed against the wall in flexion. If this occurs, there will be a large load on the lateral side of the tibial component causing it to tip into valgus. Once tipped, the bearing will move medially and normal load distribution will be restored so integration can occur.

As the symptoms tend to settle and the components integrate, it is recommended that these cases should be treated conservatively. Patients should be reassured and advised to restrict weight bearing.

Lateral compartment arthritis

In our series of 1000 cemented Phase 3 OUKAs with up to 15 years follow up, lateral progression requiring revision occurred in 25 cases (2.5% cases) at a mean of 7.0 years (range 1.9 to 11.4 years) [16]. In this series, cases with lateral progression were matched with controls but no factors leading to progression were identified. In Svard's 20-year series, the revision rate for lateral compartment OA was 2.3% [20].

Diagnosis

Pain in the knee, usually but not always on the lateral side, is the main symptom. The first radiographic sign is narrowing of the lateral compartment joint space (Fig. 11.11), and this may long precede the onset of pain. Subchondral sclerosis and disappearance of the joint space ensue. Osteophytes around the margins of the lateral compartment are very common but do not necessarily portend progressive arthritis.

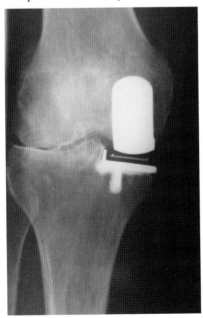

Figure 11.11 Severe lateral compartment degeneration.

Causes

Some authors have regarded arthritis of the contralateral compartment in UKA as a time-dependent consequence of the gradual, but inevitable, spread of osteoarthritis throughout the joint [21], perhaps hastened by the presence within the joint cavity of the foreign materials of the prosthesis. If this were true, there would be evidence of progressive arthritis in both the lateral and PFJ. A comparison between one year and ten year post-operative radiographs shows that this does not happen [22]. Furthermore the incidence of revision due to progression is rare (about 2.5% at 15 to 20 years) [23, 24] and revision for PFJ progression virtually never occurs. It would seem that, in general in AMOA, disease progression is arrested by OUKA [24] suggesting that the underlying disease is a focal mechanical problem. In the few cases when progression does occur, it is likely to relate to some issue with the indications or technique or perhaps an element of inflammatory arthritis or a low grade infection.

Most authors believe, as we do, that overcorrection of the varus deformity into valgus (Fig. 11.12) is an important cause, and many surgeons recommend aiming to leave the UKA knee in a few degrees of varus to avoid this. Choosing the postoperative tibiofemoral angle is not an option in the OUKA operation since the thickness of the bearing is selected to match the lengths of the ligaments, not to provide an arbitrary alignment of the limb. Therefore, an intact MCL is all-important if overcorrection is to be avoided.

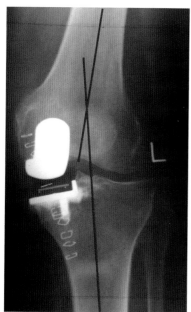

Figure 11.12 Postoperative radiograph of a knee overcorrected into valgus. Such a degree of valgus could only occur after damage to the MCL.

To minimise the risk of lateral compartment OA, we recommend valgus stress radiographs to assess the lateral compartment pre-operatively, very careful intraoperative preservation of the MCL (particularly its deep fibres) and avoidance of 'overstuffing' of the medial compartment with a thicker bearing than the ligaments will easily accommodate.

Treatment

If the symptoms warrant surgical treatment, revision to TKA is indicated. However, experienced surgeons may chose to do a lateral UKA if the medial compartment is satisfactory. We tend to open and extend the old incision and then do a lateral parapatellar approach. In our series of 27 cases with a mean follow up of four years, we have had no failures [25]. Furthermore we find that patients recover more rapidly (length of stay 2.3 days vs 4.7 days) and with less morbidity and better functional outcomes than after TKA.

Pain

Pain can be a problem and often leads to unnecessary revision.

It is most commonly encountered over the proximal tibia and is anteromedial in distribution. This type of pain is not unusual in the first six months and usually settles spontaneously. Review of our patients showed that the incidence has decreased with time and is now 2% at one year follow up [26]. In other series, it has been higher, particularly with surgical inexperience [26]. Other sites of pain are much less common. The NZJR reports pain as a cause of revision in 38% of UKA revision and data from the NJR suggests 23% of UKA revisions are for pain.

There are numerous proposed causes and many may be multifactorial. Unexplained pain is the most common presentation but there is increasing evidence [27, 28] that inappropriate indications or bone overload are the most common causes. Impingement, soft tissue irritation, cementing errors, pes anserinus bursitis or neuroma have all been implicated .

Partial thickness cartilage loss (PTCL)

It is generally thought that UKA is best used in young patients with early arthritis. We strongly disagree with this and recommend that the OUKA is only offered to patients with bone-on-bone arthritis. Cadaveric studies have shown that asymptomatic PTCL is common [29]. So, if a patient has pain and PTCL, the PTCL is not necessarily the cause of pain. In a study [30] comparing the outcome of patients with PTCL and matched patients with bone exposed (BE) or bone loss (BL), it was found those with PTCL had worse outcome scores and greater variability than BE and BL (OKS 36 (SD 10) v 43 (SD 4) & 43 (SD 5) respectively). Furthermore, 21% of the PTCL group were worse or had no substantial improvement (ΔOKS<6) after the surgery, whereas all patients in the BE and BL groups reported substantial improvement (Fig. 11.13). In the study, there were four complications, all of which were pain related and all occurred in the PTCL group [30]. Although some patients with PTCL do well with OUKA, a sizeable proportion do not. Until it can be predicted which will do well, it is sensible to avoid doing UKA in patients with PTCL. In the future, it may be possible to predict which will do well with a bone scan or MRI, but as yet this has not been shown to be possible. It is therefore important to be able to distinguish between those with PTCL and those with bone-on-bone. We do this with a series of radiographs including standing AP, varus stress or Rosenberg. If there is preserved joint space on these views, we would then do an arthroscopy and only proceed to OUKA if exposed bone is seen on both sides of the joint. If there is not bone-on-bone, we would treat the patients conservatively. The pain either tends to improve or, if the arthritis worsens, a UKA can be performed.

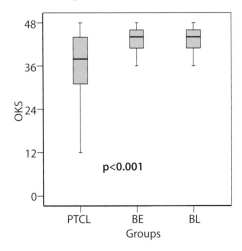

Figure 11.13 Comparison of post-operative OKS in matched patients with Partial Thickness Cartilage Loss (PTCL), Bone Exposed (BE) and Bone Loss (BL).

Niinnemaki *et al.* [31] in a series of 113 OUKA from a Finnish centre found that the re-operation rate was directly related to medial joint space on standing AP radiographs before surgery. The greater the joint space prior to surgery, the higher the re-operation rate after surgery. If it was ≤2 mm, then the re-operation rate was six times lower than when the medial joint space was more than 2 mm. If the joint space was normal, the re-operation rate was about 70% (Fig. 11.14).

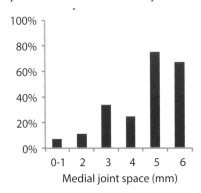

Figure 11.14 Re-operation rate according to pre-operative medial joint space width.

Bone overload

Both cadaveric studies [28] and finite element analysis (FEA) studies [27] have shown that, following UKA, the tibial strain increases anteromedially below the tibial component (Fig. 11.15). This may explain why anteromedial pain occurs postoperatively and why the pain settles as remodelling occurs and the strain returns to normal. The FEA demonstrates a 60% increase in strain with a perfect tibial resection. There is a further increase in strain with a deep vertical cut, a medial vertical cut and a deep tibial resection [11]. Clearly surgeons should take all measures to avoid these errors. The Microplasty instrumentation was designed to help address these issues.

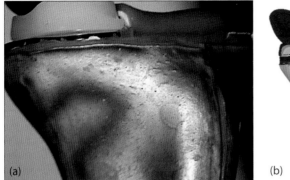
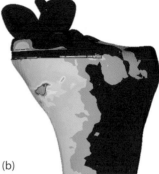

(a)　　　　　　　　　　　　　　　　　　　　　　(b)

Figure 11.15 (a) Cadaveric and (b) FEA studies showing increased strain anteromedially below the tibial component where pain often occurs [27, 28].

Cementing errors

Cementing errors are a common cause of pain. They may result in loose bodies (Fig. 11.16), soft tissue irritation from medial overhang, a tight flexion gap, and impingement.

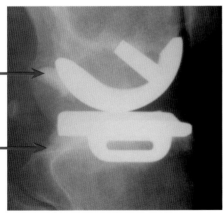
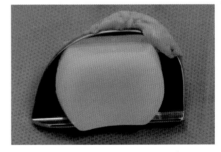

Figure 11.16 Radiograph and retrieved specimen from a patient with pain from cementing errors. Too much cement was used resulting in the tibial component not fully seating, a loose body, and bearing impingement.

Component overhang

We performed a study to assess the impact of tibial component overhang [32]. We found that medial overhang of more than 3 mm was associated with pain and poor function that tended to get worse with time. Presumably this was due to irritation of medial soft tissues (Fig. 11.17). The tibial component increases in size parametrically by 2 mm so overhang of 2 mm or more can be avoided by selecting the appropriate component size or redoing the vertical cut further laterally.

Anteromedial femoral component overhang may also cause pain and should be avoided.

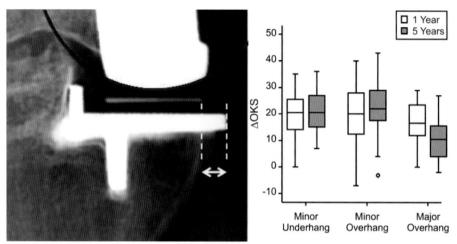

Figure 11.17 The relationship between overhang and change in OKS. Major overhang is more than 3 mm and minor overhang less than 3 mm.

Anterior impingement

Anterior impingement of the bearing against the femur in extension can occur if there is inadequate removal of anterior femoral bone. This can cause pain in extension and tends to develop with time as the fixed flexion contracture corrects.

Prevention

It is important the surgeon is aware of the cause of pain and takes the following steps to prevent it.

1. The operation is reserved for bone on bone arthritis
2. The surgeon must be meticulous with the technique, particularly relating to the tibia:
   (a) The tibial component should be supported all around its periphery by cortical bone
   (b) Care should be taken to avoid overhang, impingement, medial or deep tibial resection
3. The patient should be warned before surgery that early pain is common and, if it occurs, they should restrict their activity. The pain almost always settles spontaneously, but this may take a year.

Investigation

Radiographs are the most useful investigation: Ideally, an AP radiograph aligned with the tibial component (screened) should be obtained. This should be compared to the postoperative screened view. Physiological radiolucencies must be ignored as they are not a source of pain [33]. If femoral component loosening is suspected, lateral views at 0° and 90° should be obtained and examined carefully to determine if there is movement of the component (see Fig. 11.9) [17].

Radionuclide bone scans are not helpful and are often misleading. They are likely to be 'hot' for many years even if the patient is asymptomatic. If the pain is lateral, an MRI scan is useful as it may identify a meniscal tear. An ultrasound guided aspiration can be helpful to exclude infection.

Arthroscopy has a limited use in the management of these patients. This should not be undertaken before a year but can be useful if lateral meniscal lesions, cement loose bodies, impingement or chondral flaps in the PFJ are suspected.

Treatment of unexplained pain

The temptation for early revision should be avoided. We believe that, in general, the threshold for revision is too low. As a result, many patients are revised early for unexplained pain in all national registries. In most patients revised for unexplained pain, the pain does not improve. For example, in our retrieval study 75% of patients who were revised to TKA and had no mechanical problems identified at operation had no improvement in symptoms [18].

Patients should be treated conservatively as their pain tends to settle spontaneously. We recommend that patients should be warned that they are likely to have some pain for three to six months and that there is a small chance it may take one or even two years to fully settle. If patients have pain we advise them to decrease their level of activity and use a walking stick. If the pain is focal it is worth trying a steroid injection. If the pain persists beyond six months and the patient is becoming anxious, it is worth requesting a second opinion from a surgeon who is experienced with the OUKA, as they will tend to reassure the patient which is very helpful.

Limited motion

Knee movements are usually recovered rapidly, particularly since we have used a small incision without dislocation of the patella. Early flexion need not be encouraged since it occurs spontaneously in most patients. Occasionally, however, manipulation under anaesthesia has been employed if the knee has not recovered 90° flexion at six weeks. In these cases, unlike manipulation of a stiff joint after TKA, there are no adhesions in the suprapatellar pouch that need to be ruptured and the knee flexes fully with the application of little force.

Extension improves spontaneously after OUKA and seldom lacks more than 2°–3° at the end of the first year. If a fixed flexion deformity persists, it is usually because osteophytes in the roof of the notch or on the tibia in front of the ACL insertion have not been removed at the time of surgery.

Recurrent haemarthrosis

This is a rare complication of OUKA, as it is of TKA. The haemarthroses are usually of sudden onset and sometimes acute enough to demand aspiration for relief of pain. Each episode is usually short-lived, interfering with function for a few days, and subsiding spontaneously, but recurring, often several times.

Cause

The probable cause is recurrent mechanical damage to hypertrophic synovium. It is a vicious circle and recurrent haemarthrosis leads to a friable hypertrophied synovium which in leads to recurrent haemarthrosis.

Management

If a blood-clotting disorder is excluded, the prognosis for spontaneous cessation of the episodes is good. All drugs that interfere with blood clotting, such as aspirin and warfarin, should be stopped. If recurrent haemarthrosis persists, the treatment is difficult and it is worth arranging an angiogram and embolisation. Occasionally, an arthroscopy without tourniquet with synovectomy and coagulation of bleeding points helps. If the articular cartilage is destroyed or if the symptoms persist and become intolerable, conversion to TKA and synovectomy will be necessary.

Implant fracture

We are not aware of any cases in which the tibial component has fractured. There have been a few cases in which there have been fractures of the femoral component. These have almost all occurred when the femoral component has been used with the fixed bearing Vanguard M tibia. The fractures tend to occur just posterior to the 6 mm peg and are probably the result of inadequate posterior support.

Fourteen instances of fracture of an OUKA bearing have been reported in the literature [12,14]. We have also been told about a few other fractures. Fracture usually, but not always occurs with the thinnest (3.5 mm) bearings and is associated with impingement, resulting in increased wear. Treatment is by replacement with a new bearing usually one size bigger, and addressing the impingement.

The cause of bearing fracture is discussed in detail in Chapter 2. From a surgical point of view, the common factor was wear caused by impingement. The surgeon should ensure that impingement does not occur.

Results of revision surgery

The national registers have shown that the re-revision rate after a UKA to UKA revision is higher than a UKA to TKA revision. Therefore, the general recommendation is that UKA should be revised to TKA. However, there are certain circumstances when a UKA to UKA revision should be considered as the patient recovers quicker, with less morbidity and a better functional outcome. These include replacing a bearing for a dislocation; a lateral or medial UKA for disease progression; and implanting a new component for loosening with minimal bone loss.

The results of conversion of OUKA to TKA have been reported in a number of studies and are variable [34-37]. If there is a mechanical cause for the failure, such as disease progression, component loosening, recurrent dislocation, or damage to deep fibres of the MCL, and there is not substantial bone loss, the conversion to a primary TKA is straightforward. The tibial resection should be at the level of the top of the medial defect. The remaining defect, which is contained, can be filled with cement or bone graft from resected bone. A 14 or 16 mm tibial bearing is usually needed. The results tend to be as good as those of a primary TKA.

If there is no mechanical cause for the pain then, although the conversion to a primary TKA is straightforward, the results are poor. The typical case is a patient with early arthritis and partial thickness cartilage loss who is treated with a UKA. The UKA does not relieve the pain and the surgeons misinterpret the physiological radiolucency as indicative of loosening. At revision surgery, although the tibia is secure, it is easily removed when hit hard so it is recorded as 'loosening' in the registry. The conversion to TKA does not relieve the pain and further re-revision may be done. The message is clear – do not implant an OUKA for partial thickness disease and do not revise unless there is a definite mechanical problem.

If there is severe bone loss, for example following tibial plateau fracture, a two stage revision for infection, a deep tibial resection or gross ligament instability, then a revision TKA with stems, augments and increased constraint will be necessary. The results of this type of surgery may be similar to the results of revision TKA.

References

1. Liddle AD, Judge A, Pandit H, Murray DW. Determinants of revision and functional outcome following unicompartmental knee replacement. *Osteoarthritis Cartilage* 2014; **22**(9): 1241-50.

2. The NJR Board. 11th Annual Report of the National Joint Registry for England, Wales and Northern Ireland, 2014.

3. Pandit H, Jenkins C, Gill HS, Barker K, Dodd CA, Murray DW. Minimally invasive Oxford phase 3 unicompartmental knee replacement: results of 1000 cases. *J Bone Joint Surg Br* 2011; **93**(2): 198-204.

4. Sloper PJ, Hing CB, Donell ST, Glasgow MM. Intra-operative tibial plateau fracture during unicompartmental knee replacement: a case report. *Knee* 2003; **10**(4): 367-9.

5. Berger RA, Nedeff DD, Barden RM, Sheinkop MM, Jacobs JJ, Rosenberg AG, Galante JO. Unicompartmental knee arthroplasty. Clinical experience at 6- to 10-year followup. *Clin Orthop Relat Res* 1999; (**367**): 50-60.

6. Swanson AB, Swanson GD, Powers T, Khalil MA, Maupin BK, Mayhew DE, Moss SH. Unicompartmental and bicompartmental arthroplasty of the knee with a finned metal tibial-plateau implant. *J Bone Joint Surg Am* 1985; **67**(8): 1175-82.

7. Yang KY, Yeo SJ, Lo NN. Stress fracture of the medial tibial plateau after minimally invasive unicompartmental knee arthroplasty: a report of 2 cases. *J Arthroplasty* 2003; **18**(6): 801-3.

8. Pandit H, Murray DW, Dodd CA, Deo S, Waite J, Goodfellow J, Gibbons CL. Medial tibial plateau fracture and the Oxford unicompartmental knee. *Orthopedics* 2007; **30**(5 Suppl): 28-31.

9. Rudol G, Jackson MP, James SE. Medial tibial plateau fracture complicating unicompartmental knee arthroplasty. *J Arthroplasty* 2007; **22**(1): 148-50.

10. Seeger JB, Haas D, Jager S, Rohner E, Tohtz S, Clarius M. Extended sagittal saw cut significantly reduces fracture load in cementless unicompartmental knee arthroplasty compared to cemented tibia plateaus: an experimental cadaver study. *Knee Surg Sports Traumatol Arthrosc* 2012; **20**(6): 1087-91.

11. Pegg EC, Dodd CA, Murray DW, Pandit H. Conservative tibial resection and vertical cut minimise risk of tibial plateau fracture after UKR. British Association for Surgery of the Knee Annual Meeting. Telford, UK; 2015.

12. Berger RA, Meneghini RM, Jacobs JJ, Sheinkop MB, Della Valle CJ, Rosenberg AG, Galante JO. Results of unicompartmental knee arthroplasty at a minimum of ten years of follow-up. *J Bone Joint Surg Am* 2005; **87**(5): 999-1006.

13. Goodfellow JW, O'Connor JJ, Shrive NG, inventors; Endoprosthetic knee joint devices. British Patent Application 1534263. 1974..

14. Tibrewal S, Pandit H, McLardy-Smith P, Tibrewal SB, Murray DW. Posterior dislocation of the Oxford knee meniscal bearing: a treatment option. *J Orthop Traumatol* 2014; **15**(1): 59-62.

15. Hang JR, Stanford TE, Graves SE, Davidson DC, de Steiger RN, Miller LN. Outcome of revision of unicompartmental knee replacement. *Acta Orthop* 2010; **81**(1): 95-8.

16. Pandit H, Hamilton TW, Jenkins C, Mellon SJ, Dodd CA, Murray DW. The clinical outcome of minimally invasive Phase 3 Oxford unicompartmental knee arthroplasty: a 15-year follow-up of 1000 UKAs. *Bone Joint J* 2015; **97-B**(11): 1493-500.

17. Monk AP, Keys GW, Murray DW. Loosening of the femoral component after unicompartmental knee replacement. *J Bone Joint Surg Br* 2009; **91**(3): 405-7.

18. Psychoyios V, Crawford RW, O'Connor JJ, Murray DW. Wear of congruent meniscal bearings in unicompartmental knee arthroplasty: a retrieval study of 16 specimens. *J Bone Joint Surg Br* 1998; **80**(6): 976-82.

19. Liddle AD, Pandit H, O'Brien S, Doran E, Penny ID, Hooper GJ, Burn PJ, Dodd CA, Beverland DE, Maxwell AR, Murray DW. Cementless fixation in Oxford unicompartmental knee replacement: a multicentre study of 1000 knees. *Bone Joint J* 2013; **95-B**(2): 181-7.

20. Svard, U. and Price, A. 20-year survival & 10 year clinical results of the Oxford medial UKA. Presentation. 73rd Annual AAOS Meeting. Chicago, IL. 2006

21. Dejour H, Dejour D, Habi S. Prothese Unicompartimentale du Genou. *Cahier Enseign SOFCOT* 1998; **65**: 156-9.

22. Weale AE, Murray DW, Crawford R, Psychoyios V, Bonomo A, Howell G, O'Connor J, Goodfellow JW. Does arthritis progress in the retained compartments after 'Oxford' medial unicompartmental arthroplasty? A clinical and radiological study with a minimum ten-year follow-up. *J Bone Joint Surg Br* 1999; **81**(5): 783-9.

23. Liddle AD, McGrath C, Pandit H, Pegg E, Dada O, Mellon SJ, Spiegelberg BGI, Dodd CA, Murray DW. Predictors of arthritis progression following mobile-bearing

unicompartmental knee replacement: A case-control study. British Association for Surgery of the Knee annual meeting. Leeds, UK; 2013.

24. Svard UC, Price AJ. Oxford medial unicompartmental knee arthroplasty. A survival analysis of an independent series. *J Bone Joint Surg Br* 2001; **83**(2): 191-4.

25. Dodd CAF. Tips for preoperative assessment before UKA. ESSKA; Amsterdam; May 2014.

26. Gulati A. Outcome after medial unicompartmental knee replacement. DPhil. Oxford: University of Oxford; 2013.

27. Pegg EC, Walter J, Mellon SJ, Pandit HG, Murray DW, D'Lima DD, Fregly BJ, Gill HS. Evaluation of factors affecting tibial bone strain after unicompartmental knee replacement. *J Orthop Res* 2013; **31**(5): 821-8.

28. Small SR, Berend ME, Ritter MA, Buckley CA. Bearing mobility affects tibial strain in mobile-bearing unicompartmental knee arthroplasty. *Surg Technol Int* 2010; **19**: 185-90.

29. Emery IH, Meachim G. Surface morphology and topography of patello-femoral cartilage fibrillation in Liverpool necropsies. *J Anat* 1973; **116**(Pt 1): 103-20.

30. Pandit H, Gulati A, Jenkins C, Barker K, Price AJ, Dodd CA, Murray DW. Unicompartmental knee replacement for patients with partial thickness cartilage loss in the affected compartment. *Knee* 2011; **18**(3): 168-71.

31. Niinimaki TT, Murray DW, Partanen J, Pajala A, Leppilahti JI. Unicompartmental knee arthroplasties implanted for osteoarthritis with partial loss of joint space have high re-operation rates. *Knee* 2011; **18**(6): 432-5.

32. Chau R, Gulati A, Pandit H, Beard DJ, Price AJ, Dodd CA, Gill HS, Murray DW. Tibial component overhang following unicompartmental knee replacement--does it matter? *Knee* 2009; **16**(5): 310-3.

33. Gulati A, Chau R, Pandit HG, Gray H, Price AJ, Dodd CA, Murray DW. The incidence of physiological radiolucency following Oxford unicompartmental knee replacement and its relationship to outcome. *J Bone Joint Surg Br* 2009; **91**(7): 896-902.

34. Berend KR, George J, Lombardi AV Jr. Unicompartmental knee arthroplasty to total knee arthroplasty conversion: assuring a primary outcome. *Orthopedics*. 2009 Sep;32(9)

35. Martin JG, Wallace DA, Woods DA, Carr AJ, Murray DW. Revision of unicondylar knee replacements to total knee replacement. *The Knee* 1995; **2**:121-5.

36. Saldanha KA, Keys GW, Svard UC, White SH, Rao C. Revision of Oxford medial unicompartmental knee arthroplasty to total knee arthroplasty - results of a multicentre study. *Knee* 2007; **14**:275-9.

37. Wynn Jones H, Chan W, Harrison T, Smith TO, Masonda P, Walton NP. Revision of medial Oxford unicompartmental knee replacement to a total knee replacement: similar to a primary? *Knee* 2012;**19**:339-43.

12

The Lateral Side

Lateral unicompartmental OA is a relatively rare disease said to account for about one eighth of all unicompartmental arthritis [1]. However, the incidence may be higher because it is a disease of flexion and is commonly missed on standing AP radiographs. To identify lateral OA reliably, either a valgus stress radiograph in 45° flexion or a Rosenberg view is necessary. The clinical results of UKA in the lateral compartment have sometimes been worse than in the medial compartment [2] and sometimes better [3]. Some early papers reported results of series containing both medial and lateral operations as if they were essentially the same, but the normal anatomy and the pathological lesions of the two compartments are very different so the surgical techniques are different.

Anatomy and kinematics

The soft tissues of the lateral side of the knee are a complex arrangement of static and dynamic stabilisers whose primary function is to provide stability in varus angulation, anteroposterior translation of the tibia and internal/external rotation (Chapter 3).

The stabilising effect of the LCL is very different to that of the MCL. The latter provides stability throughout the full range of movement and therefore dislocation of a mobile bearing is rare (Chapter 9). Conversely, the LCL is tight only in extension. All of its fibres are slack beyond 12° flexion (Chapter 3) and, by 90°, 5 - 10 mm of distraction is possible in the lateral compartment. An MRI study showed that, in flexion under valgus and varus load, the medial compartment opens an average 2 mm whereas the lateral opens 7 mm (see Figs. 1.10 and 6.1) [4]. Dislocation of the mobile bearing is therefore a potential problem in mobile bearing lateral UKA.

The lateral collateral ligament (LCL) is round and cordlike, usually between 59 and 74 mm in length. It arises from the lateral epicondyle of the femur (from a fovea posterior to the apex of a bony ridge). It inserts distally into the apex of the fibular head as a conjoint tendon with the biceps femoris tendon [5].

Dynamic stability is provided by popliteus, the ileo-tibial tract and the extensor mechanism to keep the lateral articular surfaces in contact during activity.

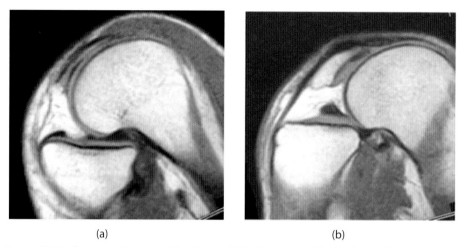

(a)   (b)

Figure 12.1 In the normal knee, in high flexion (a) in the medial side the femoral condyle is on top of the tibia; (b) in the lateral side the femoral condyle subluxes off the back of the convex tibial plateau. (Dr Y Kadoya, personal communication).

The medial plateau is larger than the lateral and is slightly concave whereas the lateral plateau is convex (Fig. 12.1). The lateral meniscus is more mobile than the medial meniscus, and its excursion during flexion–extension and axial rotation is greater than that of the medial meniscus. In high flexion (>120°), the lateral femoral condyle rolls over the posterior lip of the lateral plateau onto the posterior surface of the tibia (Fig. 12.1(b)), taking the posterior horn of the meniscus with it. By contrast, the posterior excursion of the medial meniscus is much less and the medial condyle and its meniscus, stay on the upper surface of the tibia (Fig 12.1 (a)).

Iwaki et al. [6] amongst others has shown much more movement in the lateral compartment (up to 20 mm) compared to medial side (8 mm) although the difference does depend on the loading conditions (Chapter 3) [7].

Pathology

The pattern of cartilage and bone erosion seen in anteromedial arthritis is not found on the lateral side [8]. Medial unicompartmental OA is a disease of extension whereas lateral unicompartmental OA is a disease of flexion. On the lateral side, the cartilage and bone erosions tend to begin in the central part of the tibial plateau which is in contact with the femur at about 45° flexion. On the femoral side, there is a kissing lesion at about 45° flexion. The lesion then expands both anteriorly and posteriorly. As a result there is usually some retained cartilage on the femur in extension and 90° flexion [9].

Gulati et al. [9] reported the patterns of osteoarthritis (OA) in both medial and lateral unicompartmental OA of the knee. Forty patients with medial and 20 with lateral unicompartmental knee osteoarthritis were studied to determine the location of full thickness cartilage lesions. Intra-operatively, the distance between

margins of the lesion and reference lines were measured. The femoral measurements were transposed onto lateral radiographs to determine the relationship
between the lesion site and knee flexion angles. Both tibial and femoral lesions
were significantly (p<0.01) more posterior in lateral OA than medial OA. In medial
OA, the lesion centre was, on average, at 11° (SD 3°) of flexion, whereas in lateral
OA it was at 40° (SD 3°). The smallest medial femoral lesions were near full extension and, as they enlarged, they extended posteriorly. The smallest lateral femoral
lesions extended from 20° to 60° flexion. As these lesions enlarged, they extended
both anteriorly and posteriorly. There was a well-defined relationship between the
site of the lesions and their size, suggesting that they develop and progress in a
predictable manner (Fig. 12.2). The relationship was different for medial and lateral
OA, suggesting that different mechanical factors are important in initiating the different types of OA. The lesions in medial OA occur in extension, perhaps initiated
by events occurring at heel strike [10]. The lesions in lateral OA begin at flexion angles
above those occurring during the single leg stance phase of the gait cycle, so activities other than gait are likely to induce lateral OA.

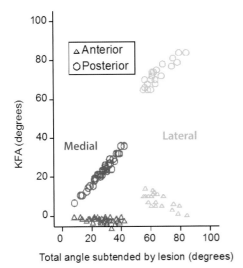

Figure 12.2 The site (Knee Flexion
Angle (KFA)) of the anterior (triangle)
and posterior (circle) extent of the full
thickness lesion compared to its length in
medial OA (red) and lateral OA (green).

History and development of the Lateral Oxford UKA

The mobile bearing OUKA has worked well in the medial compartment but the
results of lateral arthroplasty have been marred by dislocation of the bearing. Dislocation is primarily due to the lax lateral ligament in flexion. Over the years, lateral
OUKA has been successively improved but the dislocation rate still remains higher
than the medial side.

Initially both the standard Phase 1 and Phase 2 OUKA components were used
for lateral and medial unicompartmental replacement and both were implanted
through a medial parapatellar approach with patellar dislocation. Due to the

high dislocation rate, modifications to implant and technique were introduced. It was observed that the popliteus tendon sometimes wrapped around the bearing postero-laterally, tending to dislocate the bearing into the intercondylar space (Fig. 12.3). Therefore the tendon was routinely divided.

The entrapment of the medial bearing was 3 mm at the back and 5 mm at the front. The reason for the 3 mm entrapment at the back was that this was found to be the largest amount of entrapment that would allow the bearing to be inserted medially. However, on the lateral side, more entrapment could be used because of the lax ligaments. A symmetrical bearing, with entrapment of 5 mm posteriorly as well as anteriorly, was introduced. Unfortunately, despite these changes, the dislocation rate remained high. In 1996, Gunther *et al.* published the results of 53 Phase 1 and Phase 2 Oxford Knees implanted in Oxford [11]. The survival at 8 years was 76% (see Fig. 12.6 'early'). The main reason for the poor survival was that the dislocation rate was 10%. The survival with disease progression or implant loosening as failure was similar to that achieved on the medial side. As the dislocation rate was unacceptably high, it was recommended that the mobile bearing should not be used in the lateral side and a fixed bearing device should be used instead. However, if the problem of dislocation could be addressed, the results would be expected to be similar to those achieved on the medial side.

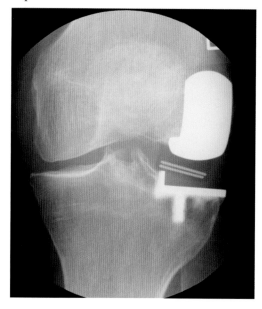

Figure 12.3 Lateral bearing dislocated onto the medial wall of the tibial component.

A radiographic study comparing knees that had and had not dislocated found that those that had dislocated were associated with a high lateral joint line [12]. This suggests that the dislocations were caused either by overstuffing the knee with the bearing too tight in extension, or by over-milling the distal femoral condyle and thus making the bearing too tight in flexion. It was therefore decided that the technique should be changed: the femoral component was implanted approximately anatomically to ensure that the distal femur was not over-milled and the bearing thickness was selected in extension so as to ensure the knee was not overstuffed. Usually, in lateral compartment OA, there is relatively little damage to the femoral condyle in full extension and 90° flexion, therefore it is straightforward to implant the femoral component anatomically by using instrumentation to ensure its surface is positioned where the retained articular cartilage was distally in full extension and posteriorly at 90° flexion. This ensures that the knee has the normal tightness in extension and the normal laxity in 90° flexion. In addition, a short lateral parapatellar approach was used without dislocation of the patella. Also, because it was observed that the bearing tended to track medially in extension, the vertical tibial saw cut was internally rotated by making it through the centre of the patellar tendon, and touching the medial side of the lateral femoral condyle. A clinical trial was undertaken using these surgical principles.

For the trial, Phase 3 femoral components were used together with Phase 2 tibial components (which were a more appropriate shape for the lateral tibial plateau) and symmetrical bearings with 5 mm entrapment at the front and back. Sixty-five components were implanted. There were three dislocations giving a 5% dislocation rate and a survival at four years of 98% (see Fig. 12.6 'flat')[13].

This dislocation rate of 5% was still unacceptably high so further modifications were made to the implant. It was observed that, with the Phase 3 components, although normal laxity of the knee was achieved in 90° flexion, in high flexion the knee became very tight and rollback was restricted. It was felt that the reason for this was that in the native knee, the femur tended to drop down on a normal convex tibial plateau (Fig. 12.1(b)), whereas this could not happen with a flat tibial component. It was therefore decided to use a convex tibial component. The surface of the component was spherical to achieve full congruity with a biconcave meniscal bearing in all positions (Fig. 12.4).

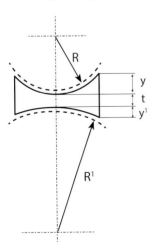

Figure 12.4. Diagram of the domed tibial design for lateral arthroplasty with a bi-concave meniscal bearing. The entrapment is increased compared to the flat tibia by distance y¹. Both articular surface pairs are spherical.

A study by Baré *et al.* [14] demonstrated that the optimal radius for the tibial sphere was about 75 mm. Cadaver studies were undertaken which demonstrated that normal rollback was achieved with the domed tibia (Fig. 12.5) and that the rollback was greater than with the flat tibia. The biconcave bearing (Fig. 12.4) increases the entrapment and, in theory, for a straight AP dislocation it should increase the entrapment from 5 mm to 7 mm.

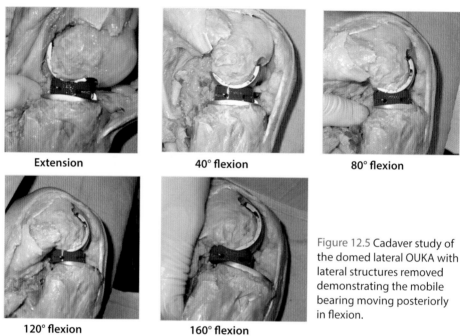

Extension   **40° flexion**   **80° flexion**

120° flexion   **160° flexion**

Figure 12.5 Cadaver study of the domed lateral OUKA with lateral structures removed demonstrating the mobile bearing moving posteriorly in flexion.

A clinical trial was undertaken by the two designer surgeons, using domed components and a modified surgical technique designed for the Phase 3 implants. At eight years in a series of 265 consecutive implants, a total of 13 knees (4.9%) had re-operations [15]. Four knees (1.5%) were reoperated for dislocation. Two were primary dislocations giving a primary dislocation rate of 0.8%. The remaining two were secondary to trauma. In both cases, when the knee was explored to reduce the dislocation, ligament damage was seen. Figure 12.6 shows that the survival and dislocation rate has progressively improved during the various developments of the lateral OUKA. With the domed lateral, while the dislocation rate is still higher than on the medial side we believe it is low enough for experienced surgeons to use the device.

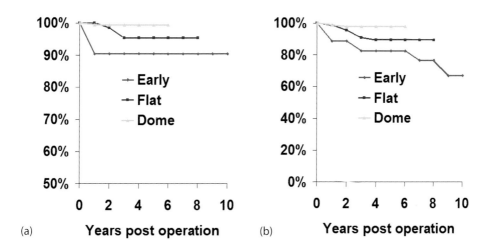

Figure 12.6 (a) Dislocation and (b) survival from the three iterations of the lateral OUKA.

Indications

As the number of lateral unicompartmental replacements we have done is relatively small, we do not have clearly defined indications for lateral OUKA supported by strong data. Instead, we tend to base the indications on the indications for medial OUKA. We believe the requirements for a successful lateral unicompartmental arthroplasty are as follows:

➤ **Bone-on-bone osteoarthritis in the lateral compartment**. This is best demonstrated by a Rosenberg view with the knee flexed to 45° or a valgus stress radiograph with the knee at 45° (Fig. 12.7). Standing AP radiographs often underestimate the disease severity.

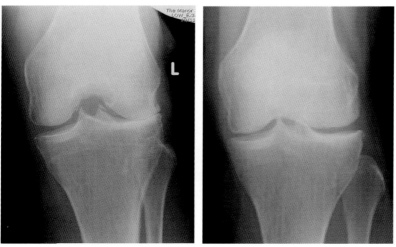

Figure 12.7 (a) Valgus stress radiograph taken at 45° flexion showing lateral OA with bone-on-bone. (b) This is not shown by a standing weightbearing radiograph taken in extension.

➤ **Full thickness cartilage in the medial compartment.** This is best demonstrated by a varus stress radiograph (Fig. 12.9). Although some believe that a Rosenberg is an adequate way of assessing the medial compartment, there is no evidence that this is the case. During the surgery it is difficult, if not impossible, to visualise the medial compartment. If there is any concern about its condition, it may be sensible to do an arthroscopy at the beginning of the procedure.

➤ **There should be a correctable intra-articular deformity**. This is best demonstrated by a varus stress radiograph (Fig. 12.9) which should show that the lateral joint space is of normal thickness or thicker.

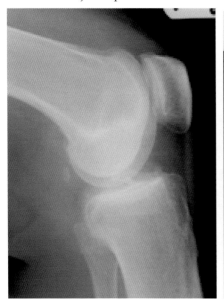 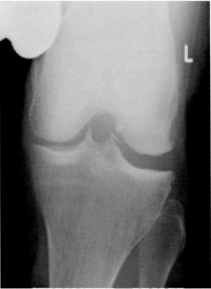

Figure 12.8 Lateral weight bearing.   Figure 12.9 Varus stress 40° flexed.

➤ **Anterior cruciate ligament**. The ACL should be intact. We do not know a good way of determining the status of the anterior cruciate in lateral OA from radiographs. We would therefore make the decision at operation having seen the status of the anterior cruciate.

➤ **No contraindications**. Like the medial side, we would ignore age, activity, obesity and chondrocalcinosis. We would also ignore the patellofemoral joint unless there was substantial damage with grooving and bone loss.

Surgical technique domed lateral UKR

The setup

The set up is the same as for medial OUKA using the leg holder (see Fig. 7.4). The hip is abducted. The thigh is supported so the hip is flexed 30 – 40°. This should allow the knee to hang flexed at 100 – 110°. The thigh support should avoid the popliteal fossa. It should be possible to flex the knee to about 135°.

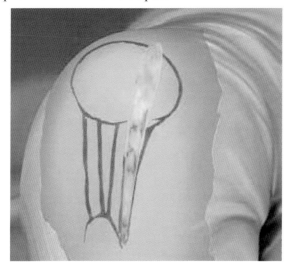

Figure 12.10 Skin incision for lateral parapatellar approach (left knee).

Incision

The incision is made over the junction of the central and lateral third of the patella and begins at the level of the superior pole of the patella and extends down to, and just lateral to, the tibial tubercle (Figs. 12.10 & 12.11). The retinacular incision is made around the lateral side of the patella and down beside the patella tendon. The anterior lateral portion of the tibia is exposed and Gerdy's tubercle and the attachment of the ilio-tibial tract identified. The incision is extended proximally around the patella and up into the extensor mechanism. Generous excision of the fat pad is required. If there is concern about the status of the ACL, this is assessed by pulling it with a hook. Osteophytes are removed from around the lateral condyle, the intercondylar notch, the anterior tibia and in front of the ACL on the tibia. If there are osteophytes on the lateral side of the patella, these are removed.

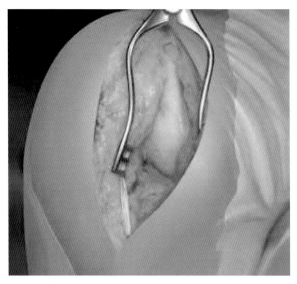

Figure 12.11 The lateral parapatellar approach.

Vertical cut

The bearing tends to move more medially with extension so the vertical cut has to be internally rotated to prevent impingement between the bearing and the wall. This is difficult to achieve if the saw cut is made lateral to the patellar tendon, therefore the cut is made through the centre of the patellar tendon (Fig.12.12). The position of the saw cut cannot be seen and is done by feel. It should rest against the medial side of the lateral condyle, and should be directed towards the ipsilateral ASIS. The cut is advanced to the depth of saw with a 7° slope similar to that used on the medial side. There should be no risk of tibial plateau fracture because the cut is made over the tibial shaft.

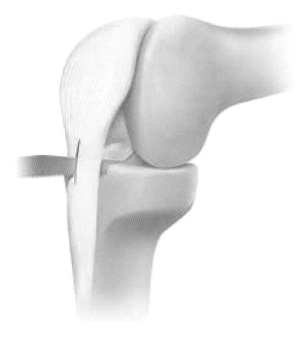

Figure 12.12 Vertical cut.

Horizontal cut

In general, more bone is removed from the lateral tibial plateau than during medial OUKA because the domed tibial component is thicker than the flat. The extramedullary sawing jig is applied in the same manner as for the medial side with the slope set at 7°. The jig is placed parallel to the tibial crest. The cut is made just below the top of Gerdy's tubercle, usually 2 – 3 mm below the defect. The Z-retractor (curly-whirly retractor) is used to protect the soft tissues.

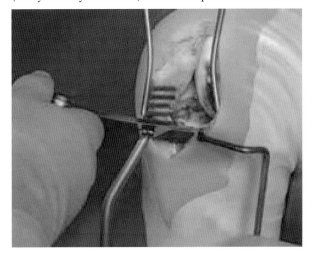

Figure 12.13 **Horizontal cut.**

An assessment is made to ensure that an adequate resection has been undertaken by inserting an appropriate tibial template and a 3 mm feeler gauge. The knee is then brought into full extension to assess the ligament tension. If the gap in extension is too tight, then the tibia is recut 2 mm distally by removing the shim from the sawing jig and repeating the horizontal cut. The final bearing thickness is selected in full extension so that the gap in full extension with the tibial template in place is an estimate of the final bearing thickness.

Femoral preparation

This is fundamentally different to the medial philosophy (Chapters 6 and 7). On the lateral side, ligament balance is impossible because the LCL is slack in flexion. The aim is to place the femoral component anatomically. The cartilage in lateral OA is relatively preserved at 0° and 90° flexion [9]. The technique therefore aims to position the implant flush to the condyle surfaces at 0° and 90° flexion. This is achieved using the standard femoral sawing jig, referencing from the posterior cartilage for AP position and by milling with a 4 spigot for distal positioning.

Femoral drill guide

Operator disorientation is quite common with this step of the procedure and malpositioning of the femoral component can occur. The aim is to position the 6 mm hole in the centre of the condyle parallel to the mechanical axis and flexed about

5°. Positioning of the IM rod is critical. The entry hole is made about 1 cm above and 0.5 cm lateral to the lateral border of the notch (Fig. 12.14). The IM rod is then inserted. A line is drawn down the centre of the condyle to aid anatomical positioning.

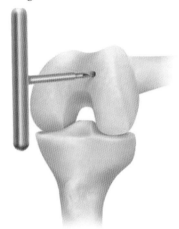

Figure 12.14 **Entry hole for left femur.**

We recommend that the Microplasty femoral drill guide is used with the lateral adapter. However, if this is not available, the Phase 3 lateral guide can be positioned parallel to the IM rod using the extramedullary rod as an extra guide.

An appropriate sized femoral component is selected based on gender and height. This is usually one size smaller than that used for the medial condyle. The medial tibial spoons can be used to help estimate the femoral component size. The appropriate femoral drill guide is set to fill the flexion gap. The lateral adapter is applied and clamped in place. This flexes the femoral component about 5° relative to the IM rod. The femoral drill guide is inserted in the knee and linked to the IM rod. The guide is adjusted so the 6 mm hole is central or slightly lateral on the femoral condyle. It is important that the femoral component does not overhang anterolaterally. It should therefore be confirmed that the femoral drill guide does not overhang anterolaterally. If it does, it should be internally rotated or moved slightly medially. When the drill guide is satisfactorily positioned, the small and large drill holes are made.

Femoral condyle preparation

The posterior saw guide is used in the standard manner to remove posterior femoral bone, thereby accurately restoring the joint line and positioning the femoral component anatomically in the AP direction. The meniscus is then removed. The next step is to place the femoral component anatomically which is usually achieved by milling using the 4 spigot. Baseline milling is therefore undertaken using 0 spigot. The gaps are then measured to ensure the flexion gap is at least 4 mm larger than the extension gap, which is nearly always the case. The distal femur is then milled with 4 spigot.

There are two caveats:

1. If the flexion gap is less than 4 mm larger than the extension gap after primary milling, then a smaller spigot should be used. The surgeon may need to recut the tibia.
2. If the flexion gap is very loose after the second milling, then a 5 spigot can be used but never more.

Final preparation

The aim of the final step of preparation is to select the bearing thickness in extension to restore the ligament tension and leg alignment to normal. Currently a one-peg femoral component should be used. A two-peg component with rounded anterior edges is available and can be used.

The surgeon must ensure that all impingement is prevented. Any posterior femoral osteophytes are removed with the chisel and slotted anti-impingement guide. The anterior mill <u>must not</u> be used on the lateral side as this will remove too much bone and the patella can jam in the defect, causing the knee to lock in flexion. The surgeon should do a trial reduction with an appropriate size of bearing to confirm that the bearing does not impinge on bone anteriorly. If there is anterior impingement, a small amount of bone should be removed from in front of the femoral component to prevent this. Care must be taken not to remove too much anterior femoral bone due to the risk of the patella jamming in the defect.

It is also important to ensure the bearing does not jam against the wall in full extension. If a thin dissector put between the bearing and the wall cannot easily be removed in full extension, the vertical cut will need to be repeated 2 mm more medially. If during trial reduction the bearing subluxes forward in high flexion and there is no posterior impingement, then the popliteus tendon should be divided. This may help prevent dislocation.

Final tibial preparation

The final tibial preparation is similar to that of the medial side.

The template must be flush with the posterior cortex and should not overhang in the region of Gerdy's tubercle. The cemented keel cut saw is used to prepare the keel slot. The cement pick should be used to clear out the bottom of the keel slot.

Careful cementation is then undertaken. Care must be taken to remove all retained cement. Definitive bearing assessment is now undertaken. A bearing that is just gripped in full extension is ideal. This will be loose in flexion. If it is difficult to insert the bearing from the front, it may be inserted antero-laterally. Routine closure is undertaken. Closure of the capsule tends to tighten the flexion gap.

Fixed bearing

In view of the high dislocation rate, our current recommendation for surgeons is to use the fixed bearing components, at least when beginning with lateral UKA. The

Fixed Lateral Oxford (FLO) prosthesis (see Fig. 12.15) has been recently introduced and can be used on the lateral side with the same instrumentation (Microplasty and adapter) and the same surgical technique.

The wear of the FLO is expected to be similar to other fixed bearing UKA but an order of magnitude greater than the mobile UKA.

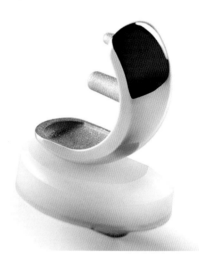

Figure 12.15 Fixed Lateral Oxford (FLO).

Results

Domed lateral UKA

Weston-Simons et al. [15] in 2014 reported the results of the first 265 domed lateral OUKA implanted by the two designer surgeons. These were all implanted for isolated disease of the lateral compartment and were prospectively and independently assessed. In this series, the mean age of patients at surgery was 64 years (range 32 to 90). At a mean follow-up of four years (0.5 to 8.3) the mean final OKS was 40 (SD 7.4). A total of 13 knees (4.9%) had re-operations, of which four (1.5%) were for dislocation. All dislocations occurred in the first two years. Two (0.8%) were secondary to significant trauma that resulted in ruptured ligaments, and two (0.8%) were spontaneous. In four patients (1.5%), the UKA was converted to a primary TKA. Survival at eight years, with failure defined as any revision, was 92.1% (95% CI 81.3 to 100).

There have been four independent studies of the domed lateral OUKA, which have confirmed that good results can be achieved (Table 12.1). In 2012 Streit et al. [16] reported on the results of their first 50 domed lateral UKRs in 50 patients with a mean follow up of 3 years (minimum 2 years) and no patient lost to follow up. There were three dislocations (6.1% (95% CI 2.0 to 17.9)). Survival using revision for any reason and aseptic revision was 94% (95% CI 82 to 98) and 96% (95% CI 85 to 99) at three years, respectively. The mean Oxford knee score was 43 (SD 5.3), the mean Objective American Knee Society score was 91 (SD 13.9) and the mean Functional American Knee Society score was 90 (SD 17.5). The mean maximum flexion was 127° (range 90° to 145°).

Schelfaut et al. [17] in 2013 described a cohort of 25 patients with a minimum follow-up of 1 year who underwent lateral UKA with the domed Oxford. One bearing dislocation occurred 4 months post-surgery. The OKS improved in all patients from a preoperative mean of 23.3 (range 8 to 40, SD 8.4) to a postoperative mean of 42.1 (range 23 to 48, SD 6.7). General patient satisfaction at a mean follow-up of 20 months was excellent in 84 %, good in 12 % and fair in 4 %.

Also in 2013, Altuntas et al. [18] described a total of 64 knees, in 58 patients, after a domed tibia, mobile bearing lateral UKA with a minimum 2-year follow-up. The mean follow-up period was 38 months (range 24 to 61, median 36). There were four knees that underwent further surgery for any reason. Two patients required revision of the implant (3.1%). There were no cases of bearing dislocation in this series. The mean pre-operative OKS was 24 (range 9 to 36) and the mean post-operative score was 42 (range 23 to 48 p<0.0001).

Table 12.1 Dislocation rates in four independent series of domed lateral arthroplasties.

Author	Year	No. of Knees	Mean FU in months	No. of dislocations	Dislocation rate
Streit [16]	2012	50	36	3	6.2%
Altunas [18]	2012	68	38	0	0%
Schelfaut [17]	2012	25	20	1	4%
Marson [19]	2013	12	35	1	8%
Weston-Simons [15]	2014	265	48	4	1.5%
Sum/average		430	43	9	2%

The combination of the modified surgical technique and new design with a domed tibial component appears to have reduced the early dislocation rate. It is however still higher than in the medial compartment. There is also variation in the reported dislocation rates in the published series with the surgeons doing larger numbers having a lower dislocation rate (Table 12.1). Although there are no significant difference in rates, it does suggests that the dislocation rate is influenced by surgical experience and technique.

Gulati et al. [20] carried out a radiographic evaluation of surgical factors affecting bearing dislocation. Aligned post-operative anteroposterior knee radiographs of seven knees that had dislocated and 87 control knees were compared. All bearing dislocations occurred medially over the vertical wall of the tibial component into the intercondylar notch (Fig. 12.2). Knees that dislocated tended to be overcorrected compared with those that did not dislocate:, they were in 2° less valgus (p = 0.019) and the tibial components were positioned 2 mm more proximal (p < 0.01). Although the relative position of the centre of the femoral component and the tibial component was the same (p = 0.8), in the dislocating group the gap between the edge of the femoral component and the top of the wall in flexion was 3 mm greater (p= 0.019) suggesting that the components were internally rotated.

This study confirmed the findings of the previous study that to minimise the risk of dislocation, the knee should not be overstuffed [12]. This is best achieved by selecting the bearing thickness that just tightens the ligaments in full extension. In addition, the size of the gap between the femoral and tibial components through which the bearing dislocates should be minimised. We used to rotate the femoral component internally so as to minimise the risk of anteromedial overhang, this however increases the size of the gap. It therefore seems sensible to implant the femoral component in neutral rotation. This is best achieved by using the micro-plasty femoral drill guide. We have therefore modified the technique to include this. It should however be noted that this is a recent change so we do not have any outcome data and therefore cannot be certain if it helps decrease the dislocation rate. There is always a concern that a change to the technique may worsen the results.

The management of a dislocated bearing

Dislocations commonly occur medially over the wall of the tibial component, but can occur in other directions such as anteriorly, posteriorly or laterally. A medial dislocation should really be considered to be a subluxation as the knee may continue to function well and the patient may not be aware of the problem. A dislocation may reduce spontaneously when the patient is anaesthetised or can occasionally be reduced by manipulation. More commonl,y however, the old incision has to be opened and the bearing retrieved under direct vision. A careful exploration is undertaken to identify any potential causes for bearing dislocation, for example, impingement, component loosening, bowstringing of popliteus or ligament injury. A trial bearing is inserted to aid assessment, and the retrieved bearing is inspected for evidence of impingement. These problems are addressed as required, and a new bearing, usually one size thicker, is inserted. Recurrent dislocation is unlikely but can occur.

We have introduced a technique to prevent recurrent medial dislocation [21]. The aim is to decrease the gap between the femoral and tibial components through which the bearing dislocates. Two 3.5 mm AO screws about 24 mm in length are inserted under direct vision just medial to the tibial wall one third and two thirds of the way back (Fig. 12.16). They are angled posteriorly and medially. The screws are advanced until their heads sit on top of the wall, thus acting as an extension of the wall. They are tightened so that they do not overhang the wall laterally and therefore will not touch the bearing. A trial reduction, using a bearing that is just tight in extension, must be carried out. The knee is put through a full range of movement and the screw heads are observed to ensure that they do not hit the femoral component or the bearing. If the screws touch the bearing, they should be tightened. If they touch the femoral component they should be removed. A definitive bearing is then inserted.

Weston-Simons *et al.* [21] in 2011 reported on seven cases using this technique. One recurrent dislocation was identified months after the stabilisation of the bearing with screws. During exploration, it was found that the lateral collateral ligament was stretched and slack, presumably because the bearing had been dislocated for an extended period (over 6 months) before the original dislocation was treated. As a result, the tibial component was revised to a fixed bearing component. In all the other cases, this technique has prevented further dislocations. The patients recover quickly and the range of movement is regained rapidly. The clinical outcome scores, both objective as well as functional, are as good as those without bearing dislocation.

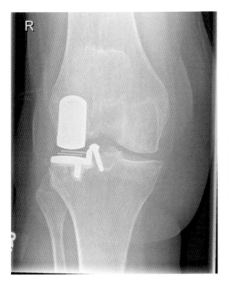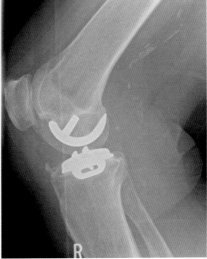

Figure 12.16 A postoperative anteroposterior and lateral radiograph of a reduced lateral meniscal bearing illustrating screw position and alignment [21].

References

1. Jamali AA, Scott RD. Lateral unicompartmental knee arthroplasty. *Techniques in Knee Surgery* 2005; **4**(2): 79-88.

2. Scott RD, Santore RF. Unicondylar unicompartmental replacement for osteoarthritis of the knee. *J Bone Joint Surg Am* 1981; **63**(4): 536-44.

3. Jonsson GT. Compartmental arthroplasty for gonarthrosis. *Acta Orthop Scand Suppl* 1981; **193**: 1-110.

4. Tokuhara Y, Kadoya Y, Nakagawa S, Kobayashi A, Takaoka K. The flexion gap in normal knees. An MRI study. *J Bone Joint Surg Br* 2004; **86**(8): 1133-6.

5. Takeda S, Tajima G, Fujino K, Yan J, Kamei Y, Maruyama M, Kikuchi S, Doita M. Morphology of the femoral insertion of the lateral collateral ligament and popliteus tendon. *Knee Surg Sports Traumatol Arthrosc* 2015; **23**(10): 3049-54.

6. Iwaki H, Pinskerova V, Freeman MA. Tibiofemoral movement 1: the shapes and relative movements of the femur and tibia in the unloaded cadaver knee. *J Bone Joint Surg Br* 2000; **82**(8): 1189-95.

7. Freeman MA, Pinskerova V. The movement of the normal tibio-femoral joint. *J Biomech* 2005; **38**(2): 197-208.

8. Harman MK, Markovich GD, Banks SA, Hodge WA. Wear patterns on tibial plateaus from varus and valgus osteoarthritic knees. *Clin Orthop Relat Res* 1998; (352): 149-58.

9. Gulati A, Chau R, Beard DJ, Price AJ, Gill HS, Murray DW. Localization of the full-thickness cartilage lesions in medial and lateral unicompartmental knee osteoarthritis. *J Orthop Res* 2009; **27**(10): 1339-46.

10. Gill HS, O'Connor JJ. Heelstrike and the pathomechanics of osteoarthrosis: a pilot gait study. *J Biomech* 2003; **36**(11): 1625-31.

11. Gunther T, Murray DW, Miller RK, Wallace D, Carr AJ, O'Connor JJ, McLardy-Smith P, Goodfellow JW. Lateral unicompartmental arthroplasty with the Oxford meniscal knee. *Knee* 1996; **3**(1-2): 33-9.

12. Robinson BJ, Rees JL, Price AJ, Beard DJ, Murray DW, McLardy Smith P, Dodd CA. Dislocation of the bearing of the Oxford lateral unicompartmental arthroplasty. A radiological assessment. *J Bone Joint Surg Br* 2002; **84**(5): 653-7.

13. Pandit H, Jenkins C, Beard DJ, Price AJ, Gill HS, Dodd CA, Murray DW. Mobile bearing dislocation in lateral unicompartmental knee replacement. *Knee* 2010; **17**(6): 392-7.

14. Bare JV, Gill HS, Beard DJ, Murray DW. A convex lateral tibial plateau for knee replacement. *Knee* 2006; **13**(2): 122-6.

15. Weston-Simons JS, Pandit H, Kendrick BJ, Jenkins C, Barker K, Dodd CA, Murray DW. The mid-term outcomes of the Oxford Domed Lateral unicompartmental knee replacement. *Bone Joint J* 2014; **96-B**(1): 59-64.

16. Streit MR, Walker T, Bruckner T, Merle C, Kretzer JP, Clarius M, Aldinger PR, Gotterbarm T. Mobile-bearing lateral unicompartmental knee replacement with the Oxford domed tibial component: an independent series. *J Bone Joint Surg Br* 2012; **94**(10): 1356-61.

17. Schelfaut S, Beckers L, Verdonk P, Bellemans J, Victor J. The risk of bearing dislocation in lateral unicompartmental knee arthroplasty using a mobile biconcave design. *Knee Surg Sports Traumatol Arthrosc* 2013; **21**(11): 2487-94.

18. Altuntas AO, Alsop H, Cobb JP. Early results of a domed tibia, mobile bearing lateral unicompartmental knee arthroplasty from an independent centre. *Knee* 2013; **20**(6): 466-70.

19. Marson B, Prasad N, Jenkins R, Lewis M. Lateral unicompartmental knee replacements: early results from a District General Hospital. *Eur J Orthop Surg Traumatol* 2014; **24**(6): 987-91.

20. Gulati A, Weston-Simons S, Evans D, Jenkins C, Gray H, Dodd CA, Pandit H, Murray DW. Radiographic evaluation of factors affecting bearing dislocation in the domed lateral Oxford unicompartmental knee replacement. *Knee* 2014; **21**(6): 1254-7.

21. Weston-Simons JS, Pandit H, Gill HS, Jackson WF, Price AJ, Dodd CA, Murray DW. The management of mobile bearing dislocation in the Oxford lateral unicompartmental knee replacement. *Knee Surg Sports Traumatol Arthrosc* 2011; **19**(12): 2023-6.

Appendix:

Mathematical models of the knee

Introduction

Mathematical models make it possible to calculate the values of quantities which are difficult or impossible to measure and provide insights which are not obtained from experiment alone. They are a necessary adjunct to the experimental method, but are not a common feature of biological or clinical research. A model is based on a series of assumptions or hypotheses about the way a physical system works. It is validated by comparing its predictions with independent experimental measurement. Reasonable validation then gives confidence in the assumptions on which the model is based and in the predictions of quantities which cannot be measured. The purpose in presenting our models here is to explain the differences between unloaded and loaded motion described in Chapter 3.

Many mathematical models of the natural knee [1-3] and of knee replacement have been proposed [4-6]. They have usually modelled the movement of the joint under load. We have found it easier to model the mobility of the knee in the absence of load, then the stability of the knee under load but in the absence of movement, and then to combine both to study activity, i.e. movement under load.

Three-dimensional model of knee mobility

The model (Fig. A1) explains the coupling of axial rotation to flexion and, more generally, how the joint achieves a range of unresisted passive mobility [7]. The model was formulated using the assumptions that the articular surfaces medially and laterally remain continuously in contact without interpenetration during passive flexion and that single fibres within each of the two cruciates and the MCL remain isometric. These five constraints to motion, when acting together, reduce the six possible degrees of freedom of the bones to one, so that axial rotation is coupled to flexion. The calculated coupling of axial rotation to flexion required to satisfy these assumptions agrees well with measurements described in Chapter 3 (Fig. A2).

Pictures of the model in extension and at 45° and 90° flexion (Fig. A1) show that during flexion the articular surfaces of the femur roll and slide on the surfaces of the tibia while the femur rotates externally on the tibia. The three isometric ligament fibres rotate about their insertions into the tibia. The sliding and rolling of the surfaces and the rotation of the ligament fibres are accomplished without tissue deformation and therefore without generating resistance to motion.

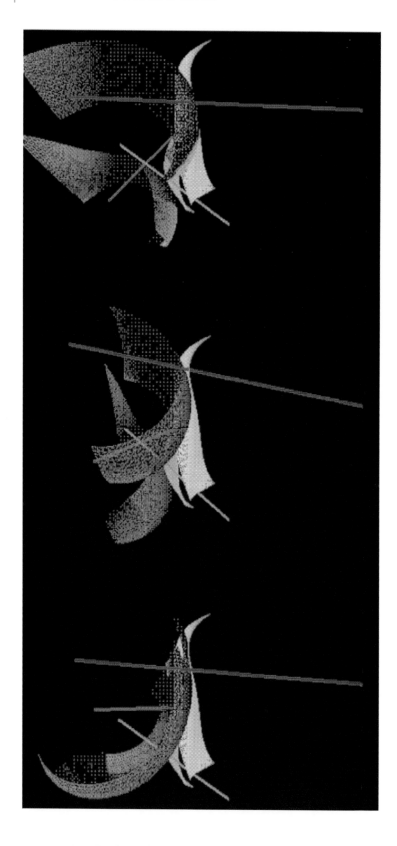

Figure A1 Three-dimensional model of knee mobility at extension, 45° flexion, and 90° flexion. The brown shells are the surfaces of the model femoral condyles, the yellow shells are the surfaces of the tibial plateaux, and the red, green and blue lines are the isometric fibres of the ACL, PCL, and MCL, respectively.

An animation of the model (Animation 1) can be found on the website accompanying this book, www.oxfordpartialknee.com, and demonstrates how the surfaces of the bones move on each other. The axial rotation of the surfaces of the femoral condyles can best be appreciated by watching the movements of their posterior edges.

The predictions of the model are sensitive to the choice of its parameters: (1) the shapes of the articular surfaces and (2) the positions of the points of origin and insertion of the isometric ligament fibres. If spherical femoral condyles and flat tibial surfaces are chosen, the result is greater anteroposterior movement of the contact points on the tibia in both compartments and larger values of coupled external femoral rotation. The model also demonstrates the important role of the MCL, and the absence of a role for the LCL, in guiding passive motion. If the model MCL is placed on the lateral rather than the medial side, obligatory internal rather than external rotation of the femur occurs during flexion, a result that is unlikely to be deduced except by modelling.

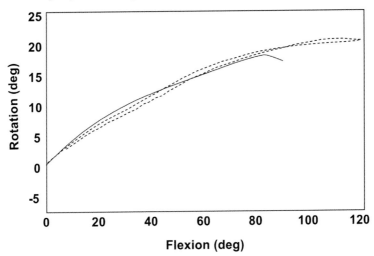

Figure A2 External rotation of the femur plotted against flexion angle. The solid line calculated from the three-dimensional model of mobility (Fig. A1) matches well the experimental curves of Figs. 3.2 and 3.3 (dotted lines).

Two-dimensional model of the knee: the four-bar linkage

Mobility

The rolling and sliding movements of the femur on the tibia are more clearly seen in the simpler two-dimensional four-bar linkage model of Figure A3 (website, Animation 2) [8-11]. The figure shows the femur flexing on a fixed tibia with lines representing the extensor and flexor muscles. The distal surface of the femur has separate curves representing (1) the sulcus of the trochlea, anteriorly, in contact with the patella, and (2) the distal and posterior facets of the condyle in contact with the tibia. The model tibial articular surface is flat, a two-dimensional compromise between the slightly concave medial and slightly convex lateral plateaus of the human knee (see Fig. 12.1). Lines representing the isometric fibres of the two cruciates, rotating about their insertions on the tibia, and lines joining their attachments on the two bones form a crossed four-bar linkage [12]. The two-dimensional model separates the kinematics of the joint in the sagittal plane from the effects of coupled axial rotation.

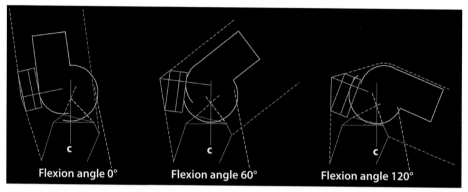

Flexion angle 0°   Flexion angle 60°   Flexion angle 120°

Figure A3 Two-dimensional four-bar linkage model of the knee in which isometric fibres in the ACL (dashed) and PCL (dashed white) guide the rolling and sliding movements of the femur on the tibia during passive flexion–extension. The point of contact C between the articular surfaces of the bones lies on the perpendicular to the tibial plateau through the intersection of the ligament fibres. Muscle tendons are shown as single lines. The rectangular model of the patella is held between the quadriceps and patellar tendons (dashed green). The hamstrings tendon and the gastrocnemius tendon are shown by pink and blue dashed lines, respectively.

The flexion axis of the joint passes through the point of intersection of the isometric ligament fibres (the 'instant centre' of the linkage) and moves backwards relative to the tibia during flexion, and forwards during extension. The point of contact between the femoral condyle and the flat tibial surface of the model always lies on the perpendicular to the tibial plateau through the flexion axis and therefore also moves backwards on the tibia during flexion and forwards during extension (as indicated by the vertical lines marked C in Fig. A3). The femur rolls as well as slides on the tibia; it rolls backwards (while sliding forwards) during flexion, and rolls forwards (while sliding backwards) during extension. The calculated value of the slip ratio (movement of the contact point on the tibia divided by its movement on the femur) varies between 0.2 and 0.4, similar to the range of values estimated by Feikes [13] for the intact cadaver knee (Fig. 3.8). The model contact point moves backwards 11 mm over 120° flexion, similar to the mean value of the average movement of the contact point in human knees estimated by Feikes, Table 3.1 [13].

Therefore the model describes the average behaviour of the two compartments without axial rotation. The isometric ligament fibres keep the articular surfaces continuously in contact, and the articular surfaces keep the ligament fibres just tight. Unresisted passive flexion and extension can occur without tissue deformation because the isometric fibres rotate about their insertions on the bones without stretching, and the articular surfaces roll and slide on each other without indentation.

The directions of the model ligaments, the lengths of the lever arms of the flexor and extensor muscles, and their variation with flexion angle agree well with measurements on cadaver human knee specimens made by Hertzog and Read [11, 14].

Ligament kinematics

The architecture of the ACL and PCL ligament arrays has been described by Friederich et al. [15] and Mommersteeg et al. [16] (see Figs. 3.11 & 3.12), and the model's cruciate ligaments (Fig. A4) are based on those studies. The attachment areas are shown as straight lines, with a definite arrangement between the point of origin of an individual fibre and its point of insertion (fibre mapping). Tight fibres are shown as straight lines, and slack fibres are shown buckled.

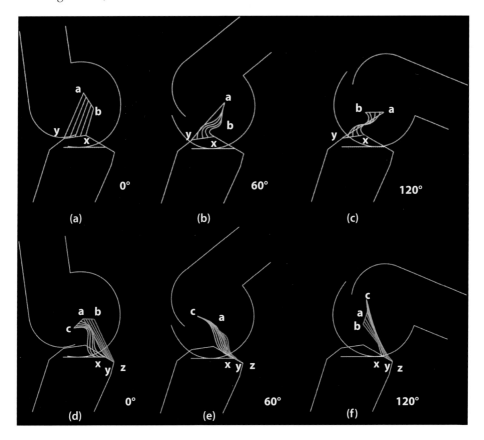

Figure A4 Model knee with arrays of fibres representing the ACL and two bundles of the PCL, attached to the femur along **ab** and **cab** respectively. (At 60°, the attachment point **b** of the PCL lies under the fibres and is not visible. See website, Animation 3.)

The fibres of the model ACL are straight, almost parallel, just tight in extension, and attached to the femur along the line *ab* (Fig. A4(a)). The PCL is modelled as two bundles of fibres attached to the femur along the lines *ca* and *ab*, with the anterior bundle being slack and the posterior bundle just tight in extension (Fig. A4(d)). Five representative fibres are drawn in the ACL and in each bundle of the PCL, but the mathematics assumes a continuous distribution of fibres along each attachment line. The most anterior ACL fibre *ay* and the most anterior of the PCL posterior bundle *ay* are the isometric fibres of Figure A3, and the relative motion of the bones is the same in both figures.

During flexion of the joint to 120°, the femoral attachment areas of both ligaments rotate through the same 120° relative to the tibia, appearing to pivot about the insertions of the isometric fibres. As a result, the ligaments change their shapes. In both ligaments, fibres originating along the attachment line *ab* are more or less parallel in extension but are crossed on each other at 120°. Cross-over occurs when the attachment line *ab* lies along the isometric fibre *ay*. This occurs at about 70° flexion for the ACL and 60° flexion for the posterior fibres of the PCL (see website, Animation 3).

Fibres passing behind the intersection of the isometric fibres slacken during flexion and tighten during extension. Fibres passing in front of the intersection of the isometric fibres tighten during flexion and slacken during extension. Prior to cross-over, points of origin and insertion in the ACL and in the posterior bundle of the PCL approach each other during flexion, and fibres slacken. After cross-over, these points depart from each other and fibres tighten. The anterior fibres of the model PCL pass in front of the intersection of the isometric fibres and tighten during flexion as its femoral attachment area *ac* rotates away from the tibia. They are just tight and straight at 120°. Thus, most ligament fibres are slack in most positions of the unloaded joint. No fibres are stretched.

The changes in shape of the model ACL are very similar to those reported in the cadaver human knee using Röntgen stereometric analysis [17] and to the sketches of Friederich *et al.* [18] (see Fig 3.12) and Girgis *et al.* [19]. The shape changes of the model PCL are similar to the sketches of Brantigan and Voschell [20], and the patterns of fibre slackening and tightening predicted by the model are quantitatively similar to those measured in cadaver knees [21–25]. These comparisons with experiment serve to validate the model and the assumptions on which it is based.

Animation 4 on the website is of a knee model with arrays of fibres representing all four principal ligaments, including the two cruciates of Figure A4. Many observers agree that all fibres within the LCL become slack once flexion begins [23, 27, 28]. This is because the fibres always lie behind the flexion axis of the joint.

The behaviour of the model MCL demonstrates one of the deficiencies of a two-dimensional model. The fibres of that ligament cover the intersection of the two isometric cruciate fibres so that the flexion axis of the joint passes through the ligament. As a result, the most anterior of the superficial fibres of the model MCL stretch during passive flexion. However, the two-dimensional model does not account for obligatory axial rotation. The associated forward movement of the femoral attachment area of the MCL relative to the tibia, as seen in the three-dimensional model in Figure A1 (and in Animation 1 on the website), slackens these stretched fibres and allows unresisted flexion. This feature of the two-dimensional model prompted the development of the three-dimensional model and the incorporation of an isometric MCL fibre in addition to the cruciates (see Chapter 3.)

Discussion

The rolling of the femur on the tibia during passive flexion–extension is required to minimise ligament strain in the unloaded knee and allow unresisted passive movement. Predictions of the mathematical models of passive motion compare well with measurements made on cadaver specimens in our own and other laboratories, validating the principal assumptions underlying the models, i.e. that the human knee behaves as a mechanism during passive motion, guided by the articular surfaces in contact and by isometric fibres within the cruciates and the MCL. Every implantation of an Oxford prosthesis which succeeds in matching the 110° flexion gap to the 20° flexion gap when the bone surfaces are distracted by gap gauges is evidence of ligament isometricity. The slack model LCL in the flexed knee is believed to explain the high rate of bearing dislocation in lateral OUKA (see Chapter 12).

These concepts have recently been challenged by Freeman [29], without confronting the many experimental validations of the models but on the grounds that the PCL is (apparently) slack in flexion, an argument advanced by Strasser in 1917 [30] in a criticism of the first description of the four-bar linkage model given by Zuppinger in 1904 [31]. All fibres of a ligament cannot be isometric unless they all originate on or pass through the flexion axis of the joint. Slackness of most fibres does not preclude the isometry of some. The isometric fibres within the PCL lie within the body of the ligament and are difficult to observe visually. Nonetheless, the shapes of the model ligament in extension and flexion shown in Figure A4 are very similar to those shown in Section 8 of Freeman's booklet [29], and are consequences of the isometricity of some fibres, not an argument against it. The changes of fibre length in the PCL predicted by the model are very similar to those described by Wang and Walker [23] and by Covey *et al.* [25]. Freeman also shows how the PCL is readily deflected sideways by a transverse force. But even a very tight rope, like a bowstring, offers little resistance to transverse motion of a point in the middle of its span. A better demonstration of the function of the PCL is to show how its slack fibres are systematically recruited to resist backward movement of the tibia relative to the femur when the knee is appropriately loaded.

Stability of the loaded joint

Figure A5 shows how the model ACL responds when the tibia is moved backwards and forwards relative to the femur (as in a drawer test) at a fixed flexion angle [32,33]. With the unloaded knee flexed to 50°, all but the anterior fibres of the ACL are slack (Fig. A5(b)). When the tibia is pushed backwards 5 mm from the neutral position, the anterior fibre slackens and all other fibres slacken further (Fig. A5(a)). When the tibia is pulled forwards 5 mm from its neutral position, ACL fibres are progressively tightened and stretched to bear load (Fig. A5(c)). A 5 mm anterior translation tightens and stretches about half the model ACL (see website, Animation 5).

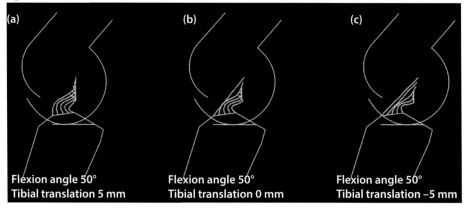

Figure A5 Fibres of the model ACL, with the knee at 50° flexion, (a) slacken and (c) tighten when the tibia is pulled backward and forward from the neutral unloaded position (b).

Figure A6 (and Animation 6 on the website) show similar diagrams of the model knee with all four ligaments modelled as arrays of fibres. Posterior translation of the tibia (Fig. A6(a)) tightens the PCL and the LCL, and slackens the ACL and the MCL. Anterior translation (Fig A6(c)) tightens the ACL and the MCL, and slackens the PCL and the LCL. The ligaments offer increasing resistance to anteroposterior displacement from the neutral position (Fig. A6(b)) as more and more fibres are recruited to bear load, giving the knee its characteristic laxity. The laxity allowed by ligament strain is further increased by indentation of the articular surfaces under load [34]. The calculation of the anteroposterior laxity of the model joint under a drawer force of 67 N by Huss et al. [34] agrees well with measurements made by Grood and Noyes [35], providing a validation of the model (see Fig. 3.21).

Discussion

The laxity allowed by stretching of the ligaments should be recovered after unconstrained unicompartmental arthroplasty which retains all the ligaments and restores them to their natural tensions. The contribution to laxity attributed to deformation of the surfaces will be lost when they are replaced by more rigid prosthetic components. However, the contribution of surface deformation in the intact joint is relatively small [34].

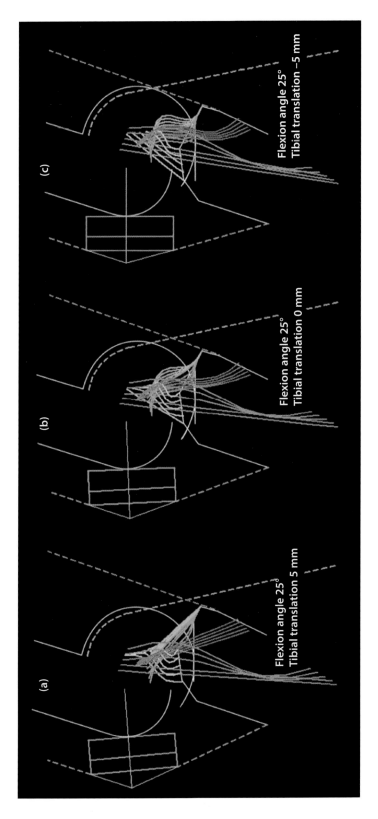

Figure A6 Model knee with arrays of fibres representing the ACL (yellow), the two bundles of the PCL (blue and green), the superficial fibres of the MCL (purple), and the LCL (red). Fibres within the PCL and LCL tighten and those within the ACL and MCL slacken when the tibia is pushed backwards (a) from the neutral position (b), and vice versa when the tibia is pulled forward (c) from the neutral position.

Mathematical model of OUKA

A two-dimensional mathematical model of OUKA created by Imran [36] explains the observed differences between passive and active flexion described in Chapter 3 .

The sequence of images in Figure A7 represents passive motion in the absence of load. Those in Figure A8 model a drawer test, with the bones at a fixed flexion angle and moved anteroposteriorly relative to each other by an external force against the resistance of the ligaments.

The model of passive motion (Fig. A7) finds the position of the femur on the tibia which minimises ligament strain. The anteroposterior position of the femur on the tibia was adjusted mathematically, as in Figure A8(b), until both cruciate ligaments had just fully slackened, with zero force in each. This condition requires rollback of the femur on the tibia and consequently, posterior translation of the meniscal bearing during flexion (see website, Animation 7).

The patterns of fibre strain in Figure A7 are very similar to those in Figure A4 which were based on the assumed presence of the two isometric fibres of Figure A3 (see Fig 3.12). Therefore, the model in Figure A7 predicts rather than assumes the presence of isometric fibres. It is emphasised that the only inputs to the model were the geometry of the arrays of fibres in extension, the positions of the prosthetic components, the femoral trochlea, and the tibial tubercle relative to the ligament attachment areas, the length of the patellar tendon, and the shape of the model patella. The positions of the bones relative to each other were then calculated using the laws of geometry and mechanics. The model of passive mobility (Fig. A7) predicts passive bearing movements very similar to those observed fluoroscopically (see Fig. 3.16).

Model of the active extension exercise

Comparison of Figures A7 and A8 shows that the anteroposterior movements of the meniscal bearing on the tibia required to tighten slack ligaments are similar in magnitude to those which occur during passive movements. These two effects are superimposed in activity and can augment or cancel each other. Figure A9 shows a model of active extension with the femur horizontal and the weight of the leg balanced by tension forces in the patellar and quadriceps tendons. In extension, the patellar tendon pulls the tibia upwards, a movement resisted by tension in the ACL (and MCL). All fibres of the ACL are shown stretched tight. The stretch of the ligament allows the femur (and the bearing) to move backwards on the tibial plateau relative to their positions in the unloaded joint. As the knee bends and the leg falls, the forces in the ACL (and MCL) diminish. At 57° (Fig. A9(b)), only the most anterior fibre of the ACL is just tight and the bearing lies close to its corresponding position in the unloaded joint. With further flexion, the PCL begins to tighten and stretch and the ACL goes completely slack, allowing the femur to move forward relative to its position in the unloaded joint. Therefore the total excursion of the bearing on the

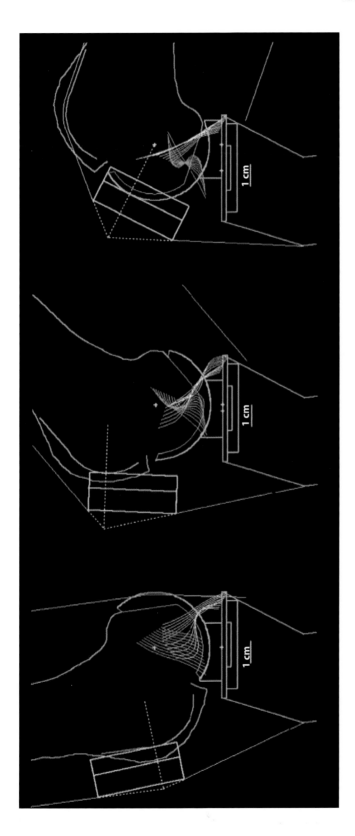

Figure A7 Model of the unicompartmental meniscal knee in situ with arrays of fibres from Fig A4 representing the ACL (green) and the PCL (white) with the extensor mechanism and hamstrings tendon of Figure A3. At each flexion angle, the position of the femur on the tibia was that which produced zero force in each cruciate ligament.

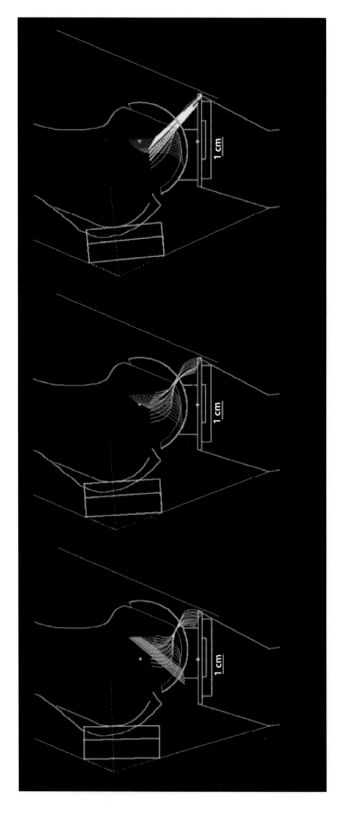

Figure A8 (a) Forward movement of the tibia from the neutral position (b) tightens the ACL and slackens the PCL. Backward movement (c) slackens the ACL and tightens the PCL (see website, Animation 8).

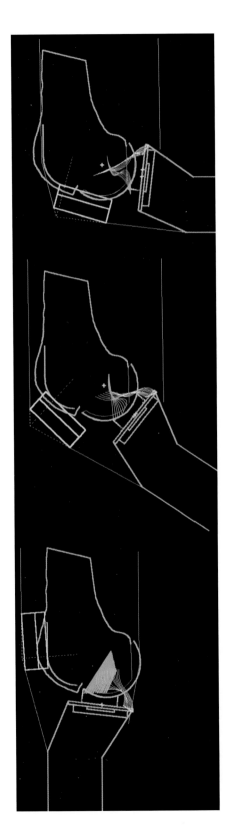

Figure A9 Model of active flexion–extension when the weight of the leg is balanced by tension in the patellar tendon. In extension (a), the tibia is pulled anteriorly relative to the femur; the ACL is stretched, and the PCL is slack. At 57°, all fibres of both ligaments are just slack. At 90°, the PCL has begun to tighten. The excursion of the meniscal bearing on the tibia is reduced compared with passive flexion (Fig. A7) (see website, Animation 9).

tibia is much reduced compared with passive motion, because of the stretching of the ligaments. While this two-dimensional model does not account for axial rotation and does not therefore predict exactly the observed pattern of bearing movement during active extension–flexion (see Figs. 3.28 and 3.29), it demonstrates the effects of ligament strain and explains the differences between active and passive motion observed fluoroscopically.

In the unloaded state, the meniscal bearing moves to that position which minimises ligament strain, requiring rollback of the femur on the tibia. Under load, the bearing moves to the position required to balance ligament and muscle force components parallel to the tibial plateau. These criteria are different and the movements of the bearings are also different. This analysis validates the assertion we made in 1978 that 'the components [of a knee prosthesis] should allow and should not resist the movements demanded by the soft tissues' [37]. This criterion can also be satisfied by unconstrained two-component designs but at the expense of excessive wear. The fully congruent meniscal bearing meets the criteria of both minimum wear and minimum constraint.

Ligament mechanics

The patterns of ligament strain during passive motion can be modelled with or without the assumption of isometry, with similar results. Because of these isometric fibres, the width of the gap between the femoral and tibial components of the prosthesis in the medial component remains constant over the range of passive flexion and can be filled with a rigid meniscal bearing of the appropriate thickness.

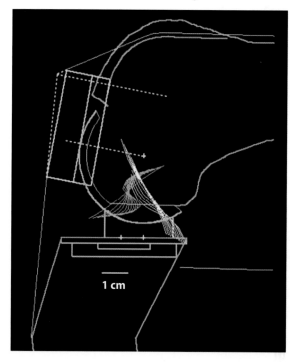

1 cm

Figure A10 Model knee at 99° flexion when patellar contact is about to transfer from the trochlea to the femoral component. The perpendiculars to the surfaces of the patella at the two contact points are parallel.

The patellofemoral joint

The model patella used in our two-dimensional models [10] is shown as a rectangle in Figures A3, A6, A9, and A10 with two straight-line articular surfaces parallel to its anterior surface. In addition to a circle defining the sulcus of the trochlea, Figures A7–A10 contain a more anterior curve outlining the flanges of the trochlea.

The most posterior surface of the model patella, representing the median ridge of the human patella, makes contact with the femoral trochlea at extension and over most of the flexion range. The more anterior surface represents the medial and lateral facets of the patella. Patellofemoral contact occurs near the distal pole of the patella in extension (Figs. A3(a) and A7(a)), and moves proximally (Figs. A3(b) and A7(b)) with increasing flexion. Eventually, contact moves onto the medial and lateral facets of the patella, and onto the femoral condyle (Fig. A3(c)) or the femoral component (Fig. A7(c)). The median ridge (the anterior articular surface) then passes into the intercondylar notch and lies proximal to the articular surface of the femur.

The predicted movement of the contact area on the model patella is very similar to that observed in the human knee (see Fig. 5.1) [38]. The patella rolls proximally as it slides distally on the femur during knee flexion, ensuring that the line of action of the patellofemoral contact force always passes through the intersection of the patellar and quadriceps tendons, a condition necessary for mechanical equilibrium of the patella [10].

A number of the predictions of patellofemoral behaviour from this model agree well with independent measurements [39]. The quadriceps tendon is shown as a line extending proximally from the proximal pole of the model patella (Figs. A3, A6, A7–A10). At high flexion angles (>85°), it wraps around the trochlea to form the tendofemoral joint, as described by Bishop and Denham [40]. The angle between the quadriceps and the patellar tendons, called the patella mechanism angle, diminishes with increasing knee flexion. The variation of this angle as calculated from the model agrees well with measurements by Buff et al. [41]. The angles between each of the tendons and the line of action of the patellofemoral force are not equal, and as a result the tension forces in the two tendons are not equal [42]. The variation of the ratio of the tendon forces with flexion angle calculated from the model agrees well with measurements [40–44].

The instant of transition from trochlear contact to condylar contact is shown in Figure A10, with the model knee drawn at 99° flexion. Contact is about to move from the trochlea onto the femoral component. The patella is held anteriorly on the trochlea until its medial and lateral facets overlie the femoral component. The anterior edge of the femoral component is bypassed and is never in contact with the patella, so that there is no danger of the type of impingement described by Hernigou and Deschamps [45] (see Fig 5.2) as a common complication of fixed-bearing polycentric unicompartmental arthroplasties.

The models of the intact and replaced joints both demonstrate changes in PTA with flexion similar to those observed in living patients (see Fig. 3.27) with complete restoration of function. This may be a reason why revision of an OUKA for patellar problems is rare.

Conclusion

Experimental and mathematical studies of the mobility and stability of the normal knee show that each requires interaction between the articular surfaces and the ligaments.

The joint achieves its mobility because the surfaces can roll and slide on each other while the ligaments rotate about their origins and insertions on the bones. The articular surfaces keep some fibres of the ligaments just tight over the range of movement, while the ligaments keep the surfaces just in contact. These interactions require no tissue deformation and give the joint its range of unresisted motion, leading to the coupling of axial rotation to flexion angle and to femoral rollback.

The joint achieves its stability because the articular surfaces resist indentation under compressive forces and the ligaments resist elongation under tensile forces. As load increases, the indentations and elongations continue and the contact areas adjust until the ligament forces balance the applied loads and muscle forces. This mechanism gives the joint its characteristic laxity, requiring rapidly increasing applied loads to move the bones from their passive positions.

In activity, motion occurs under load and the mechanisms which control mobility and stability are combined.

All these features of natural mobility and stability can be restored to a satisfactory extent by retaining all ligaments and implanting fully unconstrained prosthetic components which allow but do not resist the movements required by the soft tissues. Polyethylene wear can be minimised by the use of fully conforming mobile meniscal bearings. Exact reproduction of the shapes of the natural articular surfaces is not required. The balance between restoration of function and resistance to wear is achieved by the use of spherical and flat articular surfaces on the metal components with an interposed fully conforming meniscal bearing to give a ligament compatible arthroplasty.

References

1. Crowninshield R, Pope MH, Johnson R, Miller R. The impedance of the human knee. *J Biomech* 1976; **9**: 529–35.

2. Andriacchi TP, Mikosz RP, Hampton SJ, Galante JO. Model studies of the stiffness characteristics of the human knee joint. *J Biomech* 1983; **16**: 23–9.

3. Blankevoort L, Huiskes R. Validation of a three-dimensional model of the knee. *J Biomech* 1996; **29**: 955–61.

4. Sathasivam S, Walker PS. Optimization of the bearing surface geometry of total knees. *J Biomech* 1994; **27**: 255–64.

5. Sathasivam S, Walker PS. A computer model with surface friction for the prediction of total knee kinematics. *J Biomech* 1997; **30**: 177–84.

6. Sathasivam S, Walker PS. Computer model to predict subsurface damage in tibial inserts of total knees. *J Orthop Res* 1998; **16**: 564–71.

7. Wilson DR, Feikes JD, O'Connor JJ. Ligaments and articular contact guide passive knee flexion. *J Biomech* 1998; **31**: 1127–36.

8. O'Connor JJ, Shercliff TL, Biden E, Goodfellow JW. The geometry of the knee in the sagittal plane. *J Engng Med, Proc Inst Mech Eng [H]* 1989; **203**: 223–33.

9. Zavatsky AB, O'Connor JJ. A model of human knee ligaments in the sagittal plane. Part 1: Response to passive flexion. *J Engng Med, Proc Inst Mech Eng [H]* 1992; **206**: 125–34.

10. Gill HS, O'Connor JJ. Biarticulating two-dimensional computer model of the human patellofemoral joint. *Clin Biomech* 1996; **11**: 81–89.

11. Lu T-W, O'Connor JJ. Lines of action and moment arms of the major force-bearing structures crossing the human knee joint: comparison between theory and experiment. *J Anat* 1996; **189**: 575–85.

12. Hall AS. *Kinematics and Linkage Design*. Englewood Cliffs, NJ: Prentice-Hall, 1961.

13. Feikes JD. The mobility and stability of the human knee joint. DPhil Thesis, University of Oxford, 1999.

14. Herzog W, Read LJ. Lines of action and moment arms of the major force-carrying structures crossing the human knee joint. *J Anat* 1993; **182**: 213–30.

15. Friederich NF, Muller W, O'Brien WR. [Clinical application of biomechanic and functional anatomical findings of the knee joint]. *Orthopäde* 1992; **21**: 41–50.

16. Mommersteeg TJ, Blankevoort L, Huiskes R, Kooloos JG, Kauer JM, Hendriks JC. The effect of variable relative insertion orientation of human knee bone–ligament–bone complexes on the tensile stiffness. *J Biomech* 1995; **28**: 745–52.

17. van Dijk R, Huiskes R, Selvik G. Roentgen stereophotogrammetric methods for the evaluation of the three dimensional kinematic behavior and cruciate ligament length patterns of the human knee. *J Biomech* 1979; **12**: 727–31.

18. Friederich NF, O'Brien WR. Anterior cruciate ligament graft tensioning versus knee stability. *Knee Surg Sports Traumatol Arthrosc* 1998; **6**(Suppl 1): S38–42.

19. Girgis FG, Marshall JL, Monajem A. The cruciate ligaments of the knee joint. Anatomical, functional and experimental analysis. *Clin Orthop* 1975; **106**: 216–31.

20. Brantigan OC, Voshell AF. The mechanics of the ligaments and menisci of the knee joint. *J Bone Joint Surg [Am]* 1941; **23-A**: 44–66.

21. Sidles JA, Larson RV, Garbini JL, Downey DJ, Matsen FAI. Ligament length relationships in the moving knee. *J Orthop Res* 1988; **6**: 593–610.

22. Sapega AA, Moyer MA, Schneck C, Komalahiranya N. Testing for isometry during reconstruction of the anterior cruciate ligament. *J Bone Joint Surg [Am]* 1990; **72-A**: 259–67.

23. Wang C, Walker PS. The effects of flexion and rotation on the length patterns of the ligaments of the knee. *J Biomech* 1973; **6**: 587–96.

24. Amis AA, Dawkins GPC. Functional anatomy of the anterior cruciate ligament: fibre bundle actions related to ligament replacements and injuries. *J Bone Joint Surg [Br]* 1991; **73-B**: 260–7.

25. Covey DC, Sapega AA, Sherman GM, Torg JS. Testing for 'isometry' during posterior cruciate ligament reconstruction. *Trans Orthop Res Soc*; 1992; **17**; 665.

26. Meister BR, Michael SP, Moyer RA, Kelly JD, Schneck CD. Anatomy and kinematics of the lateral collateral ligament of the knee. *Am J Sports Med* 2000; **28**: 869–78.

27. Rovick JS, Reuben JD, Schrager RJ, Walker PS. Relation between knee motion and ligament length patterns. *Clin Biomech* 1991; **6**: 213–20.

28. Robinson B. Dislocation in mobile bearing lateral unicompartmental arthroplasty. DPhil Thesis, University of Oxford, 2002.

29. Freeman MAR. *Tibiofemoral Movement*. London: British Editorial Society of Bone and Joint Surgery, 2001.

30. Strasser H. *Lehrbuch der Muskel und Gelenkmechanik. III Band: Die untere Extremitart*. Berlin: Springer-Verlag, 1917.

31. Zuppinger H. *Die Active Flexion im Umbelasteten Kniegelenk*. Weisbaden: Bergmann, 1904.

32. Zavatsky AB, O'Connor JJ. A model of human knee ligaments in the sagittal plane. Part 2: Fibre recruitment under load. *J Engng Med, Proc Inst Mech Eng [H]* 1992; **206**: 135–45.

33. Lu TW, O'Connor JJ. Fibre recruitment and shape changes of knee ligaments during motion: as revealed by a computer graphics-based model. *J Engng Med, Proc Inst Mech Eng [H]* 1996; **210**: 71–9.

34. Huss RA, Holstein H, O'Connor JJ. The effect of cartilage deformation on the laxity of the knee joint. *J Engng Med, Proc Inst Mech Eng [H]* 1999; **213**: 19–32.

35. Grood ES, Noyes FR. Diagnosis of knee ligament injuries: biomechanical precepts. In: Feagin JA Jr (ed) *The Crucial Ligaments: Diagnosis and Treatment of Ligamentous Injuries about the Knee*. New York: Churchill Livingstone, 1988; 245–85.

36. Imran A. Mechanics of the ligament deficient knee. DPhil Thesis, University of Oxford, 1999.

37. Goodfellow J, O'Connor J. The mechanics of the knee and prosthesis design. *J Bone Joint Surg [Br]* 1978; **60-B**: 358–69.

38. Goodfellow J, Hungerford DS, Zindel M. Patello-femoral joint mechanics and pathology. 1: Functional anatomy of the patello-femoral joint. *J Bone Joint Surg [Br]* 1976; **58-B**: 287–90.

39. O'Connor J, Shercliff T, FitzPatrick D. Mechanics of the knee. In: Daniel D, Akeson W, O'Connor J (ed) *Ligaments: Structure, Function, Injury and Repair*. New York: Raven Press, 1990.

40. Bishop R, Denham R. A note on the ratio between tensions in the quadriceps tendon and infrapatellar ligament. *Eng Med* 1977: **6**; 53–4.

41. Buff HU, Jones LC, Hungerford DS. Experimental determination of forces transmitted through the patello-femoral joint. *J Biomech* 1988; **21**: 17–23.

42. Maquet P. *Biomechanics of the Knee*. Berlin: Springer-Verlag, 1976.

43. Ellis MI, Seedhom BB, Wright V. Forces in the knee joint whilst rising from a seated position. *J Biomed Eng* 1984; **6**: 113–20.

44. Huberti HH, Hayes WC, Stone JL, Shybut GT. Force ratios in the quadriceps tendon and ligamentum patellae. *J Orthop Res* 1984; **2**: 49–54.

45. Hernigou P, Deschamps G. Patellar impingement following unicompartmental arthroplasty. *J Bone Joint Surg [Am]* 2002; **84-A**: 1132–7.

Index

CONTENTS

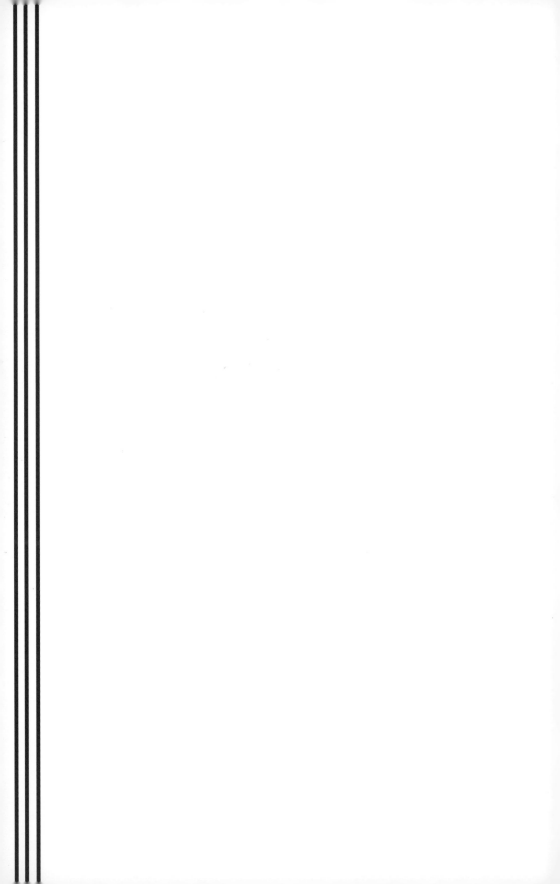

1

FATHER AND SON AT DAYTONA

The 1993 Daytona 500 was winding down, and superstar driver Dale Earnhardt, the five-time series champion, was in the lead. He was leading a line of cars in the historic race that included rookie Jeff Gordon, Dale Jarrett, Geoff Bodine, and Hut Stricklin.

With three circuits remaining around the 2.5 mile–long Daytona International Speedway, Dale Jarrett, the son of two-time **NASCAR** champion Ned Jarrett, stormed past Gordon and was side by side with "The Intimidator" Earnhardt, best known for his dominating, aggressive driving style. Bodine guided his Ford Thunderbird behind Jarrett's Chevy, creating what is called a two-car **draft**. In stock car racing, two cars running nose to tail can run faster than one car alone because of the way they cut through the wind. Gordon then eased his Chevrolet Lumina on the bumper of Earnhardt's car to form a pack of four cars clustered together, running at speeds of nearly 200 miles per hour.

With less than a lap remaining in the Great American Race—stock car racing's equivalent of the Super Bowl—four cars were in a position to win the coveted trophy. The cars of Jarrett and Earnhardt touched momentarily, although the skilled drivers averted a full-scale collision. The draft created by Jarrett and Bodine, however, proved too much for Earnhardt and Gordon. Pushed by Bodine, Jarrett pulled ahead going into the final corner.

In the broadcast booth high above the speedway, Dale's father, Ned, a member of CBS's on-air team, got an instruction from the broadcast's producer, Bob Stenner. During all live broadcasts, producers talk to their on-air people through small devices in the broadcasters' ears. Normally the conversations are about upcoming commercials, instant replays, or what the broadcaster should say about a certain driver's on-track position. But this time, the instructions were different. Through his earpiece, Jarrett heard Stenner say, "Ned, root your son home."

Jarrett, who had silently been working out his son's strategy, was now free to say what he was thinking. His colleagues in the broadcast booth went silent. CBS turned cameras on both Jarretts, the father in the broadcast booth and the son on the track. "Come on, Dale! Go baby, go!" Ned Jarrett shouted, rising to his feet and shaking his fists in the air. "He's going to make it! Dale Jarrett's going to win the Daytona 500!" Dale Jarrett held onto the lead and beat Earnhardt across the finish line by .19 seconds, less than two car lengths.

In the practice of sports journalism, the broadcaster, commentator, or reporter should never be part of the story; cheering for any of the participants is a major "no-no." Broadcasters must remain objective and impartial at all times. And for Jarrett, who during his racing

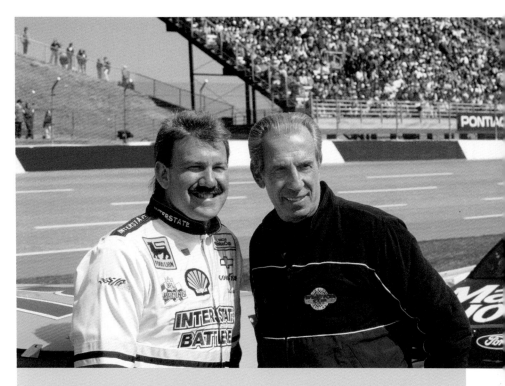

NASCAR champions Dale Jarrett (*left*) and his father, Ned Jarrett, pose for a picture during the 1993 racing season. As a CBS announcer at the Daytona 500, Ned cherished the moment when he was able to root for his son from the broadcast booth.

career became known as "Gentleman Ned" for his calm demeanor on and off the track, this sort of outburst was highly unusual.

"I'm not the real emotional type. I'm not Dick Vitale," Ned said, referring to the legendary and usually loud basketball announcer. "But this was something different. It's the greatest feeling I can have, the greatest feeling I've ever had, no doubt." He continued, "Any accomplishment that I had winning any of my races or those two championships do not mean nearly as much as this does."

Television sports critics, who in most other cases would lambaste a broadcaster for rooting for a player, embraced Jarrett's CBS performance as something to be cherished. It was a sports moment that would be hard to match. "Stenner asked the others to back off and told me to do the call, he said, 'Be a father.' That got me pumped up. I got a little more emotional. It was a natural father's reaction, I think," Jarrett explained.

TRADITION ON THE TRACK

In a way, Dale Jarrett's win in stock car racing's most prestigious event brought full circle a racing journey started by Ned Jarrett back in the 1950s, when he debuted as a local driver in North Carolina. That trek brought Ned Jarrett fame, fortune, and a child who had now won the Daytona 500. Ned Jarrett had earned two championships and 50 career wins, but he had never won the Daytona 500. Dale had now proven he could make it in the sport in which his father had made such a mark three decades earlier.

After emerging from his car, Dale spoke to his father on a two-way radio: "You came so close when you ran out of gas in '63," he told his dad. "I got this one for you and all the family." The win was only the second in Dale Jarrett's career, and the first for car owner Joe Gibbs, who earlier in his life had won three Super Bowls as coach of the Washington Redskins. "I had three things going for me," Dale said. "I had a good car, good luck, and God on my side. . . . That's what it takes to win the Daytona 500."

Although his father retired when Dale was just a kid, Dale Jarrett had been around racing, or at least influenced by the sport in some way, just about all of his life. "I sat in my dad and mom's car when I was eight and nine years old, pretending I was driving in the Daytona 500," Dale said. "Of course, I

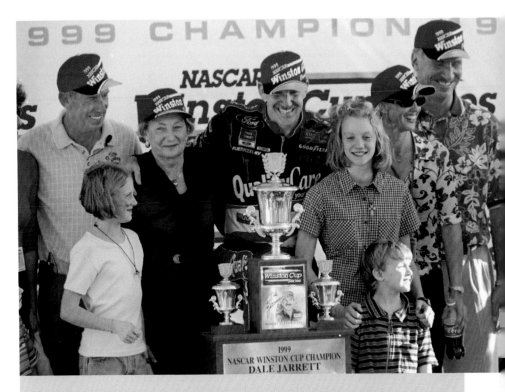

Jarrett family members celebrate Dale's winning of the 1999 NASCAR Winston Cup Series. (*From left*) two-time Winston Cup champion Ned Jarrett; Dale's daughter Karsyn (age 9); Ned's wife, Martha; Dale Jarrett; Dale's daughter Natalee (11); son Zachary (5); wife, Kelly; and brother, Glenn Jarrett.

won every time back then. Now, I really have won it." After leaving the sport in 1966, Ned Jarrett remained a racing broadcaster and track promoter in North Carolina. Dale's older brother, Glenn, had also raced for a while, although he eventually turned to broadcasting as a career.

PARENTAL GUIDANCE

Dale's parents had originally tried to steer him away from racing. He was a multisport star, and they hoped he would pursue professional golf full time. But it was no use. Dale

DRIVING FOR A BIGGER AUDIENCE

NASCAR started in 1949, but it wasn't until 1979 that the Daytona 500 or any other stock car race was carried live from start to finish on broadcast television. Until then, racing coverage had been limited to short snippets carried on other sports shows such as ABC's *Wide World of Sports*.

CBS carried the 1979 Daytona 500, airing it during a raging snowstorm on the East Coast that gave the telecast a huge, homebound audience. And what a race they got. Legendary driver Richard Petty won, but a crash involving Bobby Allison and Cale Yarborough was the event imprinted in the minds of viewers. The two men emerged from their cars and started a fight in the infield, becoming the unforgettable "stars" of the 1979 event.

Despite the fight, the telecast was strong enough to get other broadcasters looking at NASCAR events as money-making television programming. It took another decade to get all NASCAR races covered from start to finish. Today, every top-level NASCAR race airs live on a major network, with more than 18 million people watching at least a portion of the Daytona 500 each year.

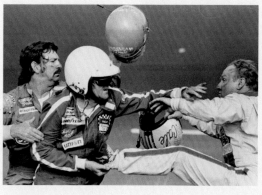

Bobby Allison *(in white helmet)* holds the foot of Cale Yarborough after Yarborough kicked him following an argument during the 1979 Daytona 500.

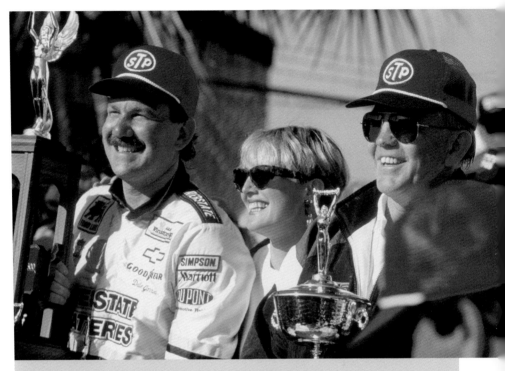

Dale Jarrett (*left*) accepts the trophy and celebrates his 1993 Daytona 500 victory with his wife, Kelly, and car owner Joe Gibbs.

pursued his dream, and although he had to overcome some lean years, he grew to be included among an elite bunch of drivers.

"I've gone back and watched the replay of my father's call three times," Dale said a few weeks after his 1993 win. "For a few minutes, the Jarretts took over national television. It's a day I'll never forget." Neither will Ned. He was as proud as a peacock over his son's accomplishment. "You never know how your kids are going to turn out, so you try to set examples and help them along the way," Ned once told a reporter. "We've been extremely fortunate that ours have turned out so well. We've been blessed in that sense."

2

THE EARLY DAYS

Ned Jarrett was born on October 12, 1932, in Newton, North Carolina, a small town northwest of Charlotte. Like most kids in Newton, Jarrett grew up on a farm. His father, Homer, ran the family-owned sawmill, which turned raw trees into usable lumber for the rapidly growing region. In 1932, Herbert Hoover was president of the United States and the formation of the National Association for Stock Car Auto Racing (NASCAR) was still 16 years away. Stock car racing was also in its infancy. There was no formal organization to oversee the sport as there is today. What loosely organized races existed were predominantly in the South. And, in fact, stock car racing's roots are directly tied to the trends and laws of the time in the United States.

Ned Jarrett was born a year before the United States government lifted its ban on the manufacture, transportation, and consumption of alcohol. From 1920 to 1933, the government banned the sale of alcoholic drinks such as beer, wine, and liquor. Despite the legal risks, the lure of tax-free money, combined with public demand, led many people to make alcohol in secret operations. People who manufactured illegal liquor were called "bootleggers" or "moonshiners." The equipment they used to produce the alcoholic beverages were called "stills," and were located in the woods throughout the South. To get their products from the stills to their customers, moonshiners hired drivers who would use cars to move the liquor. These "runners" souped up their cars by stripping them of any unnecessary interior weight: seats were removed to make room for the bottles of alcohol, and the engines were finely tuned. In addition, they tried to make their cars faster than those of the police, just in case they got caught driving down a road with a carload of the illegal product.

A SPORT AND A DRIVER ARE BORN

When they weren't hauling liquor, moonshine runners often raced against each other. It is not surprising that two men standing around talking about how fast their cars were would eventually race against each other to prove who was really the fastest. These incidents led to organized races, which were often held in open fields. When people realized that fans would pay to see the races, organized stock car racing was born.

Ned's parents got him interested in racing as a child. His father, however, was not overjoyed with the sport's image. In addition to the moonshine business, the sport was hurt by shady promoters who often ran off with the prize money before the race was over, leaving the participants empty handed. And because the races were run on dirt tracks, the drivers, fans, and everyone else usually left the event covered with dust.

The sport of racing moved to improve its image in 1948, when William Henry Getty France and a group of race

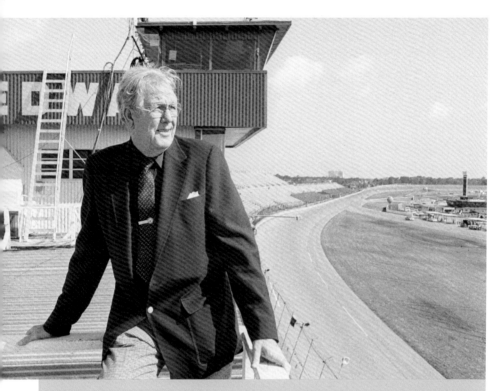

Motor sport legend Bill France Sr. looks out at the Daytona International Speedway from the top of the grandstand in February 1983. France started out holding stock car races on the beach in Daytona, Florida, before building the track in 1969.

promoters from around the country formed the National Association for Stock Car Auto Racing, or NASCAR. Their mission was to improve conditions for the fans, clean up the sport overall, and provide a national umbrella organization, or governing body, to oversee all aspects of the sport. Five years later, when Ned Jarrett was 21, he joined with another local race fan named John Lentz. Together they worked on a race car that was basically a beefed-up street vehicle.

In the early days of racing, the cars used were stock cars, which meant that they had to be those available at the typical car dealer's showroom. The technology then was nowhere near as advanced as it is today, with drivers sitting in carefully crafted cockpits framed with steel tubing (called a **roll cage**) and padding to limit the potential for injury—or worse—in the case of a horrible crash. When Ned Jarrett started racing, there were no seat belts, no roll cages, and no special racing tires. Most racers back in the early days drove their own cars to the track and removed the headlights and taillights before the race. If they didn't wreck the cars, when the race was over, they replaced the missing parts and drove the cars home.

With Lentz driving and Jarrett working on the car, the team made its debut in 1953 at the brand new Hickory Motor Speedway in Hickory, North Carolina. Ned's father

NASCAR GROWS

In the early days of NASCAR racing, the sport was much different than it is today. When Ned Jarrett began his driving career, in 1953, Herb Thomas won NASCAR's top title by driving in 37 races and winning 12 times. In the years that followed, the number of official NASCAR events would balloon to nearly 60, giving drivers many chances to race.

In the beginning, the top drivers made most races, but there were many more drivers who raced only when the series came to a track near their hometowns. In 1973, however, NASCAR officials changed the process and limited the number of events each season. In 2004, there were 36 points races in NASCAR's top series in addition to two non-points races, which kept the teams on the road upwards of 40 weeks that year and gave them very few weekends off during the season.

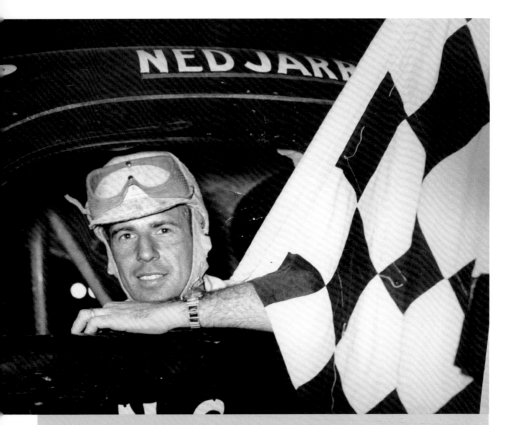

Ned Jarrett is shown holding the checkered flag early in his career when he started racing at the Hickory Motor Speedway in Newton, North Carolina.

was still adamant that his son not get mixed up in racing, and Ned was just as adamant that he would race. "I just simply didn't discuss it," Ned said. "I didn't think that much about it and I didn't think it would make that much difference." Ned and his father finally came to a compromise: Ned could be a partner in the car as long as he did not drive. But on the night they were to run their first race, Lentz got sick. The other members of the team didn't look any farther than Jarrett as a replacement. He and Lentz had the same build, and with a helmet on, few could tell it wasn't Lentz behind the wheel.

Jarrett entered the race as Lentz and finished tenth in the 50-lap event. "I thought I was in good physical condition, having grown up on a farm, but I was so tired afterward that I had to be helped out of my car," Jarrett said. "Later, I learned the mental strain had really worn me out. Once I learned to relax, I didn't get so tired."

His tiredness notwithstanding, Jarrett fell in love with driving, even though it was under another man's name. Jarrett kept racing under his assumed name, but found it was hard to keep his identity secret. He ran under Lentz's name nearly a dozen times before he got his first win. And, because he had promised his father that he wouldn't be driving at all, the victory celebration was subdued. "Finally, I lucked out and won," Jarrett said. "And living in a small community, it got back to him." Because his earlier warnings had gone unheeded, Homer Jarrett gave in and told his son he could continue racing, this time under his own name. With this, Ned Jarrett's racing career officially began. At the same time, the building blocks of NASCAR were coming together as well.

3

⬛⬛⬛⬛⬛⬛⬛

NED JARRETT'S RACING CAREER

Ned Jarrett's success at the Hickory Motor Speedway instilled in him a sense of great confidence. Though never a hard charger, Jarrett's smooth and steady style made him a consistent performer on the track. Off the track, he was known as an all-around good guy. By 1953, he was married, had a three-year-old son named Glenn, and was about to venture into the big leagues of stock car racing.

Just as Jarrett was growing as a driver, so too was NASCAR racing. The cars, still fairly close to true stock cars, were becoming more sophisticated. There were no giant changes, but instead a gradual evolution as drivers became more inventive. The minor changes included beefing up the suspension, taking out the rear passenger seats, adding primitive roll cage setups, and, most importantly, adding crude seat belt setups.

Armed with a newfound confidence, Jarrett had decided he wanted to race with the men competing on NASCAR's Grand National series, which was a forerunner of the current NASCAR/Sprint Cup series. He made his

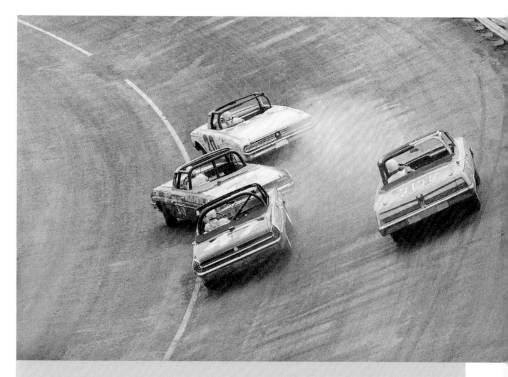

Ned Jarrett in the number 11 car (*far right*) prepares to pass Ralph Earnhardt (75) and two other racers during the 1962 Rebel 300 race at Darlington Raceway in Darlington, South Carolina. Earnhardt is starting to spin out as he attempts to pass the number 20 car.

first Grand National start on August 29, 1953, in a 100-mile race held at the Hickory Motor Speedway. He finished eleventh in a field of 12 cars. He next set his sights on a larger facility: the newly created Darlington Raceway in South Carolina. Developer Harold Brasington built the track in 1950 as the first super speedway on NASCAR's Grand National circuit.

Darlington, originally built at 1.25 miles in length and later expanded to 1.375 miles long, was the fastest track on the circuit. Its egg-shaped design was difficult for drivers to manage. The buzz that developed around the facility, later dubbed "Too Tough to Tame," proved too tough for Jarrett to resist. "I thought I was good enough to do that," he said.

He dabbled a bit in the Grand National series, picking up a race or two each year, but continued racing primarily in NASCAR's sportsman division, the equivalent of today's Busch Grand National division. He won the NASCAR Sportsman Championship in 1957 and again in 1958. Then, having mastered the short-track circuit, Jarrett graduated to the Grand National circuit full time in 1959. By then, off the track, Jarrett's family life was in full swing. His son Dale was born in 1956, and daughter Patti on August 31, 1959.

Still, Jarrett's time away from home and the time dedicated to his sport was increasing rapidly. In his first full season on the Grand National series, Jarrett started 17 events, picking up two wins and earning $3,860 in prize money. A year later, in 1960, he started 40 events, won five races, and increased his earnings to $25,438.

GENTLEMAN NED

Jarrett's off-track demeanor, combined with his on-track style, earned him the nickname "Gentleman Ned" from his competitors. His conservative driving style came out of necessity, he said. He didn't have a lot of money, so if he crashed, his racing career would end suddenly. "You either had to run up front and be dramatic, and if you broke down, okay, or be conservative," he said. "To do that, you had to take care of the equipment back then. Some people labeled you a conservative driver. I learned pretty quickly in the sport that you had to finish before you could win. I learned how to handle a car to make it last. That was the concept I chose."

He improved his performance using the steady style he developed early in his career. He also was able to boost his points totals by performing extremely well on short tracks, which at the time still played host to a majority of the events. "I was not, and am not, a speed demon," Jarrett told writer Kim Chapin in the book *Fast as White Lightning.* "I liked competition, but I wanted the car to feel comfortable . . . if it didn't, I'd slow it down enough to where it did. I didn't try to be a hero. I knew for a fact that there were plenty of people who were as physically capable as I, and maybe some more so, of turning that steering wheel and getting around the track."

Jarrett said his strength on the track was in looking ahead further than other drivers, which helped him anticipate, and often avoid, potential wrecks or other disasters. He had the lowest number of accidents among the drivers of his time. His consistency paid off in 1961 when he started 46 of NASCAR's 52 races. Although he won just one race, his string of 33 finishes in the top 10 was enough to put him ahead of Rex White to win the series championship. For his efforts, Jarrett earned a total of $41,056 for the entire year.

A SPOKESMAN FOR RACING

Despite the glory that comes with a championship, an incident off the track changed Jarrett's life forever. Following his championship, members of the Elk's Club in Newton, North Carolina, asked him to take part in their Sunday afternoon induction ceremony for incoming officers. Jarrett saw the event as a chance to prove to local leaders that race car drivers were not bad people.

He prepared for the meeting much the way he'd prepare for a race. He memorized his short speech and practiced it for days. But when he appeared before the group, he could not remember a word. "I was scared to death and it was so embarrassing," he told a reporter. "I made up my mind at that very moment that I'd do whatever it took to make myself a better person."

The next day he attended a meeting for the famed Dale Carnegie public-speaking course. He continued with the program for several months until he felt comfortable speaking in front of groups of people. Following completion of the course, Jarrett, often accompanied by his sons, set out to discuss motorsports with church groups in the South. He turned that one horrible moment in Newton into a positive force, and in the process set an example for his sons of how to deal with people. "I was 11 when Dad

SPOTLIGHT ON RACERS

Ned Jarrett was one of the first NASCAR drivers to see how important being a good public speaker was to his career. Today, however, new drivers routinely undergo media training, some before ever running their first top-level races. That's because these days, not only does a driver drive in races, but he or she is also a spokesperson for any of the products appearing on the sides of their cars.

Moreover, unlike the days when Ned Jarrett started, stock car drivers are true sports superstars. As such, they're called on to speak at events, appear on television shows, and star in commercials. It's not at all uncommon these days to see a stock car driver on the front of a box of cereal or appearing on a late-night talk show.

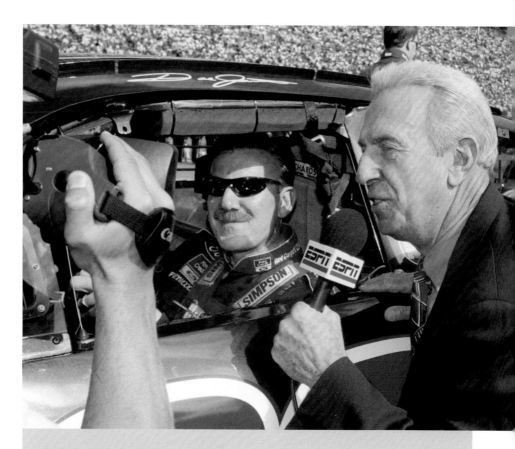

Ned Jarrett interviews his son Dale on pit row. After Ned took a public-speaking course, he built on the experience to create a new career in racing behind the microphone.

saw the light, so to speak," Glenn Jarrett said. "I remember one night we drove to a Baptist church 50 or 60 miles from home, just so he could speak. There was no pay for it. He did it to make himself better."

4

A CAREER HIGH

In the 1960s, NASCAR underwent several dramatic changes that impacted the sport both on and off the track. In 1962, Chrysler and the Ford Motor Company, both of which had pulled out of racing in the late 1950s, returned to the sport and provided financial assistance to selected teams. The involvement of these manufacturers was driven by the total dominance of the Chevrolet and Pontiac teams, which had won 18 of the first 20 races of the season. Only Richard Petty, who drove his Plymouth to victory twice, was able to defeat the Chevy and Pontiac teams. Jarrett drove a Chevrolet for team owner Bee Gee Holloway in 1961, but a few seasons later he was driving a Ford for Bondy Long.

In some ways, the automakers' direct involvement in the sport had a positive effect, while in other areas, it did not. Because the carmakers demanded wins, drivers were forced to push harder on the track than they may have wanted. And unlike today's sleek racers, the cars of the early 1960s did not run as smoothly.

This pressure to win was tough on the drivers. If they didn't win, team owners, pushed by the manufacturers, changed drivers as a means of finding on-track magic. "I don't think the average fan would realize the amount of pressure that was involved," Jarrett said. "There was always somebody that was trying to get your job, and certainly you were aware of it, but it was never anything that really bothered me to the point that I lost sleep over it. If I lost the job, well, fine. I was out there doing my best and that's all I figured anyone could expect."

Jarrett's best was better than most. In 1962, he raced in 52 events and won 6 times to earn $43,444 in prize money. He finished third in the points standings. In 1963, he drove in 53 races, won 8, and took home $45,844 in prize money to finish fourth overall. And in 1964, he logged 59 races, 15 wins, $71,925 in earnings, and finished second in the point standings.

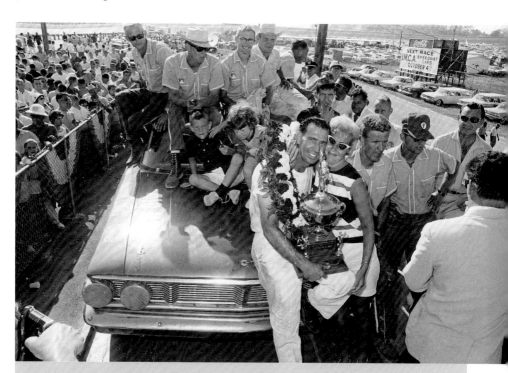

Ned Jarrett holds the Governor's Cup trophy and receives a hug from his wife, Martha, after winning the 1964 Dixie 400 race in Atlanta, Georgia.

To the general public, the sport was known for the super-speedways such as Daytona, Darlington, and Talladega—the staples of the circuit. Racing was moving away from the dirt tracks—where it all started—to the asphalt ovals. Safety was still not a major factor in the sport. Speeds were increasing, and drivers didn't wear fire suits as they do today. Most wore street pants, short-sleeved shirts, shoes, and open-faced helmets. In the late 1950s and early 1960s, drivers dipped their clothes in a fire-resistant solution that, although able to prevent injury, made the clothes uncomfortable. As a result, many drivers stopped using the liquid. Seat belts were just lap belts, similar to the ones that came with the cars. And many cars still had bench seats. 1964 was a particularly gruesome year for racing: a handful of well-known racers were killed.

The growing danger, as well as not being with his family as much as he liked, started to wear on Jarrett. NASCAR's schedule was hectic, and the stress and strain of keeping a job were tough. Also, unlike drivers of today, NASCAR's stars were not millionaires. In a single race in the 1990s, a driver could earn what Jarrett earned in all of 1964.

Still, Jarrett started the 1965 season in fine form. By mid season, he and fellow Ford driver Dick Hutcherson were ahead of all the others for the series championship. But Jarrett's season was upended just 60 laps into a race at Greenville-Pickens Speedway in South Carolina. His car died while leading the race. Despite his efforts to pull off the track, he was rammed by another car, which sent him back into traffic. His car was pummeled by others and torn apart with such force that his seat was pulled from its anchors. Jarrett suffered a serious back injury, which doctors told him would require three weeks of hospital rest and then three months of rehabilitation.

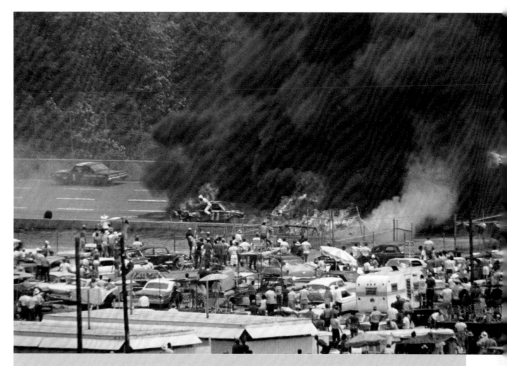

Ned Jarrett can be seen jumping from his vehicle after being involved in a fiery crash at the Charlotte Motor Speedway. In the 1960s, racing became very dangerous as speeds increased while safety precautions remained haphazard.

That wasn't what Jarrett wanted to hear. He had a race to run the following Thursday night. Jarrett doubled the therapy, and with the help of a plastic brace, he raced five days later. He used the brace for three months and despite serious pain maintained his lock on the NASCAR points lead.

THE FINAL LAPS

After his one championship, Jarrett longed for a win in the prestigious Southern 500 at Darlington. He felt that if he could win that race, his career would be complete.

The night before the race, he spoke to a Methodist Youth Fellowship group and asked the kids for their prayers. Their response gave him a sense of confidence going in: "Not that I or any other particular driver might win it," Jarrett said then, "but I went away from there with a genuine feeling that those kids were behind me, that they would say a prayer for me. It made me feel good."

Winning the race wouldn't be easy. Although Jarrett still had the points lead, Hutcherson was strong. Jarrett figured that if he were to win the Southern 500 himself, Hutcherson's car would have to falter. As luck would have it for Jarrett, Hutcherson did run into mechanical troubles after less than 100 miles, but Jarrett was still far from victory. He, too, suffered from mechanical problems as his Ford began to overheat.

Jarrett dodged several accidents that day, and one by one, his chief competitors started to fall. With 100 miles to go, Darel Dieringer and Fred Lorenzen dropped out of

MONEYMAKERS

There is perhaps no better yardstick with which to measure the success of NASCAR since Ned Jarrett retired in 1965: When Jarrett hung up his helmet after 352 races, he had earned $348,967 in total prize money, including 50 wins. For comparison, Mark Martin won $395,313 for finishing sixth at the 2005 Daytona 500, and that was just one of 36 races for the top-level driver.

Though no two contracts are exactly the same, a superstar driver can earn 40 to 50 percent of the prize winnings. This means that Martin took home more than $237,000 for one race, or two thirds of what Ned Jarrett made in his entire career.

the race, leaving Jarrett in front for the final 63 laps. Then, because of his overheating engine, Jarrett had to slow his car from an average of 134 mph to 125 mph. "I was saying a prayer every lap for the last several laps," Jarrett said after the race. "I wasn't the fastest on the track, but I was hoping those fellows who were lapping me would wear themselves out. That's what happened."

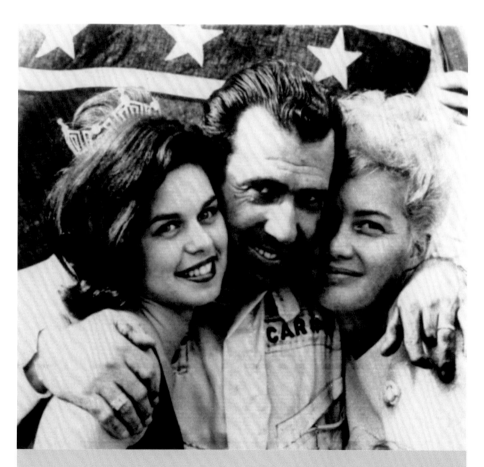

A happy Ned Jarrett squeezes his wife, Martha (*right*) and Miss Southern 500, Vicki Johnson, after winning the Southern 500 race at Darlington Raceway in 1965. The win was Jarrett's most memorable and propelled him to his second NASCAR Grand National Championship.

His win in front of some 60,000 cheering fans remains his most memorable. "It was the oldest and most prestigious at the time," Jarrett told *Winston Cup Scene*. "It was also a tough track, and the win gave me a great sense of accomplishment. It was also a real highlight for me because I won it by 14 laps—which is still a record."

Dale Jarrett, who was just nine years old at the time, vividly recalled the day. "That was a pretty special day for all of us," he said. "I remember sitting in the family grandstand in the fourth turn and watching the race and after the race we got to meet Doc and Festus from [the television series] *Gunsmoke* in **Victory Lane**. That was the highlight of the race for me. I knew it was a big race back then because about 80 percent of Camden, South Carolina, was at our house."

The Labor Day weekend win propelled Jarrett to his second NASCAR Grand National Championship. He won 13 of the 54 races he entered and took home $93,625. That season he ran a career-high 13,525 laps, representing a total of 9,121 miles.

Winning the title brought Jarrett to a career crossroads. He had met all of the goals he had set for himself. He had watched friends die in the sport he loved. And he missed his kids and his wife. Jarrett was determined to retire. "I'd set goals for myself and vowed that I'd quit when I got there," he said. "I didn't want [the fans] to remember me as a has-been. I wanted them to remember me for what I was, the reigning champion." Midway through the 1965–1966 season, while still the reigning champion, he stepped down, at the age of 34. During his career, Ned Jarrett had run in 352 races, won 50, and earned $348,967 in prize money.

5

FOLLOWING A TRADITION

Ned Jarrett left the competitive side of racing, but he never left the sport. His two championships left a legacy that continues today. And even though his sons, Glenn and Dale, were relatively young when he retired, Ned's racing experience left a permanent impression on both of them.

When he retired, Ned returned home and, with a partner, started a consulting business that helped people find franchise businesses. A franchise business is one in which a person pays a fee to a large company, such as a fast food or gas station chain, for the permission to open up a branch of that company. Jarrett paid a fee to have control of a local territory and informed interested customers about a long list of franchise businesses. "I fell in love with the concept," he said. "Unfortunately, the parent company did not perform. I saw what was happening and I got out after a year."

Jarrett never considered taking over his family's lumber business. It simply didn't interest him. Instead, he focused on enhancing his public-speaking career. In 1966, Jarrett became a financial partner in and promoter for the Hickory Motor Speedway, where he had started his racing

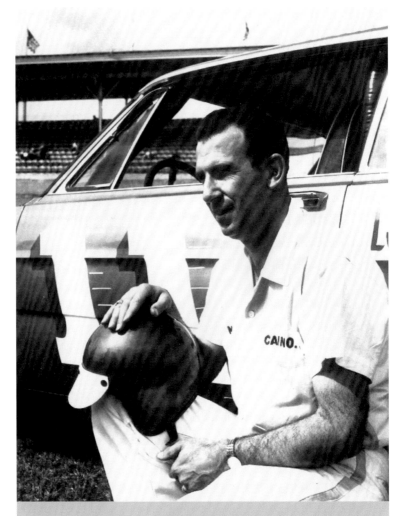

Ned Jarrett kneels by his car with his helmet in hand. This photo was taken in 1965 during Jarrett's last full year as a race car driver.

career in 1953. As promoter, he was responsible for staging races and making sure the facility ran properly.

Despite the career he had made for himself in the sport, Jarrett and his wife, Martha, tried to steer their sons away from racing. That was tough to do, however, because during his career, they had usually taken their kids to the track. The boys had fond memories of their time at the track when their father was racing. "I have a lot of memories, certainly, growing up around the sport," Dale said. "We didn't get to all of [the races], but a lot of fond memories of going to the races and being in the infield with the other families . . ." While their fathers were racing, the drivers' kids played in the infield, the center oval of grass inside the racetrack loop. Adding to the fun was the fact that the children playing there knew that at least one of them would go to Victory Lane because his or her dad had been successful on the track.

Still, Ned and Martha had seen what life on the stock car racing road could do to a family, and they were unsure, even in the 1970s, whether it was possible to make a full-time career out of racing. Job security wasn't guaranteed. If a driver did not win, he was replaced. Ned didn't want that happening to his boys.

Both Jarrett boys excelled in school and in sports. In high school, Dale was an all-conference selection in football, basketball, baseball, and golf. He was named 1975 Athlete of the Year as a senior at Newton-Conover High School, and in 1974 and 1975 he was the North Carolina High School Southern District Seven Golfer of the Year. Glenn excelled in baseball and golf as well. Following high school, Glenn went on to the University of North Carolina and then worked at the family's lumber business.

IN HIS FATHER'S TRACKS

Dale didn't talk very much about racing, recalled Ned, until he drove in his first race. He got his start in a way that mirrors Ned's entry into the sport. Dale and some friends built a car. The weekend they were to race, the mother of the young man who was to drive died. Dale took over the wheel from his friend. "After that first race he was hooked," Ned said. In 1976, Dale won a Late Model Sportsman event at Hickory when he passed the legendary Dale Earnhardt with four laps remaining in the race. A year later, when he was still just 20, Dale and some friends formed a team to run at Hickory. "He and a couple of buddies got involved," Ned said. "I didn't know about it for a time. When they got the car built they needed an engine. Dale came to me and said, 'I think I can get to drive the car if I can get an engine.'" Ned pointed his son toward some people who could get an engine for the car, and Dale's racing career was off and running.

Following his father's tracks into the sport, Dale debuted in 1977 in the Limited Sportsman division at the Hickory Motor Speedway and won the track's Rookie of the Year title for the division. Except for the pavement, it was the same track where Ned had made his debut in 1953. "I watched the early part of the race, and I thought, 'you know, he's got some potential.'" Ned said on seeing his son race for the first time.

"I always thought it was something I wanted to do, but I was 20 years old before I had the opportunity to get in a stock car," Dale told fans in an online chat session in 1997. "I had raced go-karts before, but most of my time was spent in other sports. Mostly on the golf course. But since I got in that car at Hickory, I knew that was going to be my focus for the next 20 years."

Despite their efforts to steer him in another direction, Ned and Martha Jarrett had a son in racing. "It was not that I didn't want him in racing," Ned said. "But he seemed destined for a professional sports career. A lot of people

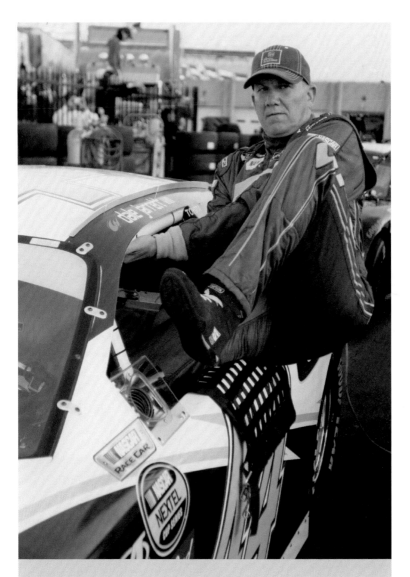

Dale Jarrett enters his vehicle before qualifying for the 2007 NASCAR Nextel All-Star Challenge race in Concord, North Carolina. Dale was a star athlete in high school and is still in good shape at the age of 51.

felt he had the potential of making it as a pro golfer. He had scholarship offers. I knew how tough it was in racing . . . "I knew the sacrifices he would have to make in racing

A FAMILY BUSINESS

Stock car racing is filled with families. Indeed, NASCAR itself is a family-owned and operated company, headed by the Frances. Chairman Brian France is the son of vice chairman Bill France Jr., who is the son of NASCAR founder Bill France.

But the family chain doesn't end there. NASCAR has been the home of several collections of brothers over the years. There have been Brett and Geoff Bodine; Terry and Bobby Labonte; and the three Wallaces—Rusty, Michael, and Kenny. And there are more sons coming along, as well. Terry Labonte's son Justin is well on his way to a top-level career. Mark Martin's son Matt has already launched a career. Lee Petty's son Richard was one of the sport's greatest drivers ever. Richard's son Kyle still races, as did Kyle's son, Adam Petty, who was killed in a crash on May 12, 2000.

if he ever were to get to the top. "I didn't want him to go through that."

"Glenn, I guess played a really big hand in me getting started and getting the opportunity," Dale once said of his brother. "He started racing when my Dad owned Hickory Speedway, and gave me the opportunity to get around race cars, and be a part of it, and learn something about them. It was fun to race with Glenn. Glenn was a good race driver."

Around the same time, Ned was planning for his own future. The same year that Dale made his debut at Hickory, Ned sold his share of the track and focused on a full-time broadcasting career. In the year of his retirement, Ned had done two radio broadcasts of local races. He also had done a few other radio broadcasts during the 1960s and 1970s.

His first attempt at television occurred in 1969, when he worked on a telecast of the Daytona 500.

In 1977, auto racing was rarely televised. No Winston/ NASCAR Cup races were carried live in their entirety, although bits and pieces were offered during ABC's "Wide World of Sports." Still, fan loyalty for the sport was growing. "I personally made the decision to build another career in racing," Ned recalled. "I'd been building a broadcast business. It was not yet a living. But I decided that this sport was heading in that direction. I believed I could build up a program for myself and make a living doing that."

A year later, Ned made his debut as part of the Motor Racing Network's live radio broadcasts of NASCAR racing. That got his foot in the door. Two years later, when CBS decided to air the Daytona 500 live from start to finish, the network called on Jarrett to offer expert analysis. He was part of NASCAR broadcasting just as the sport was getting ready to explode nationally. "Your first broadcast is similar to your early days of racing," Jarrett told a reporter, "when you have butterflies in your stomach and don't know exactly how things are going to go or what you're going to say."

Within a few years, two of the Jarretts—Dale and Glenn—were in racing and looking toward the future.

6

DIFFERENT CAREERS

The racing careers of Dale and Glenn Jarrett started off on similar paths, but differed widely later on.

After racing at Hickory, Dale landed a full-time driving job in 1982 on the newly formed Busch Grand National tour. It's not quite Winston/NASCAR Cup, but it's close. In his first year, Dale started in 29 events in the series, which uses cars similar to those in Winston Cup and runs on many of the same tracks. He earned one finish in the top five and 15 finishes in the top 10. All totaled, he won $27,261 in prize money. He won his first race in the series in 1986 at the .375-mile-long Orange County Speedway in Rougemont, North Carolina. He started on the **pole position** and averaged 95.487 mph to win. He entered the series driving for Horace Isenhower, who provided him with a luxury Glenn didn't have: cars and financial backing. Dale didn't have to worry about sinking his own money into the team, whereas Glenn, without the benefit of driving for someone else, had to fund his own operation.

Starting in 1984, Glenn became a regular in the Busch series, although he stepped down in 1988. "It became a necessity," he said. "I was funding the thing out of my pocket." At the time, Glenn was an unmarried sales representative for a company in Louisville, Kentucky. Not having to worry about supporting a family allowed him to pursue racing, although it eventually became a drain on him. He struggled with poorly performing equipment, which ultimately brought down his own on-track performance. He entered a few Winston Cup races, but was winless in both series.

Away from the track, Glenn and his father launched a Honda car dealership that demanded his time. Eventually, racing was sacrificed for business. "I had been running this deal on my own," he said. "The equipment was old and banged up. It was with all those thoughts that I decided to leave. I've regretted it ever since."

At that point the brothers' careers headed in different directions. Dale continued to drive while Glenn branched off into the business world. "The biggest difference between Glenn and Dale was that Glenn never really got any top-notch equipment," Ned said. Dale agreed: "I believe that Glenn just never got the right opportunity, which is what it's all about: getting in the right situation."

DALE PAVES HIS OWN WAY

While racing in the Busch series, Dale was looking ahead. Two years after his debut in the Busch ranks, he made his first Winston Cup start, on April 29, 1984, at Martinsville Speedway. He started the race in the twenty-fourth spot and finished fourteenth. He made two more starts that year. In 1986 he raced in one Winston Cup event, which he failed to finish. The next year, Dale landed a full-time Winston Cup ride with car owner Eric Freedlander. He ran

24 races that season, finishing twice in the top 10. He also started 27 Busch races in 1987 and won one.

By 1988, Dale's Busch racing took a back seat to the Winston Cup series. It was not an easy ride by any stretch of the imagination. He drove for three different owners in early 1988 before landing a regular job with Cale Yarborough, a legendary racer who was slowly retiring from driving. He ran 19 races for Yarborough that year and got one top 10 finish. Then, in 1989, Yarborough cut Jarrett midway through the season. Dale returned to the Busch series but struggled financially, coming near the brink of bankruptcy. He lived in his grandfather's garage apartment. "He was chasing a dream," Glenn once said of his brother. And he never gave up.

In 1990, after Neil Bonnett was injured at Charlotte, the famed Wood Brothers racing team hired Jarrett to fill in for the recovering Bonnett. He entered the deal knowing full well that if Bonnett came back, he was out of a job. But he worked hard and remained with the team the following year. Midway through the 1991 season—his second with the Wood Brothers—Dale signed a deal to drive for former Washington Redskins coach Joe Gibbs for the 1992 season. He still had to finish out the season with the Wood Brothers, though.

He entered the 1991 Champion 400 race at the Michigan International Speedway as a lame-duck driver for the Wood Brothers team. But that didn't show in his driving style. He qualified his Citgo Ford in the eleventh starting position. By lap 188, Jarrett was in fourth position, when a crash brought out a caution flag. All competitors drove into the pit areas. While others took on gas and tires, Jarrett's team opted for gas only. He exited pit road in first place.

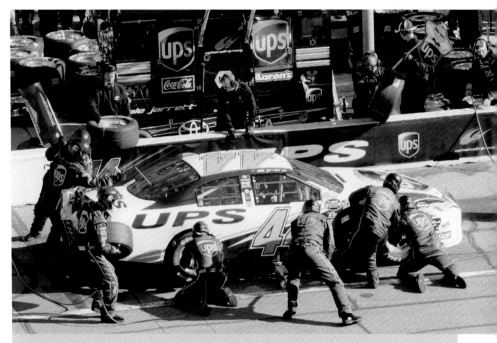

Dale Jarrett's Camry gets serviced during a pit stop at the 2007 Daytona 500. Jarrett's shrewd decisions in the pit have helped him win many races.

Davey Allison, fourth at the restart, blazed past Mark Martin's Ford and into second place, which set up a side-by-side battle with Jarrett for the final two laps of the 200-lap race. Ned Jarrett, who was working the race as part of ESPN's broadcast team, was silent. Going into the final lap, Allison's car was a nose ahead of Jarrett's. Their cars touched, sending a plume of tire smoke into the air. Jarrett held on to win by about the length of a football. "I just hope it was as good for everybody else as it was for us," Jarrett said after the race. "You just sit around and imagine these things."

In the broadcast booth, Ned was a professional. "I don't know what I did," he said later. "I'm sure I hollered, because I was so excited. With five laps to go I really got nervous, but I still did my part on TV." Once the broadcast was over, he immediately dropped his headset and headed for Victory Lane to celebrate with his son. The win was the first for Dale in his 129 Winston Cup starts. "We rubbed a couple of times there, and I hope [Allison] thought it was what he would call clean racing." Dale said. "I wasn't trying to wreck anybody. I could have gone into [turn] three and probably run him all the way to the wall. But I think I gave him just enough room to race."

GLENN GETS BACK INTO THE GAME

As Dale was winning his first Winston Cup start, his brother Glenn was making his return to the sport. After a few years out of racing, Glenn got an offer from Sports Channel America to provide **color commentary** for eight Busch Grand National races. It took some arm-twisting, but Glenn eventually was coaxed into the job. He debuted in 1990 as color analyst at a race held at Lanier Raceway in Gainsville, Georgia. "I knew it was time," he said. "I can still remember the feeling, I still have to catch my voice when talking about it. When I walked back into the garage, there they all were, my friends, the guys I used to race against. I honestly felt I'd come home. This is what I was meant to do. These are the people I like being around."

Glenn turned that eight-race opportunity into a full-blown broadcasting career. He went on to work for TBS, Jefferson Pilot Productions, and as a radio color analyst alongside racing legend Ken Squier. In the early 1990s, as Dale was winning his first Winston Cup race, Glenn joined the Nashville Network, which was starting to broadcast racing events.

DALE JARRETT MOVES ON

In 1995, after three seasons driving for Joe Gibbs, Dale Jarrett announced he would be switching teams. He had won two races with Gibbs, including the Daytona 500, and finished high in many others. But he was lured away by Robert Yates, who needed a driver to replace Ernie Irvan in his Texaco/Havoline Ford. Irvan was seriously injured in a 1994 wreck at Michigan, and it was unclear when and if he would ever return to driving. Once again, Jarrett took the job knowing there was a chance that if Irvan returned, he would be without a ride.

Dale Jarrett won one race for Yates in 1995 and earned $1,363,158. It was a difficult season, though. Irvan had been a strong competitor in the car, and Jarrett and the team struggled. That led naysayers to say Jarrett wasn't as good as Irvan. "Even though things might not have been going the way I wanted them to go, I came to realize that there was a reason for all of this," he said then. "You have to understand that even though we weren't winning races and running up front all the time, I was still doing exactly what I wanted to be doing, and that was driving a race car with a very good group of people, so there wasn't as much to be down about as people perceived."

Irvan returned later that year, putting Jarrett's 1996 season in doubt. After contemplating going out on his own, Jarrett and Yates struck a deal to form a second team. With backing from Ford, the new team debuted at the 1996 Daytona 500, and Jarrett won. He went on to win three other races, and as the season's end neared, he was in a tight points battle for the series championship. To win the title in the final event at Atlanta, he needed points leader Terry Labonte and second-place Jeff Gordon to fall out of the race early. Jarrett would need to lead almost every lap to win the race.

He knew going in that his chances of winning the title were small. "There's still a chance for us," he said before the event. "But it's a slim, slim chance, especially because we're trying to overtake two people instead of just one. Both have to have trouble at Atlanta, and we'd have to have a perfect race." His shot at the title in 1996 ended unsuccessfully, but he would return the following season with another chance at winning the title.

Jarrett entered the 1997 season brimming with confidence. Having come off a third-place finish in the Winston

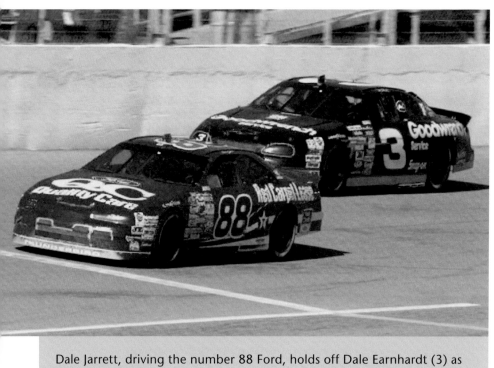

Dale Jarrett, driving the number 88 Ford, holds off Dale Earnhardt (3) as they battle down the straightaway in the 1996 Daytona 500. Jarrett went on to win the race.

Cup points standings in 1996, he and his Ford Quality Care–sponsored team had momentum on their side. He had won four races in 1996, doubling his career total for the previous 11 years of racing at NASCAR's premiere level. And he had overcome the 1995 outing, which was tough on the team.

Jarrett and his crew chief, Todd Parrott, son of legendary crew chief Buddy Parrott, had gelled as a team and were of like minds when it came to strategy on the track. Dale finished twenty-third in the 1997 season-opening Daytona 500; and by the third race of the season, he had fought back to be third overall in the points race. Then he won the fourth race of the year at Atlanta to take the points lead. "[After the first three races] dad just kept telling me to keep doing the things we were doing," he said after the win. "We were running great, things just weren't going our way, and we just had to keep doing what we were doing, and that we would get to Victory Lane." Jarrett said his father had been his biggest supporter and that it was great to have a friend who understood the business.

Dale was already talking about winning the championship, which was months away. "You start thinking about a championship at Daytona," he said. "We learned that [in 1996]. You have to race every race with that championship in mind. I think that we have the team and the people that it takes to win a championship." Jarrett, whose Winston Cup career had gotten to a shaky start, was now a contender. Over a period of a dozen years, he had risen to the top of NASCAR's ranks, a position held by his father three decades earlier.

Winning at Atlanta gave Dale a boost. Winning early in the season is important, he said. "If you can win early, you

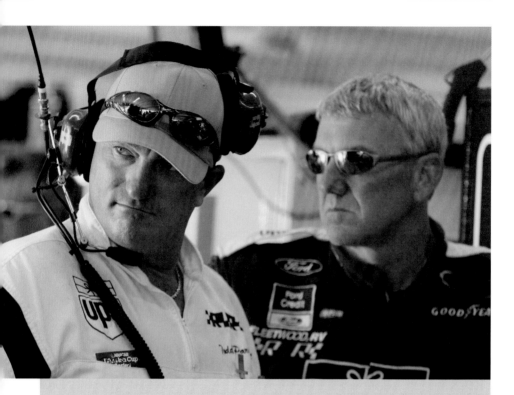

Crew chief Todd Parrott (*left*) consults with Dale Jarrett during a 2002 NASCAR Winston Cup Series race.

don't put as much pressure on yourself and they [the wins] seem to come easier, because you're just doing the things you've been doing, instead of pressing and trying to make things happen," he said. The win was also gratifying because it was the first track on the circuit where both Ned and Dale had won a race. Ned had picked up a win at Atlanta in 1964, and now Dale had etched his name into the record books.

Dale followed up his win at Atlanta with a win at Darlington and a second-place finish at the newly opened Texas Motor Speedway. He maintained his points lead

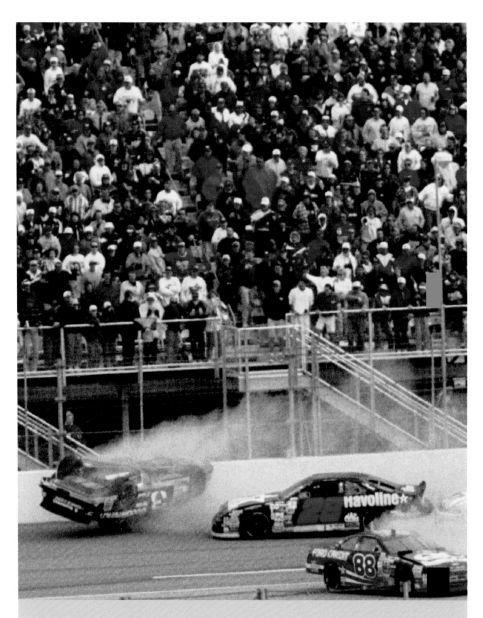

This mishap contributed to Dale Jarrett's twenty-third place finish in the 1997 Daytona 500 race. Dale Earnhardt flips over and slides upside down while Ernie Irvan (28) follows close by, and Dale Jarrett (88) spins into the infield.

until Talladega in May, when a finish in thirty-second place dropped him to third overall. As in the past, Jarrett was tough most of the season, holding onto fourth in the points for several weeks until a series of top finishes near the end put him in third, and then second, with two races to go.

He went into the next-to-last race of the year, at Phoenix, in second place, behind 1995 champion Jeff Gordon. Jarrett and his team gambled and brought a new car to Phoenix. It hadn't been raced in 1997, and it was a new design that was supposed to be better on flat tracks. The car had run in 1996, but it had been rebuilt for the Phoenix event. Nevertheless, Jarrett was going into a race on a track where

DRIVEN TO SUCCEED

Mark Martin knows well the feelings of a driver who has come close to winning a championship. Martin has finished second in the points race in NASCAR's top division a stunning four times, the latest in 2002, without ever winning the title.

In 1990, he was just 26 points behind champion Dale Earnhardt. What made that season particularly difficult for Martin was that earlier in the year his team was found with an illegal part. The team was docked 46 points by NASCAR officials.

Martin has often been asked about not winning the championship. "I really don't care what people think," he said before the 2005 Daytona 500. "Maybe I'm not good enough to win a championship, but I've won more trophies than some guys who have won two championships. Some of those guys haven't won as many races as I have, but they have championships. What have they had that I haven't? Luck."

his rival Gordon had fared well. "We're not concerned," Jarrett said. "We have to do what we can do. We can't control what they do at all. Even though you may have a good record somewhere, that doesn't always work out. You don't know what is going to happen. A flat tire can change everything. An accident certainly changes a lot of things. You just don't know what is going to happen, so we have to concern ourselves with our car and making it the best it can be."

Jarrett qualified ninth at Phoenix and won the race. That, combined with Gordon's seventeenth-place finish, left Jarrett in second place and 77 points behind, with one race to go. For the second consecutive year, Jarrett went into the season-ending race in Atlanta with a shot at the title. Following Phoenix, he and the team had two weeks to prepare for the event. "I think myself and my team are glad to have a little bit of time," he said. "We do have a lot of momentum going and a lot of confidence in our race team, but we want to make sure we're completely ready for Atlanta."

Jarrett said it was great to be able to talk about being in the championship hunt with a race to go. He was confident, too, because Gordon had the title to lose, while he could go into the race and risk everything for the win. "It is definitely more difficult to protect a lead than it is to try to come from behind," he said. "I'm sure there is some tension [in Gordon's team]." Asked why he was always so positive, Jarrett said it was important for a driver to show confidence and to have confidence in his team. "I can remember watching my dad," he said. "I remember how he handled it and what he was going through. It can be a very difficult situation if you let it be. I think what we try to do is make it a very positive experience. And that's something I did gain from my dad."

Jarrett qualified his Ford Quality Care–sponsored car in the third starting position. Gordon, who wrecked his main car in practice, started thirty-seventh. Gordon only had to finish eighteenth or better to win his second title. Jarrett didn't let that obstacle get to him, though. He raced hard and finished second, but he was still 14 points shy of the title. Gordon, three laps off the leader, finished seventeenth and won the title. "We had a tremendous season," Jarrett said. "Certainly we wanted to win the championship, but we realized we gave it everything we possibly could, and just came up a little bit short. But as far as we were concerned, as a race team, we were extremely excited about what we were able to do. We led more laps, and finished more laps and miles than anybody else out there so that says a lot about your team. We won seven races, second only to the guy who won the championship."

7

★★★★★★

LIKE FATHER, LIKE SON, LIKE GRANDSON

On March 29, 1997, Dale's son Jason, born in 1975, made his Busch Grand National debut at Hickory Motor Speedway. It was 44 years after Ned Jarrett made his debut at that same track.

Qualifying trials for the race were rained out, so Jason's starting car owners' points dictated position. He started twenty-eighth in the field of 31 cars and finished twenty-first, four laps off the lead. He earned $3,045 for the day's work. He started two other races in 1997 with an eye toward increasing the total in the future. "Jason, I'm excited about what he has in front of him here," Dale said. "We're excited for him. He's learned an awful lot about racing and race cars in a short period of time. I think that he realizes the chance that he has, and what we're doing now at DAJ Racing is trying to give him equipment that is up to his potential."

Unlike Dale and Glenn, who were young when Ned retired, Jason grew up with his dad being a top competitor in the sport. According to Ned, it should come as no surprise that Jason is

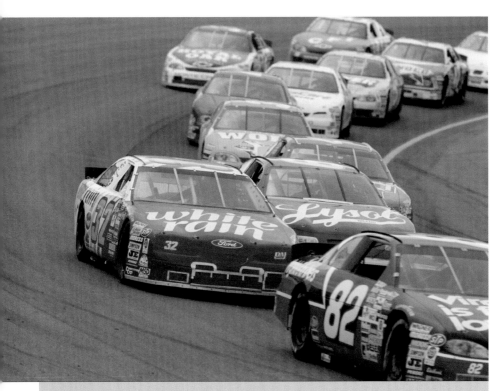

Jason Jarrett in the number 32 car fights for position during his first season in the Busch Grand National racing circuit in 1997.

pursuing a racing career. "Certainly, we had to expect that he would be interested," Ned said. "For most of his life, Dale has been racing. Dale was only 9 when I quit racing and Glenn was only 15. They were not around. Although we would take them to races, [it was never as often] as Jason was with his dad." Jason didn't show an inkling toward racing until after high school. "But once he did, he was totally engulfed with it."

A SHAKY START FOR THE THIRD GENERATION

Like his father, Jason didn't have instant success in racing. As the child of a racing star and the grandson of a racing legend, the pressure to win was incredible. If a driver with that pedigree doesn't perform, and perform early in his career, he faces inevitable comparisons with his family members. Jason Jarrett found that out the hard way.

For the 1999 season, Base Motorsports, one of the top teams on NASCAR's Busch Series, hired Jason Jarrett. Early on, he struggled on the track, and he soon found himself out of a job. "They fired me," he told a reporter. "With my inexperience, I need the very best equipment. It taught me just how tough racing can be. It built me some backbone. Dan and granddad helped me all they could to get in the Busch Series, but now it's up to me to gain skill and knowledge."

After the Base Motorsports deal fell apart, Jason drove for a Busch series team owned by his father and Brett Favre, quarterback for the Green Bay Packers. Then, in 2000, the partnership between Favre and Dale Jarrett dissolved, leaving Jason Jarrett to search for a series where he could excel and thrive.

In 2001, Jason found a home in the ARCA Re/Max series, a racing series using cars very similar to those in NASCAR's top levels. In the ARCA series, however, the level of competition varies widely between the top drivers and the bottom. Jason Jarrett was the ARCA Re/Max Rookie of the Year in 2001, a season in which he finished second in the series points standings. "I pattern my driving style after my dad, who was very smooth," Jason told the Associated Press. "You just don't have to like be like [NASCAR driver] Tony Stewart or Dale [Earnhardt] Jr. I feel maybe I'm a little too nice. Maybe it's hurt me in trying to move forward and I will continue to work on that. I'm always learning."

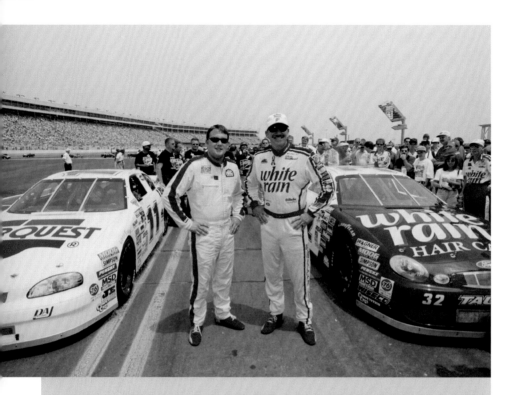

Jason Jarrett (*left*) and his father Dale Jarrett stand between their cars prior to competing in their first race together at the Charlotte Motor Speedway in 1998.

Indeed, he was third in the ARCA points in 2002 and fifth in 2004. By early 2005 he had amassed two wins in the ARCA Re/Max series and was one of the division's top drivers. Then in early 2005, he was again on the move to a different ARCA Re/Max team. In March 2005, Jason was hired to fill in for ARCA legend Bill Venturini, who was seriously injured in a crash at Daytona in February of that year. "Jason is a terrific driver," Venturini said. "He's proven he's got what it takes to be a winner. Jason has a ton of experience and will prove to be a valuable asset for our team."

STAR TRACK

The Hickory Motor Speedway refers to itself as the "Birthplace of NASCAR stars." It's hard to argue the point, considering that Ned, Dale, and Jason Jarrett all started their careers at the speedway, as did countless other top racing stars. The 2005 season marked the fifty-fifth year of racing at the track. It is the oldest professional sporting venue in North Carolina's Catawba County.

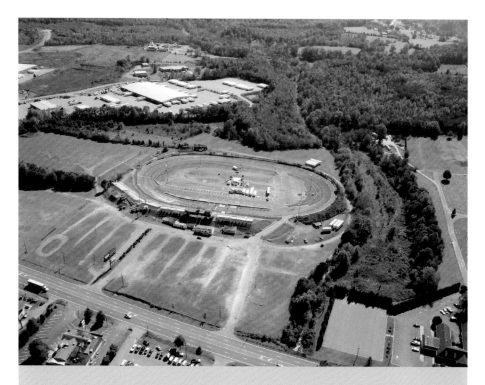

The Hickory Motor Speedway is a .363-mile track, also known as "The World's Most Famous Short Track." It opened in Newton, North Carolina, in 1951.

Working for Venturini's team was yet another step in the development of Jason Jarrett, a third-generation driver still living under the shadow of his grandfather and father. Over the years, as racing grew across the country, the pressure to succeed increased, too, making it much tougher for a driver. "I don't know if I were coming along right now, and did things the exact same way, I may have had a difficult time making it in the sport myself," Dale Jarrett said. "I'm not saying it's wrong, it's just different than when I was coming along. There are so many drivers out there willing to lay it all on the line to get noticed. Sometimes that leaves others in the wings."

8

A CHAMPIONSHIP ARRIVES, A DRIVER THRIVES

Dale Jarrett's second-place finish for the NASCAR title in 1997 inspired him. He'd lived so long trying to fit into the big shoes his father Ned had left behind that the chase for the title in 1997 proved to him and others that the victory would not be far off. A year after nearly winning it all, Jarrett, again driving for Robert Yates's racing team, finished third overall, earning $3,368,735 in total prize money for the year. The 1998 season started slowly, but Jarrett was energized and was in third place for nearly two-thirds of the year.

Drivers and teams often talk about momentum carrying over from season to season. There's something that happens within a racing team that can be very difficult to explain. It's called chemistry. Generally, a team has good chemistry when the driver, crew chief, and all other members of the team are working together, smoothly, for the betterment of the whole program. Dale Jarrett had that going into 1999. His team was together, and he was on a roll, having finished third a season before.

But the 1999 outing started off slowly. Jarrett was caught in a multi-car wreck during the season-opening Daytona 500. He finished thirty-seventh, which is the kind of finish that could sink the momentum and chemistry of a weaker, less experienced team. Not Jarrett's team, though. Indeed, Jarrett and his team rebounded, finishing second in the next race of 1999, which moved the driver up to fourteenth overall.

The momentum continued. By the tenth race of the season, he had overcome a terrible start to the season to stare his first championship dead in the eye. He was second in the points standings, although he still had a long way to go before entering the elite world inhabited by champions. By the eleventh race of the season—the Pontiac Excitement 400 at Richmond International Raceway—Jarrett was first in the standings. He never let up from there, finishing in the top 10 or better in most of the races and locking up his first title in NASCAR's top series before the final race of the season.

Despite his on-track dominance, Jarrett said it wasn't until midway through the season that he felt they were good enough to win the title. "We were running well, we were consistent, we weren't having any problems, and that's when I knew we were kind of in control of our own destiny at that time, and if we didn't mess up and do crazy things that this could happen," was what he said when he was confirmed as the titleholder.

Winning the championship in 1999 was a milestone for Jarrett and the sport of stock car racing. After 25 years

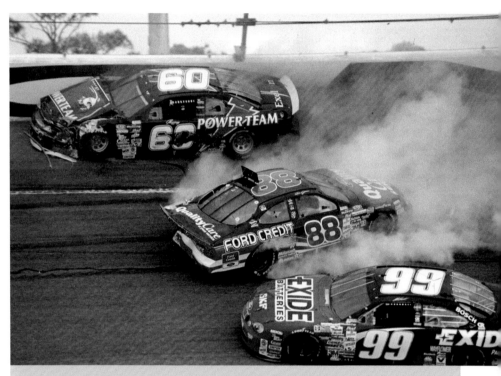

Dale Jarrett in the number 88 Ford spins as Geoffrey Bodine (60) hits the wall and Jeff Burton (99) manages to get by in a mishap at the 1999 Daytona 500. Jarrett did not let this setback spoil the momentum he had going into the 1999 season.

in the sport, he had won NASCAR's top title, joining his father in an elite group of men to be called champions. Like the winners before him, Dale Jarrett got a night to shine at the Waldorf Astoria Hotel in New York City, where NASCAR holds its annual awards banquet. "Dad, I didn't know when I got involved in this sport if I ever could achieve any of the accomplishments you did," Dale Jarrett told his father in front of a crowd of 1,400 at the December 1999 ceremony. "But it's truly an honor to be only the second father-son duo to win a NASCAR Winston Cup."

Including his race winnings and bonuses for winning the title, Jarrett earned $6,649,956 in prize money in 1999. "That's an incredible amount of money to receive for doing something I love to do," he said. "That makes my very first purse of $35 seem rather insignificant."

"I STILL LOVE TO COMPETE"

Dale Jarrett started the 2000 season by winning the Daytona 500 for the third time. He went on to finish the season in fourth place. He was fifth in the points in 2001. He fell to ninth in 2002. By 2003, Jarrett's momentum was gone, as the team finished twenty-sixth overall. And in 2004, he was fifteenth in the points.

The 2005 season was a rebuilding year for the Robert Yates team and Dale Jarrett, but it was also a time for change—again—in NASCAR. At 48, Jarrett went into the season as one of the older drivers on NASCAR's top level. He watched as some of the drivers from his generation— Rusty Wallace and Terry Labonte—were running their last races, choosing to retire or cut back rather than continue with NASCAR's grueling schedule.

Jarrett wasn't considering retirement in 2005, though. He wanted to win. And he wanted to compete. Indeed, he was the fastest qualifier at the Daytona 500. Yet, because of his time in the sport and his age, the question of his future remained. "I've seen what some of my buddies have done, but I started later than they did," Jarrett said. "I still think I can compete with anybody out there and I still love to compete." His deal with the Robert Yates racing team was through 2007. "I plan to continue for a minimum of two years and probably three years if Robert [Yates], Ford and [sponsor] UPS still want me," Dale said. "That's what I'm looking at."

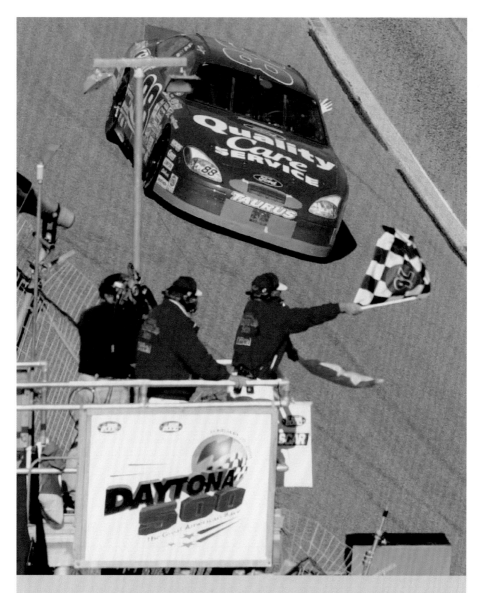

Driving the number 88 Ford Taurus, Dale Jarrett takes the checkered flag to win his third Daytona 500, in February 2000.

The relationship between Yates and Jarrett ended, however, at the end of the 2006 season. Midway through the year, as he struggled to compete on the track, Jarrett

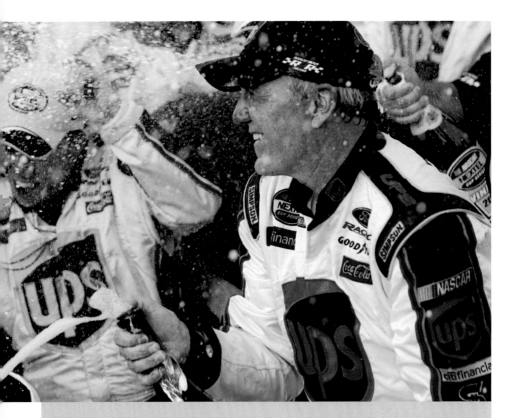

Dale Jarrett pops the cork on a bottle of champagne after winning the UAW Ford 500 NASCAR race at the Talladega Superspeedway in October 2005.

announced that he would leave Yates for a new deal with Michael Waltrip Racing in 2007. The team, owned by driver Michael Waltrip, would enter the 2007 season using Toyota Camrys, yet another historic milestone. "Dale's resume speaks for itself," Waltrip said. "To have a NASCAR champion on our team is another significant piece of the puzzle that pulls together our vision. I know his knowledge and experience will be invaluable for our start-up team with a new manufacturer, and will allow our organization to grow and succeed at a faster pace."

Leaving Yates was a "very difficult" decision, Jarrett said, in a statement explaining the move. "I feel this is a great opportunity for me to take on a new challenge and what they are building at Michael Waltrip Racing fits my plans for the future," he also said. Jarrett ended the 12-year relationship with Yates with a thirty-first place finish at the Homestead-Miami Speedway. "This certainly isn't how I wanted this day to go," Jarrett said after the race. "We made a lot of good memories here at Robert Yates Racing, and those are the ones we'll remember."

Before the start of the 2006 season, Jarrett had noted that the level of competition had changed dramatically since his 1999 title win. A bad day now at one race could damage a shot at the title. And with NASCAR's Chase for the Championship, in which only the drivers in the top 10 after the twenty-sixth race of the season are eligible for

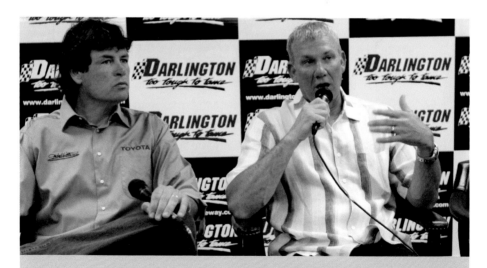

Dale Jarrett (*right*) fields questions during a news conference with Michael Waltrip. It was announced that Jarrett would join Michael Waltrip Racing in 2007 and drive a Toyota Camry.

the title, it's even tougher. "That's what makes it difficult now, you have so many teams that can make you go from a reasonable day to a really bad day with either just missing the set up or having a slight problem," he told reporters in January 2006. "I think that's why it becomes so much more difficult to get in the Chase and then from that point on, go on and win the championship." He suggested that his team at that point might be capable of finishing fifteenth in 2006 as it had in 2005. As it turned out, he finished twenty-third overall in his final season at Robert Yates racing, well behind champion Jimmie Johnson.

A LIVING LEGACY

Through it all, the Jarrett family has made its mark on racing. Whenever he decides to step down, Dale Jarrett knows he has succeeded in standing on his own as a driver. His father Ned has left broadcasting full time, but he

EDGING OUT THE COMPETITION

Dale Jarrett finished just 14 points behind Jeff Gordon in 1997, but that wasn't the closest finish ever. In fact, it was only the fifth closest in NASCAR history. The closest finish happened in 2004, the first season for NASCAR's reconfigured points race, called the Chase for the Cup. In 2004, NASCAR altered the points race so that after the twenty-sixth race, only the drivers in the top 10 were eligible for a shot at winning the championship.

The decision that year came down to the last race, in which Kurt Busch was crowned champion a mere 8 points ahead of Jimmie Johnson. The second closest points finish occurred in 1992, when Alan Kulwicki edged out Bill Elliott by 10 points.

remains a legend in the sport and a familiar face to those in the garage area at any NASCAR track. Jason Jarrett did not race in 2006, instead deciding to work for his father's racing business. Jason continues to build on the family's history in the sport.

Ned Jarrett finds a great deal of satisfaction in having a son as one of the top drivers, another son working in broadcasting, a daughter married to a top crew chief, and now a grandson racing. "It's a great feeling," he said. "I guess I'm living part of what I gave up when I quit driving through [Dale]. I have an equal feeling with Glenn and his broadcasting. I have two sons following my footsteps as a driver and the other as a broadcaster. To be able to live through them, with things I might have missed, has been wonderful."

STATISTICS

NED JARRETT (GRAND NATIONAL/NASCAR CUP SERIES)

Year	Races	Wins	Top 5 Finishes	Top 10 Finishes	Winnings ($)
1953	2	0	0	0	125
1954	2	0	0	0	25
1955	3	0	0	0	260
1956	2	0	0	0	60
1957	1	0	0	0	50
1958	0	0	0	0	0
1959	17	2	2	3	3,860
1960	40	5	15	6	25,438
1961	46	1	22	11	41,056
1962	52	6	13	16	43,444
1963	53	8	24	7	45,844
1964	59	15	25	5	71,925
1965	54	13	29	3	93,625
1966	21	0	5	3	23,255
Totals	352	50	135	54	348,967

GLENN JARRETT (WINSTON/NASCAR CUP SERIES)

Year	Races	Wins	Top 5 Finishes	Top 10 Finishes	Winnings ($)
1978	1	0	0	0	2,940
1979	2	0	0	0	2,745
1980	2	0	0	0	4,435
1981	3	0	0	0	12,650
1982	1	0	0	0	735

GLENN JARRETT (WINSTON/NASCAR CUP SERIES) (*continued*)

Year	Races	Wins	Top 5 Finishes	Top 10 Finishes	Winnings ($)
1983	1	0	0	0	1,200
1985	0	0	0	0	4,200
Totals	10	0	0	0	28,905

DALE JARRETT (WINSTON/NEXTEL/NASCAR CUP SERIES)

Year	Races	Wins	Top 5 Finishes	Top 10 Finishes	Winnings ($)
1984	3	0	0	0	7,305
1986	1	0	0	0	990
1987	24	0	0	2	143,405
1988	29	0	0	1	118,640
1989	29	0	2	3	232,317
1990	24	0	1	6	214,495
1991	29	1	2	5	444,256
1992	29	0	2	6	418,648
1993	30	1	12	5	1,242,394
1994	30	1	3	5	893,754
1995	31	1	8	5	1,363,158
1996	31	4	13	4	2,985,418
1997	32	7	11	5	3,240,362
1998	33	3	19	5	2,346,535
1999	34	4	20	5	3,590,829
2000	38	4	11	9	5,225,499
2001	36	4	12	6	4,437,644
2002	36	2	10	18	4,421,951
2003	36	1	1	7	4,121,487
2004	36	0	6	14	5,097,396
2005	36	1	4	7	4,705,436
2006	36	0	1	4	4,478,774
Totals	604	32	162	256	52,253,898

JASON JARRETT (BUSCH SERIES)

Year	Races	Wins	Top 5 Finishes	Top 10 Finishes	Winnings ($)
1997	3	0	0	0	10,695
1998	11	0	0	0	69,954
1999	9	0	0	0	145,355
2000	19	0	0	0	178,980
Totals	30	0	0	0	404,984

JASON JARRETT (ARCA RE/MAX SERIES)

Year	Races	Wins	Top 5 Finishes	Top 10 Finishes	Winnings
2000	1	0	1	1	n/a
2001	25	1	8	15	n/a
2002	22	0	8	14	n/a
2003	22	0	8	16	n/a
2004	22	1	7	11	n/a
Totals	92	1	32	57	n/a

CHRONOLOGY

1932 Ned Miller Jarrett is born on October 12 in Newton, North Carolina.

1950 Glenn Jarrett is born on August 11.

1953 Ned Jarrett enters his first NASCAR Grand National Race on August 29 at Hickory Motor Speedway.

1956 Dale Arnold Jarrett is born on November 26.

1957 Ned Jarrett wins his first of two consecutive NASCAR National Sportsman Championships.

1959 Ned Jarrett increases his schedule on the NASCAR Grand National Series; Patti Jarrett is born on August 31.

1961 Ned Jarrett wins his first of two NASCAR Grand National Championships.

1965 Ned Jarrett wins his second NASCAR Grand National title and vows to retire; wins famed Southern 500 at Darlington Raceway.

1966 Ned Jarrett retires from racing with 50 wins.

1975 Jason Jarrett is born on October 14.

1976 Dale Jarrett makes his racing debut at Hickory Motor Speedway.

1979 Ned Jarrett appears on CBS in a live flag-to-flag telecast of the Daytona 500, the first Winston Cup Race ever to air live in its entirety on television.

1982 Dale Jarrett races full time on the NASCAR Busch Grand National Series.

1984 Glenn Jarrett debuts on the Busch Series; Dale makes his first Winston Cup start.

1986 Dale Jarrett wins his first Busch race.

1987   Dale Jarrett moves into Winston Cup racing full time.

1988   Glenn Jarrett retires from racing.

1991   Dale Jarrett beats Davey Allison by eight inches to win his first Winston Cup race in the Champion 400 at Michigan International Speedway (now simply called Michigan Speedway).

1993   Dale Jarrett wins the Daytona 500; he repeats the feat in 1996.

1997   Jason Jarrett makes his Busch Series debut on March 29 at Hickory Motor Speedway and finishes twenty-first; Dale Jarrett finishes second in the Winston Cup points race.

1999   Dale Jarrett wins the Winston Cup championship.

2001   Jason Jarrett becomes a full-time racer in the ARCA Re/Max series and earns the Rookie of the Year title.

2002   Dale Jarrett finishes ninth in the Winston Cup Series; Jason Jarrett finishes third in the ARCA Re/Max Series.

2003   Dale Jarrett finishes twenty-sixth in the Winston Cup Series, breaking a seven-year streak of finishing in the top 10; Jason Jarrett finishes second in the ARCA Re/Max Series.

2004   Dale Jarrett finishes fifteenth in the Nextel Cup Series, NASCAR's newly renamed top division; Jason Jarrett finishes fifth in ARCA Re/Max Series.

2005   Dale Jarrett finishes fifteenth in the Nextel Cup Series; Jason Jarrett finishes ninth in ARCA Re/Max Series.

2006   Dale Jarrett reveals he will leave Robert Yates Racing at season's end to take a job driving for Michael Waltrip; he finishes twenty-third in the Nextel Cup Series; Jason Jarrett does not compete in ARCA Re/Max.

GLOSSARY

Color Commentary—Expert analysis and background information, such as team or player statistics and strategy; often provided by a person called the color commentator or analyst, who works with the play-by-play announcer.

Draft—Two cars running nose-to-tail can move faster than one car alone at high speeds. That two-car move is called a draft. To get around tracks such as the Daytona International Speedway, where speeds reach nearly 200 mph, cars must draft to be successful.

NASCAR—The National Association for Stock Car Auto Racing is the governing body for major stock car racing events in the United States. NASCAR oversees the NASCAR Nextel Cup, the premiere series, the NASCAR Busch Series, the NASCAR Craftsman Truck Series, and several others.

Pole position—The best place in the starting line-up, given to the car with the fastest time during the qualifying round.

Qualifying—Before every race, drivers must qualify for their starting position by running a series of laps at full speed.

Roll Cage—Inside every race car is a web of steel tubing that encases the driver's compartment. The roll cage is designed to protect the driver in a crash and absorb some of the impact of other cars.

Victory Lane—Also called the "winner's circle," this is the spot on the infield of a racetrack where the winner of a race and his team, family, friends, and admirers gather to celebrate the victory.

BIBLIOGRAPHY

Branham, H.A. *The NASCAR Vault: An Official History Featuring Rare Collectibles from Motorsports Images and Archives*. Bellevue, Wash.: Becker & Mayer Books, 2004.

Garner, Joe, and Jeff Gordon. *Speed, Guts and Glory: 100 Unforgettable Moments in NASCAR History*. New York: Warner Books, 2006.

Golenbock, Peter. *NASCAR Confidential: Stories of the Men and Women Who Made Stock Car Racing Great*. Osceola, Wisc.: MBI Publishing, 2004.

——, and Greg Fielden. *NASCAR Encyclopedia*. Osceola, Wisc.: MBI Publishing, 2003.

Jensen, Tom. *Cheating: An Inside Look at the Bad Things Good NASCAR Nextel Cup Racers Do in Pursuit of Speed*. Phoenix, Ariz.: David Bull Publishing, 2004.

Sporting News. *NASCAR Record & Fact Book 2006 Edition*. St. Louis, Mo.: Sporting News, 2006.

FURTHER READING

Allison, Liz, and Darrell Waltrip. *The Girl's Guide to NASCAR.* New York: Center Street Publishing, 2006.

Fielden, Greg, and the Auto Editors of Consumer Guide. *NASCAR Chronicle.* Wisconsin Rapids, Wisc.: Publications International, 2005.

———. *NASCAR: A Fast History.* Wisconsin Rapids, Wisc.: Publications International, 2005.

Fresina, Michael J., and Brian France. *A Week in the Life of NASCAR: A View from Within.* Chicago: Triumph Books, 2005.

Hammond, Jeff, and Geoff Norman. *Real Men Work in the Pits: A Life in NASCAR Racing.* Emmaus, Pa.: Rodale Press, 2005.

Martin, Mark, and Beth Tuschak. *NASCAR For Dummies.* Hoboken, N.J.: For Dummies, 2005.

McLaurin, Jim. *Then Junior Said to Jeff: The Best NASCAR Stories Ever Told.* Chicago: Triumph Books, 2006.

Thompson, Neal. *Driving with the Devil: Southern Moonshine, Detroit Wheels, and the Birth of NASCAR.* New York: Crown Publishing Group, 2006.

WEB SITES

www.nascar.com
NASCAR's official site is great for catching up on the latest racing news.

www.dalejarrett.com
Racing fans can browse Dale Jarrett's official site for the legendary driver's racing history and current statistics.

www.arcaracing.com
The official Web site of the Automobile Racing Club of America (ARCA) lets fans find up-to-date scheduling information and statistics for the ARCA Re/Max racing series.

www.thatsracin.com
The Real Cites news network offers an all-encompassing racing
site of NASCAR stats and schedules and Formula 1 and
Champ Car series racing.

www.espn.com
The official site of the sports broadcasting company ESPN,
offering up-to-date information for NASCAR fans and
other sports enthusiasts.

www.speedtv.com
Official site of the SPEED Channel, a cable network dedicated
to all things automotive.

msn.foxsports.com
Sports Web site of the Fox Network, where fans can browse
their favorite players and games and sign up for customized
sports updates.

www.nbcsports.com
NBC Sports news and statistics are reported on this site.
NASCAR fans can find detailed information and highlights
related to the current driving season.

PICTURE CREDITS

INDEX

ABOUT THE AUTHOR

RICHARD HUFF is an award-winning journalist whose previous books include *Behind The Wall: A Season on the NASCAR Circuit; Stock Car Champions;* and *Reality Television.* He is a deputy features editor/television and a motorsports writer for the *New York Daily News.* His work has appeared in such national publications as *Stock Car Racing, Old House Journal, Do! Magazine, Circle Track* and *Drill* magazine. He lives in Atlantic Highlands, New Jersey, with his wife Michelle, son Ryan, and daughter Paige.

WOODLAND HIGH SCHOOL
800 N. MOSELEY DRIVE
STOCKBRIDGE, GA. 30281
(770) 389-2784